Pediatric Ophthalmology and Strabismus   THE REQUISITES IN OPHTHALMOLOGY

SERIES EDITOR   **Jay H. Krachmer,** MD
Professor and Chairman
Department of Ophthalmology
University of Minnesota Medical School
Minneapolis, Minnesota

Visit our website at **www.mosby.com**

Pediatric Ophthalmology and Strabismus

THE REQUISITES
IN OPHTHALMOLOGY

KENNETH W. WRIGHT, MD
Professor, Ophthalmology and Pediatrics
University of California, Irvine School of Medicine
Irvine, California;
Physician, Research Associate, and Surgeon
Cedars-Sinai Medical Center
Los Angeles, California

PETER H. SPIEGEL, MD
Assistant Professor, Department of Ophthalmology
University of Tennessee, Memphis;
Consulting Ophthalmologist
St. Jude Children's Research Hospital
Memphis, Tennessee

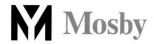 Mosby

St. Louis Baltimore Boston Carlsbad Chicago Minneapolis New York Philadelphia Portland
London Milan Sydney Tokyo Toronto

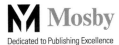

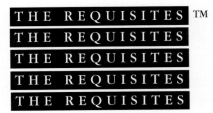

THE REQUISITES is a proprietary trademark of Mosby, Inc.

Acquisitions Editor: Kim Cox
Senior Managing Editor: Kathy Falk
Project Manager: Patricia Tannian
Senior Production Editor: Melissa Mraz Lastarria
Design Manager: Gail Morey Hudson

Mosby, Inc.
A Harcourt Health Sciences Company
11830 Westline Industrial Drive
St. Louis, Missouri 63146

Printed in the United States of America

Library of Congress Cataloging in Publication Data

Wright, Kenneth W. (Kenneth Weston)
    Pediatric ophthalmology and strabismus / Kenneth W. Wright, Peter H. Spiegel—1st ed.
      p. cm.—(Requisites in ophthalmology series)
    Includes bibliographical references and index.
    ISBN 0-323-00181-5
    1. Pediatric ophthalmology. 2. Strabismus. I. Spiegel, Peter H.
  II. Title. III. Series: Requisites series.
    RE48.2.C5 W747   1999
    618.92'0977—dc21
                                              99-34127
                                                CIP

99 00 01 02 03 GW/MV-Y 9 8 7 6 5 4 3 2 1

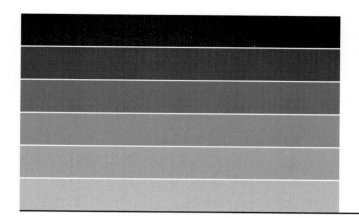

Preface

The specialty of pediatric ophthalmology involves much more than just treating "small eyes." Pediatric eye diseases require an intimate knowledge of embryology, eye development, genetics, neurovisual development, amblyopia, and strabismus. This book was written to provide a concise, yet comprehensive, overview of pediatric ophthalmology and strabismus. Many students find pediatric ophthalmology and strabismus a difficult subject to learn, and it is our goal to provide a reader-friendly textbook that is lucid and easily understood. The book covers a broad spectrum of key pediatric ophthalmology topics providing important and clinically relevant information. It is the authors' hope that this volume will be useful for ophthalmology residents, comprehensive ophthalmologists, and pediatric ophthalmologists alike.

Acknowledgments

I would like to acknowledge Tina Kiss for her help in editing and preparing the manuscript. Additional thanks to Dr. Anthony Nesburn and Discovery Fund for Eye Research for their assistance and support, and a special thanks to Cedars-Sinai Medical Center and their continuing support of academic endeavors.

Kenneth W. Wright, MD

My contribution to this book was greatly improved by many individuals in the Ophthalmology Department at the University of Tennessee, Memphis. Most important of these is Barrett Haik, who strongly supported this effort. My colleagues in Memphis critically reviewed my work and helped to keep the content focused and clinically relevant, and I am extremely grateful to them: Richard Drewry, Jr., Chris Fleming, Natalie Kerr, Peter Netland, Stephen Scoper, Chris Walton, Greg Carroll, Alessandro Iannaccone, and Eniko Pivnick. I would like to acknowledge Pat Conley, who edited many of the chapters and tightened up too many loose sentences, as well as Terry Ferguson, who assisted in preparing and organizing the manuscript. I am also grateful to Mark Greenwald, who supplied some of the clinical images, and to Mary Smith, who makes so much around here happen. Finally, I thank Ken Wright, who asked me to collaborate on this project.

Peter H. Spiegel, MD

To the students
who make our work in pediatric ophthalmology and strabismus fun.

KENNETH W. WRIGHT

To my parents
Mel and **Barbara,** *and to my brother,* **Robert.**

PETER H. SPIEGEL

The following material was borrowed from Wright KW, et al (editors): *Pediatric Ophthalmology and Strabismus,* St Louis, 1995, Mosby:

Figures	10-7	**Tables**	**Boxes**
1-6	11-3 to 11-8	1-1 to 1-3	11-1
1-7	11-11 to 11-13	6-1 to 6-3	12-1
2-1 to 2-8	11-15	8-2	12-2
2-10 to 2-15	13-1 to 13-17	18-1	19-5
3-2 to 3-4	13-19	19-2	20-2
4-1	13-21	19-4	
4-2	13-24 to 13-30	20-1	
4-5	14-1 to 14-30		
4-6	15-1 to 15-40		
4-10	16-1 to 16-9		
4-12 to 4-14	17-1 to 17-3		
5-1 to 5-10	18-3		
6-1	18-5		
6-4	19-2		
6-7	19-3		
6-9	19-6 to 19-9		
6-10	20-3		
7-1 to 7-8	20-4		
8-1 to 8-18			
9-1 to 9-9			

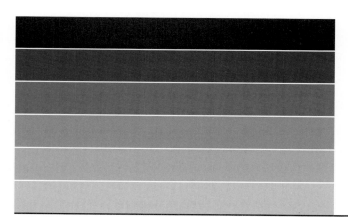

Contents

Pediatric Ophthalmology and Strabismus

THE REQUISITES IN OPHTHALMOLOGY

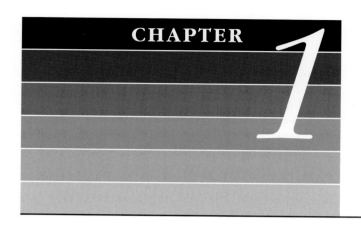

CHAPTER 1

Practical Aspects of the Pediatric Examination

In this introductory chapter, practical, basic concepts in pediatric ophthalmology are covered. First, normal ocular and visual development is reviewed. Next, a brief overview of important points to be included in the history is presented. Following this, specific suggestions for examining children of varying ages are provided. Some of these are simply in-office examination techniques, which every ophthalmologist should be able to perform, whereas others are more specialized methods. The concluding sections of the chapter cover causes of visual impairment and evaluation of children with visual impairment. Dyslexia is briefly discussed.

OCULAR AND VISUAL DEVELOPMENT

Corneal Diameters

The horizontal corneal diameter in full-term infants averages 9.8 mm, and the vertical diameter is slightly greater. However, the normal range is fairly wide, from 9.0 mm to 11.0 mm, and only eyes with measurements falling outside this range require further investigation. Much of the corneal growth occurs in the first year of life. The average adult value of 11.7 mm is reached by 7 years of age.

Globe Size and Axial Length

The anterior segment of the newborn's eye is approximately 75% to 80% of the adult size. However, the posterior segment is less than half the adult size. The volume of a normal eye more than doubles from birth to adulthood. The neonatal eye is approximately 16 mm long, compared with the typical adult length of slightly greater than 23 mm (Fig. 1-1). The majority of the required increase in axial length occurs in the first 18 months of life, after which the axial length averages 20.3 mm (Fig. 1-2). The remainder of the axial elongation may be divided into two subsequent phases. The infantile growth phase (age 2 to 5 years) accounts for about 1.1 mm of growth, and the juvenile phase (5 to 13 years) accounts for another 1.3 mm. Overall, males have slightly longer eyes than females, a difference in adults of 0.3 to 0.4 mm. The shorter neonatal eye requires greater refractive power, and this is provided in large part by the cornea. Whereas average adult keratometric powers are approximately 42.5 diopters, an average value in newborns is about 47.6 diopters.

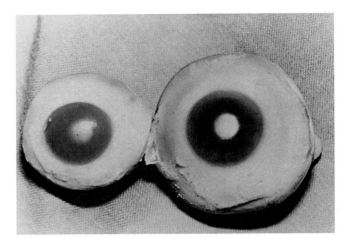

Fig. 1-1 Comparison of a globe from a neonate *(left)* with that of an adult *(right)*. (From Swan KC, Wilkins JH: *J Pediatr Ophthalmol Strabismus* 21:44-49, 1984.)

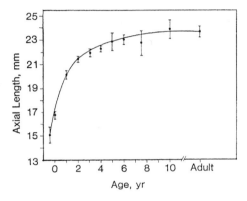

Fig. 1-2 Change in axial length from birth to adulthood. The rapid postnatal growth phase is depicted here. Axial length increases until 13 years of age, but the rate of growth slows dramatically after 3 years of age. (Modified from Gordon RA: *Arch Ophthalmol* 103[6]:785-789, 1985.)

Refractive Errors and Spectacles in Infancy

Full-term infants tend to be hyperopic at birth, with a mean refraction of +0.62 diopters. However, the range is wide. One study found 75% of infants to be hyperopic and the remainder to be myopic. Population studies show an overall trend toward increasing hyperopia until about 7 years of age. Thereafter the trend is toward myopia until adulthood.

The factors responsible for *axial elongation* and ocular growth are a subject of interest worldwide. The ability to modulate the growth of the eye and specifically to prevent or minimize high myopia could affect the lives of millions. Probably both hereditary and environmental factors play a role in the development of myopia. Some data have suggested that prolonged near work in childhood promotes the development of myopia, but the mechanism by which this occurs and the strength of this relationship have yet to be determined. Published stud-

ies have suggested that chronic atropinization (frequent atropine eyedrops) lessens the development of myopia, but the methodology of these studies has been criticized. Multiple genetic factors, rather than a single gene, are believed to influence eye growth and myopia. Caution is advised in predicting a child's final (adult) refractive error. However, although 8% to 10% of healthy children of emmetropic parents become myopic, up to half of children become myopic if both parents are nearsighted.

Many ocular diseases are associated with myopia, including albinism, choroideremia, gyrate atrophy, and retinitis pigmentosa. The most important association may be that of prematurity with myopia, particularly in eyes that have required treatment for retinopathy of prematurity. Short eyes develop in infant monkeys reared in complete darkness, whereas allowing only blurred images results in axial elongation because of posterior segment growth. This process is believed to be at least partly due to a regulating effect by dopamine at the level of the retina. Other neural transmitters may also play a role. Therefore infants who were premature should have refractions and be fitted with spectacles if they are found to have moderate or high degrees of myopia.

Astigmatism is common in infants: 71% have "against-the-rule" astigmatism, and 21% have "with-the-rule" astigmatism. However, by the age of about 6 years, most children with astigmatism have the "with-the-rule" form.

Occasionally infants require spectacles because of refractive errors. Babies who were born prematurely, as previously mentioned, may need refractive correction. Another condition requiring such correction is infantile accommodative esotropia. This entity is certainly more common than was recognized 10 years ago, and favorable results can be obtained with appropriate use of spectacles. This topic is covered further in Chapter 16.

Intraocular Pressure

Accurate measurement of intraocular pressure in infants and young children can be challenging because of poor cooperation (crying, straining) and the influence of anesthesia. Furthermore, the values may differ depending on the instrument used. Clearly the normal intraocular pressure in infants is significantly lower than in adults, falling in the range of 8 to 12 mm Hg, depending on technique. As children age, the normal pressure gradually increases. These considerations are most important when evaluating a child with possible infantile or juvenile glaucoma. In such children without elevated pressures, the physician must rely on various other signs to help establish the diagnosis (see Chapter 7).

Extraocular Muscles

The positions of the extraocular muscle insertions in infants differ significantly from those in adults (Figs. 1-3

Corneal - Limbal Distance

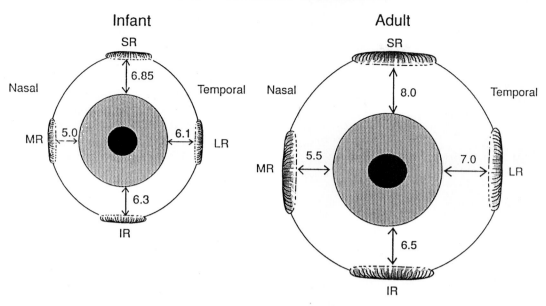

Fig. 1-3   Comparison of the corneal limbal distance in an infant eye *(left)* and an adult emmetropic eye *(right)*. (Modified from Christensen LE, Wright KW: *Surgical anatomy in color atlas in ophthalmic surgery,* Philadelphia, 1991, JB Lippincott.)

and 1-4; see Chapter 13). Because of the very small size of the neonatal globe, the insertions are closer to the limbus, but they are also much closer to the equator. The mean distance of the medial rectus insertion to the limbus is 5.1 mm in babies aged 3 months and 5.8 mm in those 6 months old. This very small difference suggests that infants with congenital esotropia undergoing bilateral medial rectus recessions at 3 to 4 months of age should not be expected to have an excessive overcorrection rate compared with those undergoing surgery later.

Retinal Maturation

The retinal vasculature develops centrifugally, from the optic nerve anteriorly, and first becomes evident in the fourth month of gestation. The vasculature of the nasal periphery is complete by the eighth month of gestation. However, the temporal retina may not become fully vascularized until a few weeks postterm. The density of cones in the newborn is about half that in the adult. Most of the increase in cone density occurs in the first 4 years of life with a corresponding improvement in visual acuity.

Visual Development

Determination of the normal visual acuity levels during maturation is challenging (see Chapter 15). The values depend in part on the technique used. The primary methods include preferential looking, visual-evoked potentials, and optokinetic nystagmus. At birth the visual acuity is in the 20/400 to 20/800 range, as determined by these methods. The presence of optokinetic nystagmus roughly parallels the results obtained with preferential looking. By age 4 months each technique suggests that the normal visual acuity is 20/200. By age 18 to 30 months an acuity of 20/20 is reached. Visual maturation, as measured with visual-evoked potentials (VEPs), occurs somewhat faster, with 20/20 visual acuity reached by age 12 months (Table 1-1). Both preferential looking and optokinetic nystagmus techniques require a motor response as part of the assessment of visual acuity. Therefore these tests are not as "pure" as those that rely on afferent information and may underestimate visual acuity. On the other hand, the measured responses when only VEPs are used are derived from the primary visual cortex, but the higher cortical regions may be important in the perceptual processes of interest.

Normal visual field development has also been studied. The monocular field of a newborn is fairly narrow, extending 28° to the right and to the left of fixation and 11° above and 16° below fixation. By 6 months of age the field approaches that of an adult.

The development of stereopsis parallels that of acuity. By 3½ to 6 months of age stereopsis can be demonstrated. Stereopsis depends on an interplay between afferent processing and a stable motor system.

By 2 months of age, fixation is well developed. Smooth pursuit is established by 2 to 3 months of age. The normal tracking of moving objects by neonates therefore consists of a series of saccades. Important visual developmental milestones are listed in Box 1-1.

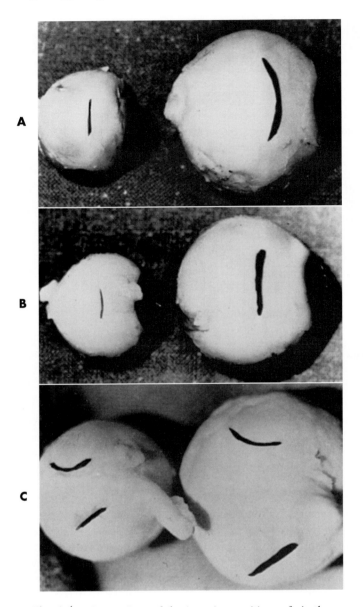

Fig. 1-4   Comparison of the insertion positions of, **A,** the medial rectus, **B,** the lateral rectus, and **C,** the superior and inferior oblique muscles in neonatal and adult emmetropic eyes. The medial rectus insertion and the lateral rectus insertion in the neonate's eye are quite close to the equator. The superior and inferior oblique insertions are much closer to each other in the neonatal eye than in the large adult eye. (From Swan KC, Wilkins JH: *J Pediatr Ophthalmol Strabismus* 21:44-49, 1984.)

HISTORY

During a patient visit a few essential historical points must be established; further information to be obtained depends on the specific situation and physical findings. As in other aspects of history taking, parents' observations tend to be reliable. The birth history (gestational age and birth weight) is noted. Any problems encountered during pregnancy, labor and delivery, or the postnatal period must be explored. For patients who were premature, it is important to determine whether examinations or treatment for retinopathy of prematurity was performed. Premature babies who see poorly may have had hydrocephalus or intracranial hemorrhage, information the parent may not volunteer unless asked. Parents should be asked how long the child was hospitalized and whether any surgeries were performed.

The examiner should determine whether any visual problems are believed to be congenital or acquired. The parents should be asked to describe the child's visual abilities. Does the child hold objects very close to see them? Can the patient localize and pick up very small objects? Do the eyes "wander"? Does the child show light aversion, eye rubbing, or night blindness? Additional information to be reviewed includes trauma and medication. Family history, particularly the presence or absence of strabismus or amblyopia, unexplained blindness or poor vision, and other ocular diseases, must be detailed to the extent of the parents' abilities.

EXAMINATION

The ability to perform an effective pediatric ophthalmologic examination can be developed with a little practice. However, even the most experienced examiner sometimes fails to obtain the required information when the patient simply will not cooperate. In such instances the patient's appointment should be rescheduled to another day. Hungry or tired babies tend to be difficult patients. The examiner should strive to work efficiently and obtain a majority of information rapidly, before the child's attention is lost.

Observation

A pediatric patient encounter should not be expected to proceed in a linear fashion. Sometimes the best information is obtained immediately on entering the room, in the instant before the child starts crying. The examiner should be polite but should direct attention to the patient as the history is obtained. The patient's visual behavior and ocular alignment should be noted. Are the examiner's movements followed? Is there a head tilt or turn? Is there an obvious developmental delay or dysmorphic syndrome?

Assessment of Visual Function in Preverbal Patients

Monocular fixation   In estimation of the visual acuity of an uncooperative or preverbal child, the descriptive terms *central, steady,* and *maintained* (CSM) are frequently used and the quality of the fixation and the following ability are noted. *Central* means that fixation appears to be made with the central fovea. If

Table 1-1   Age-related visual acuity estimates by test method

| | Age | | | | | |
Technique	Birth	2 mo	4 mo	6 mo	1 yr	Age for 20/20
Optokinetic Nystagmus	20/400	20/200	20/200	20/100	20/60	20-30 mo
Forced-choice preferential Looking	20/400	20/200	20/200	20/150	20/50	18-24 mo
Visual-evoked potential	20/400	20/60	20/60	20/40	20/20	6-12 mo

Box 1-1   Normal Visual Development

Pupillary light reaction present—30 weeks' gestation
Blink response to visual threat—2-5 months
Fixation well developed—2 months
Smooth pursuit well developed—6-8 weeks
Saccades well developed (not hypometric)—1-3 months
Optokinetic nystagmus
  1. Present at birth but with restricted slow-phase velocity
  2. Temporal to nasal monocular response better than nasal to temporal until 2-4 months
Accommodation appropriate to target—4 months
Stereopsis well developed—3-7 months
Contrast sensitivity well developed—7 months
Ocular alignment stabilized—1 month
Foveal maturation complete—4 months
Optic nerve myelination complete—7 months-2 years

fixation is not being made with the central part of the fovea, the designation *not central* should be given. Examples of visual fixation that are *not central* include amblyopia, in which fixation can wander around the center of the fovea, and dragged maculas. *Steady* means that the object of regard is held by the fovea continuously. This implies the absence of nystagmus. *Maintained* means that in a strabismic patient the eye holds fixation after the fellow eye is uncovered. *Fixation* can be graded as excellent, good, fair, or poor, and the *following* of a small object can be graded in a similar manner.

Measuring and recording visual function in this manner are far from perfect but are often sufficient. One problem is that a child can have excellent fixation and following with imperfect visual acuity. Also, because the preceding schemes do not allow precise gradations, mild differences between fellow eyes are difficult to distinguish. Children with ocular motility problems such as cranial nerve palsies and oculomotor apraxia may be er-

roneously judged to have poor vision when assessment relies on the motor system.

Fixation preference   Much critical information can be obtained simply by observing patients with manifest strabismus to determine the *fixation preference* (see Chapter 15). The examiner should determine which eye is the preferred eye for fixation and whether fixation between the eyes alternates spontaneously. Patients who spontaneously alternate fixation can be assumed not to have a clinically important difference (amblyopia) between the two eyes. If spontaneously alternating fixation is not present, the examiner must estimate how strongly the fixating eye is preferred. This is done by briefly covering the fixing eye and observing the nondominant eye while it takes up fixation. Then the patient is allowed once again to view with both eyes. If the patient immediately switches fixation back to the dominant eye, the fixation preference for the favored eye is quite strong. If the patient holds fixation with the nonpreferred eye for a few seconds, through a blink or while making pursuit movements, the *ocular dominance* is not as strong. Amblyopia treatment in strabismic patients may be deemed very successful if the child holds fixation well with the amblyopic eye or spontaneously alternates fixation. Determining fixation preference and the degree of ocular dominance is an important skill for any ophthalmologist.

Induced tropia test (vertical prism test)   Determining the presence and degree of ocular dominance in a straight-eyed patient is a greater challenge. The *induced tropia test* or *vertical prism test* can be used to determine ocular dominance in preverbal children without strabismus or in children with the monofixation syndrome. This test is useful in patients with suspected anisometropic amblyopia, or other types of monocular amblyopia. It can be performed with the patient fixating at a near or distant target. A 10- to 15–prism diopter loose prism is placed base up or base down in front of one eye as the patient views a target binocularly. If this causes both eyes to "jump," the child is presumed to have been fixating with the eye behind the prism, thus defining the dominant eye (Fig. 1-5). To check this, the ex-

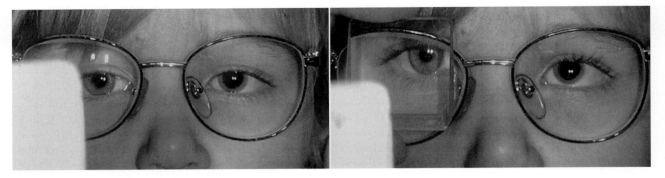

Fig. 1-5   Vertical prism test. This patient has anisometropic amblyopia of the right eye, which is being treated by atropinization of the left eye. *Left,* The eyes are straight and are directed toward a near target. *Right,* Immediately after a base-down prism is placed in front of the right eye, both eyes make upward saccades, indicating that the right eye is fixating. Since the weaker eye is now preferred, successful treatment of amblyopia is likely.

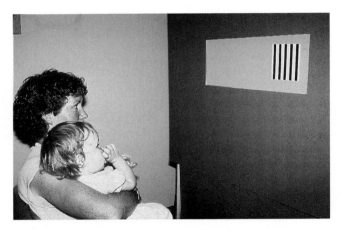

Fig. 1-6   Teller card preferential looking apparatus.

aminer removes the prism and the patient reestablishes fixation with another quick eye movement. Then the prism is placed before the other eye. The absence of induced movement once again shows that the fellow eye is the dominant eye. In some patients, placing the prism before either eye induces a conjugate refixation saccade or has no effect. Both of these results indicate no significant difference between the eyes. However, once a difference is discovered, an effort should be made to determine the depth of the asymmetry. This is performed in a fashion similar to that in patients with strabismus. While the prism is held in front of the dominant eye, that eye is briefly occluded and the nondominant eye is forced to take up fixation. On removal of the cover the quality and duration of fixation maintained with the nondominant eye are assessed. The vertical prism test can be performed in seconds and often provides important information.

Preferential looking   The *preferential looking test,*

in which Teller Acuity Cards are used, assesses the grating acuity by presenting the preverbal child with two visual stimuli. This test is first performed binocularly and then monocularly. The stimuli consist of high-contrast gratings of various spatial frequencies, along with a paired blank card. Children find the striped stimulus more visually appealing and prefer to look at it than at the blank card. To perform the test, the examiner works from behind a screen and presents the child with a test card and a control card simultaneously (Fig. 1-6). The examiner views through a peephole and assesses to which card the child directs his or her gaze. Test cards with progressively finer gratings are used until the child no longer demonstrates a preference for the test card. At that point it is assumed that the child perceives no difference between the cards and the result is given as a grating acuity in cycles per second. Then the process is repeated for the fellow eye.

Preferential looking techniques are in wide use but have well-known limitations. First, performing the test requires trained personnel and may take 20 to 30 minutes. Second, the child must cooperate. Third, although useful in the assessment of anisometropic or deprivation amblyopia, the test may underestimate strabismic amblyopia or decreased acuity caused by macular disease, in which grating acuity may be much less affected than Snellen acuity. Fourth, grating acuity cannot be precisely correlated with Snellen acuity because the range of "normal" values of grating acuity is wide.

Optotype Visual Acuity

Allen figures are simple line drawings scaled to correspond to Snellen acuity notation. These figures are useful in testing the acuity of children who do not yet know the alphabet. Either hand-held cards or projected figures may be used. Use of a single hand-held figure is preferred for younger patients because it holds their attention better. To test a child in this fashion, the examiner should start close to the patient and move backward. In young children the endpoint is more often demonstrated by a loss of attention than by an incorrect response. The disadvantage of testing acuity with a single figure is that it does not detect the crowding phenomenon. Therefore, as soon as the child is able, linear testing should be performed. Both single and linear Allen figures test only to the level of 20/30, which is adequate for children under 3 years of age.

The next step in preliterate acuity testing uses the *tumbling "E"* or the *Lantoldt "C."* These tests require the child to indicate the orientation of the optotype and may be performed with single characters or a line of optotypes. Since the patient has to indicate only by pointing in the direction the letter is oriented, shy or nonverbal children may cooperate better with these tests. The results obtained closely approximate those of Snellen acuity testing.

Once the child is literate, *Snellen letters* can be used. For most children this occurs at around 5 to 7 years of age. Some parents overestimate their children's facility with letters. Therefore, if the child performs poorly with Snellen testing, one of the methods mentioned previously should be used.

Optokinetic Nystagmus

Optokinetic nystagmus is an induced form of nystagmus, which is a normal phenomenon. The optokinetic response is generated with a moving full-field stimulus, which induces a pursuit movement. Saccadic recovery movements are made to refixate. In the clinic an optokinetic nystagmus drum *(OKN drum)* is used. The drum, which contains high-contrast stripes, is held close to the child's eye to fill the visual field and then is slowly rotated. With the standard drum, induced ocular movements imply vision of finger counting at 3 to 5 feet. However, the absence of induced optokinetic nystagmus has uncertain significance, particularly in young children. Children should be tested monocularly in both the horizontal and the vertical plane.

Pattern Visual-Evoked Potential

Pattern visual-evoked potentials *(PVEPs)* measure a summed occipital cortex response to a pattern stimulus. An alternating checkerboard pattern is typically used, allowing assessment of macular function. The important parameters of the waveform are the amplitude and the latency. Both amblyopia and organic disease can be detected by use of VEPs. The major drawbacks of PVEP testing are that special equipment and personnel are required and that the waveform amplitudes, even in normal control subjects, may vary widely. Furthermore, proper fixation and refractive correction are essential because eccentric viewing and blur produce abnormal results. The visual acuities measured with PVEP techniques reach adult values earlier than with other techniques.

Bruckner Test

The Bruckner test uses the direct ophthalmoscope and assesses the red reflexes simultaneously in both eyes. This rapid test can provide powerful information and should be part of the routine pediatric ophthalmology examination. Primary care physicians who care for children should also screen their patients in this way. In a dim room the observer views through the ophthalmoscope from a distance of approximately 1 m. The red reflexes should appear bright and equal in both eyes. Any asymmetry should be investigated further. A brighter reflex may be found in a deviating eye. A dull reflex may be found in an ametropic eye or one with a media opacity. The dimmest light with which the reflexes can be adequately visualized should be used.

Dilation, Cycloplegia, and Refraction

Adequate cycloplegia is essential for refraction of young patients. Even if the patient's fixation can be maintained in the distance during the refraction, high levels of hyperopia may not be detected without cycloplegia. A number of cycloplegic and mydriatic agents are available. The physician should keep in mind their primary actions, the time it takes for a good effect to begin, and side effects (Table 1-2). Also, in the refraction of young patients, cycloplegia is more important than wide pupillary dilation. Tropicamide is not a strong enough cycloplegic for young children. Instead, cyclopentolate, homatropine, or atropine should be used. Cyclopentolate has the most rapid onset and is our choice for routine use in the clinic. For most children 1 drop each of cyclopentolate 1% and phenylephrine 2.5% is adequate. One or two applications are given to patients with light irides; darker-eyed patients may require two or three. For patients younger than 6 months, including premature babies, cyclopentolate 0.5% is safer to use than 1%. Many examiners use a commercially available combination drop containing cyclopentolate 0.2% and phenylephrine 1%. Homatropine 5% is also effective for use in the clinic but has a prolonged duration of action (up to 3 days). Both cyclopentolate and homatropine produce maximal cycloplegia within 30 minutes to 1 hour after application. On retinoscopy a changing reflex or changing pupil size indicates incomplete cycloplegia. Patients in this situation require atropine. We suggest 1 drop of 1% atropine

Table 1-2   Cycloplegic and mydriatic agents in children

Agent	Strength (%)	Mydriasis		Cycloplegia		Side effects
		Maximum (min)	Recovery time	Maximum (min)	Recovery time	
Phenylephrine	2.5	20	2-3 hr	None		Tachycardia, hypertension
Tropicamide	0.5, 1	20-40	2-6 hr	30	2-6 hr	
Cyclopentolate	0.5, 1, 2	30-60	6-24 hr	25-75	6-24 hr	Psychosis, seizure
Homatropine	2, 5	40-90	1-3 days	30-60	1-3 days	Ataxia
Atropine	0.5, 1	30-60	7-14 days	60-180	3-12 days	Flushing, tachycardia, fever, delirium

given twice a day for the 3 days before a return visit. Punctal occlusion can be performed for 1 minute after instillation of the drops to decrease systemic absorption. The parent should be warned about signs of toxicity or allergy (Table 1-2).

Refraction of young children's eyes is a skill that requires practice and patience. A facility with loose lenses is required. Common errors include holding the trial lens too close to or too far from the eye and not controlling the working distance. For refraction of the deviating eye of a child with strabismus, temporarily patching the dominant eye allows an on-axis streak. At times a reliable refraction simply may not be obtainable. In such cases a repeat examination is recommended. Since refractions done at the Phoropter provide the most accurate determination of the cylinder axis, we use this instrument whenever possible, in preference to loose lenses. For children with good visual potential who are old enough, the retinoscopy should be refined with manifest refraction. However, in patients with amblyopia the subjective endpoint may be unclear and ophthalmologists often write the prescription based solely on retinoscopy.

Having a good working relationship with one or more opticians is useful for the physician and beneficial to patients. The ophthalmologist should be able to direct the patient to shops where the staff is comfortable dealing with babies and children. Such optical shops have a variety of pediatric frames, as well as personnel experienced in fitting children.

Fundus examination   Adequate examination of the fundus is imperative during a pediatric ophthalmology examination. The extent of the examination depends on the situation. In many instances visualization of the retinal periphery is unnecessary. However, a good view of the posterior pole, including the macula and optic nerve, is required for all patients. This can often be achieved with the child seated in a parent's lap by using an indirect ophthalmoscope with the light dimmed. The examiner can usually get a brief look in this fashion, particularly if the child is not touched. Sometimes the direct ophthalmoscope is useful if greater detail is re-

quired. If the situation dictates a more detailed view of the fundus, young children can be sedated or restrained. Older, uncooperative children may require examination under anesthesia.

VISUAL IMPAIRMENT IN INFANTS AND CHILDREN

Evaluation of Blind Infants

The cause of visual impairment in infants usually can be determined on the basis of the history and physical examination. The important historical points include family history, with special reference to consanguinity and history of blindness in other family members. Parents should be asked to describe the visual function in their infant, with particular attention to (1) differences in the night and day vision; (2) whether the visual function is stable, improving, or worsening; and (3) the presence or absence of nystagmus. The birth history, including the occurrence of perinatal anoxia, is particularly important. The gestational age, birth weight, and possible presence of retinopathy of prematurity should be determined. The presence of other medical problems may provide useful clues. For example, episodes of tachypnea and apnea in a baby with poor vision suggest Joubert's syndrome.

Structural causes, such as Peters' anomaly, microphthalmia, congenital cataracts, persistent hyperplastic primary vitreous, and optic nerve disorders, pose no diagnostic problem for the ophthalmologist. The real challenge occurs when the structure of the eye is normal or nearly so, yet the vision is poor. In these instances the most common disorders are Leber's congenital amaurosis, achromatopsia, and congenital stationary night blindness (CSNB). Less commonly, an early presentation of X-linked retinitis pigmentosa may be responsible.

Leber's congenital amaurosis is suggested by the findings of nystagmus at an early age, moderate to high degrees of hyperopia, and nonreactive pupils. Affected patients often have a normal-appearing fundus as infants.

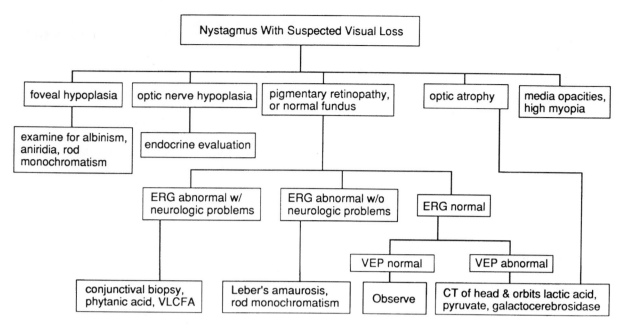

Fig. 1-7   Algorithm for the evaluation of nystagmus with suspected visual loss.

As they age, a pigmentary retinopathy, with arteriolar attenuation, develops. Achromatopsia (rod monochromatism) is suggested by light aversion, nystagmus, and paradoxical pupillary reactions. These patients have a high incidence of hypermetropia and astigmatism. The physician should suspect CSNB in children with poor night vision and paradoxical pupillary responses. Although CSNB usually comes to attention in older children, in early onset cases nystagmus may be present. The preceding entities can be distinguished with electroretinography. A suggested approach is given in Fig. 1-7.

Other causes of poor vision, usually with associated diseases or a history that points to the problem, include peroxisomal disorders, neuronal ceroid lipofuscinosis, and cortical visual impairment (cortical blindness). In cortical visual impairment, nystagmus is absent and pupil reactions are normal. Delayed visual maturation (DVM) is a term for a group of poorly understood disorders characterized by visual function that lags behind what would be expected but subsequently catches up. Hence, the diagnosis of DVM is not made until the vision improves. DVM may be an isolated defect or may be associated with systemic or ocular disease.

Evaluation of Older Children with Unexplained Visual Impairment

In many respects the evaluation of an older child with visual loss parallels that of adults. In obtaining the history, the physician must determine the pace of the visual loss, as well as whether the visual function was ever documented as normal. The general medical history should be reviewed to determine the presence of trauma, neurodegenerative disorders, and other relevant conditions. If the fundus and optic nerve appear normal, the primary diagnostic possibilities include CSNB, achromatopsia, Stargardt's disease, and early optic neuropathies, such as Leber's hereditary optic neuropathy and dominant optic atrophy.

PEDIATRIC PATIENTS WITH LOW VISION

Good vision is integral to normal cognitive and physical development. Visual impairment influences and delays global development. For instance, object permanence, knowing that something continues to exist even when it is not seen, is clearly different for a blind child than for a normally sighted one. Communication skills may be delayed because visual feedback, important in the learning of social gestures, is lacking. Visually impaired infants also may lag in motor skill development. Therefore babies and preschoolers with poor vision should be enrolled in specially designed enrichment programs.

To the greatest extent possible, children with low vision should be schooled conventionally and work independently. The role of the ophthalmologist is to determine the level of visual impairment and to prescribe low-vision aids or to refer the child to a specialist in low vision. In addition, the ophthalmologist must communicate with the patient's teachers to continually reassess the effectiveness of any aids being used.

Most children with impaired vision naturally hold material close to the face, and parents should not discourage such behavior. Because of children's high accommodative abilities, they may not require magnification. Reading materials with large print may also be useful. As the child ages, a particularly helpful tool is a stand magnifier, which is placed on a flat surface and provides a constant focus. Another useful device is a hand-held telescope. Telescopes take some practice to use effectively, but for many children their use significantly expands the visual world.

DYSLEXIA AND READING DISABILITY

Ophthalmologists are often requested to assess the eyes and the visual function of patients with subnormal reading. Such visits may be initiated by the parents of a child with poor school performance or by a pediatrician or primary care physician. *Dyslexia* may be defined as a specific primary reading defect in which the ability to read and extract information from written material is significantly lower than expected for a given patient's level of schooling and intelligence. "Reading disability" and other related terms have also been used to define this disorder. Many persons with dyslexia write poorly and show characteristic letter reversals. However, there is no single accepted definition of dyslexia and no single diagnostic test, and the cause remains unknown. Also, dyslexia appears to overlap with attention deficit hyperactivity disorder in children. About 5% to 10% of children are believed to have some form of reading disability. A familial tendency has been recognized.

The role of the ophthalmologist is to establish that the ophthalmological examination is normal and then to refer the patient for further evaluation. In 1993 the American Academy of Pediatrics, American Academy of Ophthalmology, and American Association for Pediatric Ophthalmology and Strabismus published a joint policy statement on this topic. This statement reviewed important issues related to reading disability, dyslexia, and vision. No known ocular defect accounts for dyslexia or reading disability, and no ocular treatment, including eye exercises, visual training, neurological organizational training, or the use of tinted or colored lenses, has proved effective. The use of these methods results in unwarranted expense and delays more effective treatment. The ophthalmologist should have local referral sources at hand so that a child with a reading disability is most effectively handled. Unfortunately, public school systems often lack the personnel to assess these children properly. Referral to a neuropsychologist for identification of the cognitive processing problem is a good first step. Based on these findings, an education specialist should be able to tailor learning methods to the child's particular abilities.

MAJOR POINTS

The horizontal diameter of the cornea in full-term infants averages 9.8 mm.

The average refraction in full-term infants is approximately +0.62 diopters.

The average normal intraocular pressure in infants ranges from 8 to 12 mm Hg.

The visual acuity of newborns is estimated to fall in the range of 20/400 to 20/800.

Normal visual acuity is reached by age 18 to 30 months.

The preferential looking test evaluates acuity by use of high-contrast gratings as stimuli.

In the Bruckner test the brighter reflex is often in the deviating eye.

The common ocular disorders responsible for decreased vision with a normal-appearing fundus are Leber's congenital amaurosis, achromatopsia, and congenital stationary night blindness.

SUGGESTED READINGS

Birch EE: Visual acuity testing in infants and young children, *Ophthalmol Clin North Am* 2(3):369-389, 1989.

Ferrell KA: Your child's development. In Holbrook MC, ed: *Children with visual impairments,* Bethesda, Md, 1996, Woodbine House.

Gordon RA, Donzis PB: Refractive development of the human eye, *Arch Ophthalmol* 103:785-789, 1985.

Hoyt CS, Nickel BL, Billson FA: Ophthalmological examination of the infant: developmental aspects, *Surv Ophthalmol* 26(4):177-189, 1982.

Lambert SR, Kriss A, Taylor D: Delayed visual maturation: a longitudinal clinical and electrophysiological assessment, *Ophthalmology* 96(4):524-529, 1989.

Olitsky SE, Nelson LB: Reading disorders in children, *Ophthalmol Clin North Am* 9(2):309-315, 1996.

Policy statement: learning disabilities, dyslexia, and vision; a joint statement of the American Academy of Pediatrics, American Association for Pediatric Ophthalmology and Strabismus, and American Academy of Ophthalmology, *Ophthalmology* 100(12):1867-1869, 1993.

Roland EH, Jan JE, Hill A, et al: Cortical visual impairment following birth asphyxia, *Pediatr Neurol* 2:133-137, 1986.

Sokol S, Hansen VC, Moskowitz A, et al: Evoked potential and preferential looking estimates of visual acuity in pediatric patients, *Ophthalmology* 90(5):552-562, 1983.

Tongue AC, Cibis GW: Brückner test, *Ophthalmology* 88(10): 1041-1044, 1981.

Wright KW, Walonker F, Edelman P: 10-Diopter fixation test for amblyopia, *Arch Ophthalmol* 99:1242-1246, 1981.

Zipf RF: Binocular fixation pattern, *Arch Ophthalmol* 94: 401-405, 1976.

Lid Malformations and Lesions

In this chapter a range of pediatric eyelid problems are discussed, including congenital malformations, ptosis, and congenital and acquired lesions affecting the pediatric eyelid.

CONGENITAL EYELID AND EYELASH DISORDERS

Embryology

Surface ectoderm, neural crest cell mesenchyme, and mesoderm all contribute to eyelid development. Upper and lower eyelid buds, visible by the sixth week of ges-tation, develop from corresponding precursors called frontonasal and maxillary processes. The eyelid buds elongate, grow toward each other, and fuse at about 12 weeks' gestation to cover the eye. Their gradual separation is usually complete by the sixth or seventh month. Surface ectoderm gives rise to skin and conjunctiva; neural crest cells develop into the tarsus and other structures; and the eyelid musculature is derived from the mesenchyme.

Cryptophthalmos

Cryptophthalmos is a rare condition in which the eyelids remain fused, usually with abnormal globe development. The severity of the condition may vary, but in the complete form, epidermis covers a microphthalmic eye, and there is no discernible eyelid fissure or lashes. The skin may be fused to the underlying cornea. The brow is usually absent and the hairline lowered. In less severe forms, partially formed eyelids and conjunctival sacs are present. Cryptophthalmos may be unilateral or bilateral, and autosomal recessive inheritance has been described. The association with syndactyly constitutes Fraser syndrome. Treatment is individualized, depending on severity, but good visual outcomes are uncommon.

Ankyloblepharon

In ankyloblepharon, there is complete or partial fusion of the eyelids, but the underlying globe generally is not affected. Ankyloblepharon filiform adnatum is a variant in which fine skin tags connect the eyelids.

Euryblepharon

This condition, first described by Desmarres, is caused by the lateral canthus being situated too far inferiorly, causing a widening of the lateral palpebral fissure

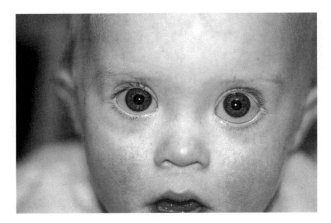

Fig. 2-1   Euryblepharon.

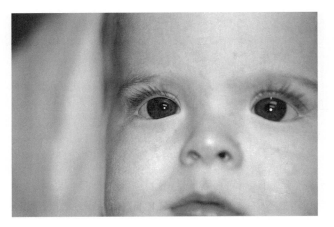

Fig. 2-2   Epiblepharon.

(Fig. 2-1). Thus it can be confused with congenital ectropion. It may occur sporadically or be inherited in an autosomal dominant fashion. Typically, the condition is bilateral and symmetrical. Treatment may require skin grafting and lateral canthoplasty, as the lower lid skin may be deficient.

Epiblepharon

Epiblepharon is an inward turning of the lashes (usually of the lower eyelid) caused by poor attachment of the inferior eyelid retractors to the skin. Thus the inferior lid crease is poorly formed (Fig. 2-2). Usually, damage to the cornea does not result, and the anatomic relationship between the lid and the eye normalizes as the face matures. However, if corneal damage such as abrasions or pannus occur, surgical repair should be performed. Excision of a strip of skin with or without orbicularis can properly orient the lower eyelid; some surgeons will pass deeper sutures to attach the lower lid retractors to the skin. Epiblepharon is common in Asian persons.

Ectropion

An outward turning of the lower eyelid is uncommon as an isolated congenital anomaly. When present there are usually associated defects such as scarring and shortening of the skin resulting from trauma or infection. Ectropion is a frequent complication of ichthyosis.

Entropion

In congenital entropion, an inward turning of the lower eyelid is caused by an abnormal tarsus. The lids also may turn in with enophthalmos and microphthalmos. Corneal damage is more likely in entropion than in epiblepharon.

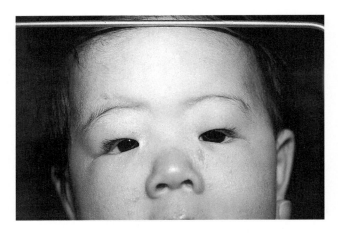

Fig. 2-3   Epicanthus tarsalis.

Epicanthus

Epicanthus refers to a fold of skin over the medial canthus that runs between the eyelids. It is usually bilateral. The most common form is epicanthus palpebralis, in which the skin folds equally involve the upper and lower lids. Epicanthus palpebralis is of clinical importance because it frequently creates the appearance of esotropia (pseudoesotropia). In epicanthus inversus, the skin folds are more prominent in the lower eyelids and may be part of the blepharophimosis syndrome (see the following discussion). Epicanthal folds more prominent in the upper lids are called epicanthus tarsalis (Fig. 2-3). Epicanthus tends to become less prominent as the nasal bridge matures.

Blepharophimosis Syndrome

Blepharophimosis means small eyelids, but most practitioners use the term *blepharophimosis syndrome* to refer to a congenital, autosomal dominant, variably ex-

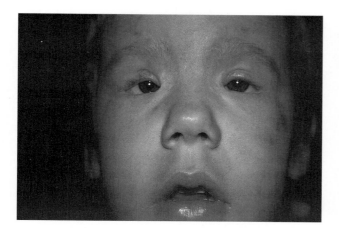

Fig. 2-4   Blepharophimosis syndrome.

pressive condition consisting of four main features. These are blepharophimosis, a vertical and horizontal narrowing of the eyelid fissures; ptosis; telecanthus; and epicanthus inversus (Fig. 2-4). Most often, the levator function is poor, and the upper eyelid creases are absent. Frontalis suspension may therefore be required early in life. Such surgery may require revision as the child matures. Since repair of telecanthus often changes the eyelid position, it should be done before ptosis surgery.

Distichiasis

In distichiasis, an accessory row of eyelashes arises from or near the meibomian orifices (Fig. 2-5). The row may be complete or incomplete, but usually the cilia are normal and do not damage the cornea. However, if required, the lashes can be treated by surgical excision or selective cryoablation.

Coloboma

Congenital full-thickness defects of the eyelids involving the lid margin most often involve the medial aspect of the upper eyelid. Lid colobomas occur as part of an ocular or systemic condition or as a sporadic and isolated finding. In Goldenhar's syndrome, the upper lid is often affected (Fig. 2-6); in Treacher-Collins syndrome, the lateral lower eyelid is involved. Colobomas affecting the globe may also be seen in otherwise isolated cases.

PTOSIS

The list of the causes of congenital ptosis and acquired ptosis in children is long, but the few most common causes, covered in the following discussion, account for most cases.

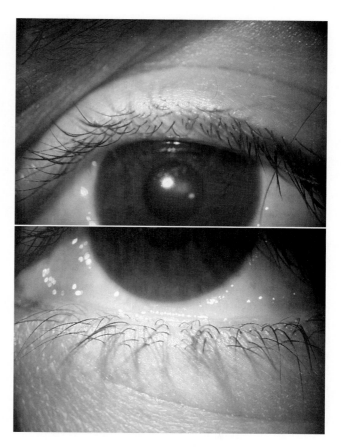

Fig. 2-5   Distichiasis. Multiple rows of lashes are present in the upper and lower eyelids.

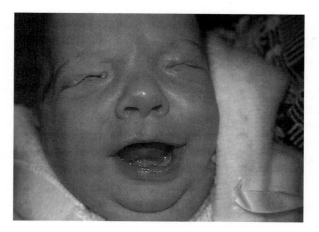

Fig. 2-6   Upper eyelid colobomata in Goldenhar's syndrome.

Congenital Ptosis

Ophthalmologists frequently encounter infants with unilateral or bilateral ptosis, which is isolated and not associated with craniofacial disorder, neurologic deficit, mass, or trauma. This type of congenital ptosis is usually

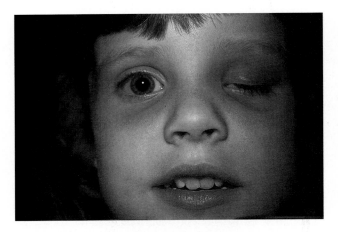

Fig. 2-7 Congenital blepharoptosis caused by levator maldevelopment.

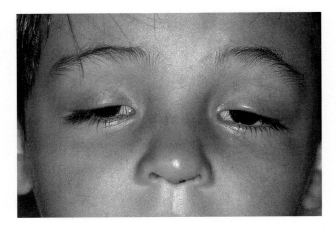

Fig. 2-8 Bilateral levator dysgenesis-type ptosis. Note brow elevation.

due to maldevelopment of the levator complex (Figs. 2-7 and 2-8). The terminology can be confusing. Many practitioners really mean levator dysgenesis-type ptosis when they use the term *congenital ptosis,* but such usage is imprecise, because there are obviously a number of types of congenital ptosis. The keys to successful management of these patients are to correctly classify the ptosis, to recognize and treat accompanying amblyopia, and to accurately grade the eyelid's function to permit the most effective surgical repair.

Isolated congenital ptosis resulting from a localized dysgenesis of the levator muscle is unilateral in 75% of cases. Occasionally, a family history can be obtained, but most cases are sporadic. Histologic examination demonstrates fibrous and fatty material instead of the usual striated muscle fibers. It is not known why this occurs, but it is remarkable that the adjacent superior rectus muscle is spared in most instances. The fibrous levator explains the classic clinical findings that are present in most cases. Ptosis occurs because the eyelid is weak and inelastic. In downgaze, the lid does not fall completely because of its stiffness ("lid lag"). Finally, the upper lid crease is absent in severe cases but better formed in milder cases.

Examination of these patients begins with observation. Obviously, infants with marked ptosis require prompt surgical intervention to prevent amblyopia. Older children, who can control their head movements, often will adopt a chin-up head position to obtain binocular vision. However, contrary to traditional teaching, amblyopia may still be present in these patients. Next, the examiner must confirm the diagnosis by evaluating the ocular motility, checking for eyelid masses, and so on. Following this evaluation, the presence of Bell's reflex is checked, particularly when contemplating surgery. Incomplete eyelid closure often accompanies "successful" congenital ptosis surgery. The Bell's reflex was

absent or abnormal in 15% of normal patients in one study; overly aggressive lid elevation in these patients risks the health of the cornea. Finally, an accurate assessment of degree of ptosis and levator function is made, which can be difficult in young children.

Many schemes have been proposed to guide the surgeon's choice of or extent of surgery, but most take into account the *degree of ptosis* and *levator function* as the main variables. Thus, if there is mild ptosis with good levator function, a small levator resection is performed. Moderate amounts of ptosis with poor levator function require very large levator resections. Marked ptosis with poor levator function is repaired with frontalis slings, and so on. Textbooks of oculoplastic surgery provide tables to guide the degree of surgery to be done, but effectiveness will vary depending on technique and surgeon. Unpredictable results may be expected in patients with mild ptosis and poor levator function. Other particularly difficult situations include highly asymmetric ptosis and congenital dehiscence of the levator. Finally the published tables generally apply to isolated congenital ptosis and not to Horner's syndrome, synkinetic ptosis, and cases with extraocular muscle dysfunction.

Marcus Gunn Jaw-winking

The Marcus Gunn jaw-winking phenomenon occurs in 5% to 10% of all congenital ptosis patients. This is a congenital, abnormal, synkinetic movement, whereby stimulation of the internal or external pterygoid muscle causes elevation of the affected ipsilateral eyelid, which is usually ptotic. In most cases, neural impulses that normally would stimulate the external pterygoid muscle instead reach and cause contraction of the levator palpebrae superioris. This synkinesis is best demonstrated by having the patient move the jaw to the opposite side, but widely opening the mouth or moving the jaw forward

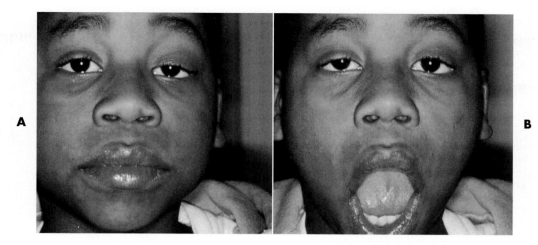

Fig. 2-9   Marcus Gunn jaw-winking. **A,** Notice left eyelid ptosis. **B,** The ptosis improves when the mouth is opened.

will also elevate the affected eyelid (Fig. 2-9). The internal pterygoid may instead be involved, but more rarely. Here, clenching the teeth will elevate the eyelid.

Marcus Gunn jaw-winking is one example of pathologic synkinetic movements with which the ophthalmologist must be familiar. Other examples of synkinetic movements are Duane's retraction syndrome, synergistic divergence, aberrant reinnervation of the third nerve, and acquired facial nerve synkinesis. The pathogenesis of the Marcus Gunn jaw-winking phenomenon is uncertain. It may be due to an insult *in utero*, an exaggeration of the normal synkinesis that is usually inapparent or both. Jaw-winking usually becomes evident in infancy during feeding, with the eyelid moving in synchrony with sucking. Occasional bilateral cases are seen, but most are unilateral and neurologically isolated. The degree of ptosis in the resting position may vary from mild to quite severe and will, of course, dictate the need for treatment. When required, a frontalis suspension with disinsertion of the levator is usually performed.

Oculomotor Palsy

Isolated ptosis as the first manifestation of a third nerve paresis is extraordinarily rare. Thus it is usually a straightforward task to determine that a third nerve problem is not responsible for a ptosis by demonstrating normal ocular motility and pupillary reactions. Congenital third nerve palsies vary in severity, and various extraocular muscles can be affected to differing degrees, producing unusual motility patterns (Fig. 2-10).

Certain features of congenital oculomotor palsies are noteworthy. A sizable percentage are a result of birth trauma (with or without the use of obstetric forceps); in these, partial or complete recovery is likely. Aberrant reinnervation is also frequently seen in congenital third

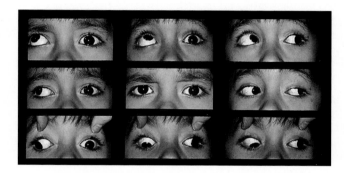

Fig. 2-10   Partial congenital right third nerve palsy.

nerve palsies, causing the pseudo von Graefe sign, pupillary miosis, and so on. The cyclic oculomotor palsy (oculomotor paresis with cyclic spasms) is a congenital palsy in which spontaneous, 10-to-30 second episodes of improved function of a paretic third nerve occur. The brief resolution of ptosis, lessening of the exotropia and pupillary miosis, will occur about every 1 to 3 minutes and persist throughout life. Finally, neurologic deficits such as hemiparesis can accompany congenital third nerve palsies.

Acquired third nerve palsies in childhood also may be classified according to the presence or absence of other neurologic deficits. Most isolated cases are probably post-viral or migrainous. Only a few cases of aneurysms, causing oculomotor paresis in children have been reported. Nonisolated third nerve palsies occur in trauma, with meningitis, with CNS tumors, and so on.

Horner's Syndrome

Damage to or dysfunction of the oculosympathetic pathways causing ptosis, pupillary miosis, and decreased sweating on the side of the problem is referred to as Horner's syndrome. Practically speaking, the complete triad is often absent, with the anhidrosis being by far the least consistent sign. Total loss of function of the sympathetically innervated Mueller's muscle causes mild ptosis, usually 2 to 3 mm. Remember that the lower eyelid also contains sympathetically innervated muscle. Therefore the *lower* lid can sometimes be seen to elevate about 1 mm as a result of decreased sympathetic activity. To bring this out, have the patient slowly elevate his gaze until the inferior limbus of an eye reaches the lower lid margin; this provides an easy landmark with which to compare the two sides. Although such lower lid elevation "upside-down ptosis," or "inverse ptosis" is not always present, we feel that it is a highly specific and under-appreciated sign of sympathetic dysfunction.

The pupil signs are possibly more reliable than the eyelid signs in diagnosing Horner's syndrome. One finds an anisocoria greater in darkness than in the light, which is due to the affected pupil's deficient dilation in the dark. Other characteristics are *dilation lag* in which the affected pupil shows prolonged (though incomplete) dilation in darkness, and poor dilation after instillation of topical cocaine. A more detailed description of pharmacologic testing in suspected Horner's syndrome is presented elsewhere in this series.

It is useful to distinguish between congenital and acquired cases in children. In most cases of isolated congenital Horner's syndrome, no specific etiology is found (Fig. 2-11). The majority of the remaining cases are caused by peripartum injury to the sympathetic plexus that envelops the ascending internal carotid artery. Uncommonly, congenital tumors cause compression, or there are other associated congenital defects. The most frequent causes of acquired Horner's syndrome in children are neuroblastoma (caused by a compressive lesion in the neck), trauma, and brainstem processes such as tumors, hemorrhages, and trauma. Iris heterochromia, with the affected iris lighter, is common in congenital cases and rare in acquired cases.

EYELID LESIONS

Molluscum Contagiosum

Molluscum contagiosum are common eyelid tumors in children caused by a poxvirus. They appear as small, often multiple, umbilicated nodules, typically along the eyelid margin (Fig. 2-12). Histopathologic examination shows the characteristic intracytoplasmic hyaline molluscum bodies (Fig. 2-13). Shed viral particles from even very small molluscum lesions can cause a follicular conjunctivitis; this is a frequently overlooked cause of chronic conjunctivitis. Treatment with expression or curettage and diathermy is usually curative, but all of the lesions on the entire body must be found and treated.

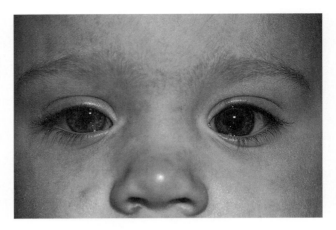

Fig. 2-11   Right congenital Horner's syndrome.

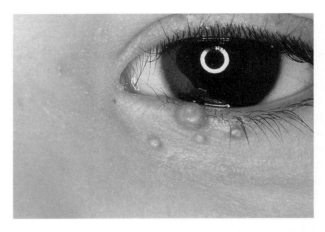

Fig. 2-12   Multiple molluscum contagiosum lesions of lower eyelid.

Viral Papillomata

Viral papillomas, or warts, are caused by human papilloma viruses, double-stranded DNA viruses that infect mucous membranes. Conjunctival lesions may appear to arise from the eyelid margins (Fig. 2-14). Papillomas can be observed or completely excised.

Chalazia

Chalazia are eyelid masses composed of lipogranulomatoses inflammation, which result from meibomian gland obstruction. They are the most common acquired eyelid masses in children and, although not dangerous, can be multiple, recurrent, and thus quite bothersome. Smaller, younger lesions often will resolve with the simple application of warm compresses for 4 to 8 weeks, but often curettage, intralesional steroid injection, or both are required. Remember that injected steroids can cause skin depigmentation (beware in dark-skinned patients!) and skin and fat atrophy.

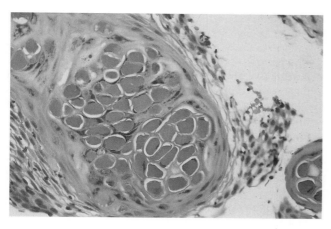

Fig. 2-13   Histopathology of molluscum contagiosum displaying eosinophilic molluscum bodies. See color plate.

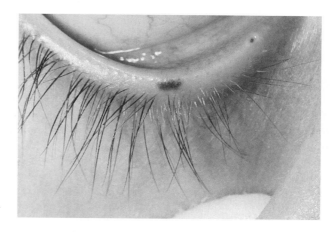

Fig. 2-15   Eyelid nevus. See color plate.

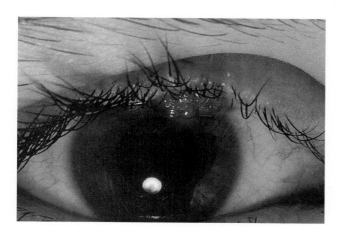

Fig. 2-14   Upper eyelid margin papilloma.

Nevi

Nevi involve the eyelids and eyelid margins just as they involve the skin elsewhere. In children, they are usually flat or slightly elevated and can grow and darken, presumably because of hormonal influences (Fig. 2-15). Junctional nevi are found in the base of the epidermis (the "junctional zone"), are usually flat, and spare the dermis. Intradermal nevi are confined to the dermis and are least likely to undergo malignant change. Compound nevi involve both the junctional zone and the dermis. "Kissing nevi," which involve adjacent regions of the upper and lower eyelids, are compound nevi. Blue nevi and cellular blue nevi occur in the deep dermis. When to excise a nevus in a child can pose a real clinical dilemma because general anesthesia is often required. Furthermore, tumor growth and darkening usually occur in the absence of malignant change. Nonetheless, in such instances we generally advocate excision.

Nevus of Ota

In nevus of Ota (oculodermal melanocytosis), there is congenital hyperpigmentation of the episclera, uvea, and skin in the regions of the first and second divisions of the trigeminal nerve. Orbital and meningeal involvement may also be present, and it is bilateral in 10% of patients. The increased pigmentation results from increased numbers of normal melanocytes. They are diffusely located in the uvea, and in the dermal layer of the skin. Asians and African-Americans are more commonly affected than whites. Involvement of the eye alone is referred to as ocular melanocytosis. Patients with nevus of Ota are at increased risk of glaucoma and melanoma. The lifetime

MAJOR POINTS

Cryptophthalmos is usually accompanied by an abnormal globe.

In euryblepharon, the temporal aspect of the palpebral fissure is wider than the nasal side.

Most cases of epiblepharon are asymptomatic and require no treatment.

The main elements in the blepharophimosis syndrome are a vertical and horizontal narrowing of the eyelid fissures, telecanthus, ptosis, and epicanthus inversus.

One fourth of congenital ptosis cases resulting from levator dysgenesis are bilateral.

Levator function and degree of ptosis determine the best surgical approach in congenital ptosis.

In Marcus Gunn jaw-winking ptosis, the external pterygoid is usually involved.

In cases of suspected Horner's syndrome, the finding of an elevated lower lid will support the diagnosis.

Molluscum contagiosum lesions may be multiple and cause a follicular conjunctivitis.

risk of an affected patient developing uveal melanoma has been estimated to be one in 400.

Other Eyelid Lesions

Neurofibromas, dermoids, and capillary hemangiomas account for the remainder of the important eyelid lesions in children. These are covered in the discussion of orbital disease, Chapter 4.

SUGGESTED READINGS

Al-Hazzaa SAF, Hidayat AA: Molluscum contagiosum of the eyelid and infraorbital margin: a clinicopathologic study with light and electron microscopic observations, *J Pediatr Ophthalmol Strabismus* 30:58-59, 1993.

Balkan R, Hoyt GS: Associated neurologic abnormalities in congenital third nerve palsies, *Am J Ophthalmol* 97:315-319, 1984.

Beyer-Machule CK, Johnson CC, Pratt SG, et al: The Marcus-Gunn phenomenon: a review of 80 cases (an update), *Orbit* 4:15-19, 1985.

Gupta SP, Saxena RC: Cryptophthalmos, *Br J Ophthalmol* 46: 629-632, 1962.

Jordan R: The lower-lid retractors in congenital entropion and epiblepharon, *Ophthalmic Surg* 24:494-496, 1993.

Keipert JA: Euryblepharon, *Br J Ophthalmol* 59:57-58, 1975.

Kodsi SR, Younge BR: Acquired oculomotor, trochlear, and abducent cranial nerve palsies in pediatric patients, *Am J Ophthalmol* 114:568-574, 1992.

McCord Jr CD: The correction of telecanthus and epicanthal folds, *Ophthalmic Surg* 11:446-456, 1980.

Noda S, Hayasaka S, Setogawa T: Epiblepharon with inverted eyelashes in Japanese children: I. Incidence and symptoms, *Br J Ophthalmol* 73:126-127, 1989.

Sauer C, Levinsohn MW: Horner's syndrome in childhood, *Neurology* 26:216-220, 1976.

Sellar PW, Bryars JH, Archer DB: Late presentation of congenital ectropion of the eyelids in a child with Down syndrome: a case report and review of the literature, *J Pediatr Ophthalmol Strabismus* 29:64-67, 1992.

Sullivan TJ, Clarke MP, Rootman DS, et al: Eyelid and formix reconstruction in bilateral abortive cryptophthalmos (Fraser syndrome), *Aust N Z J Ophthalmol* 20:51-56, 1992.

Weinstein JM, Zweifel TJ, Thompson HS: Congenital Horner's syndrome, *Arch Ophthalmol* 98:1074-1078, 1980.

Wilson ME, Johnson RW: Congenital ptosis: long-term results of treatment using lyophilized fascia lata for frontalis suspensions, *Ophthalmology* 98:1234-1237, 1991.

Wolfley D: Excision of individual follicles for the management of congenital distichiasis and localized trichiasis, *J Pediatr Ophthalmol Strabismus* 24:22-26, 1987.

CHAPTER 3

Lacrimal System

Most lacrimal system disease in children involves the lacrimal drainage system. Up to 6% of babies have clinically evident nasolacrimal duct obstruction. Diagnosis and treatment of nasolacrimal duct obstruction (NLDO) is first covered in this chapter, followed by a discussion of a related entity, dacryocystocele. Less common anomalies of the nasolacrimal drainage system and disorders lacrimal gland are then briefly discussed.

EMBRYOLOGY AND ANATOMY OF THE LACRIMAL SYSTEM

The nasolacrimal duct arises from a cord of ectodermal tissue that becomes enveloped in the mesoderm of the infolding naso-optic fissure. By the sixtieth day of gestation, canalization has started, progressing from the upper end downward. Often the process is not complete at birth, and a residual membrane at the distal opening, the valve of Hasner, persists. Pathologic study has shown this to be the case in the majority of term babies.

The lacrimal gland arises at about 40 to 45 days gestation, budding from conjunctival tissue. Two distinct lobes ultimately form, the orbital lobe and the palpebral lobe. These share a common secretory duct that passes through the palpebral lobe and empties superotemporally in the conjunctival fornix. Tear production is pre-

sent at birth but becomes clinically evident in the first few weeks of life.

The puncta are 0.3 mm diameter openings to the lacrimal drainage system, beyond which are the ampullae of the canaliculi. The canaliculi course vertically for 2 mm and then turn and extend 8 to 10 mm (the commonly given adult measurement) toward the lacrimal sac. In 90% of systems, the upper and lower canaliculi merge into a common canaliculus before merging with the lacrimal sac. The lacrimal sac lies in the bony lacrimal fossa, which is formed by the nasal process of the maxilla and the lacrimal bone. The adult lacrimal sac is about 10 to 12 mm in length, and at its inferior end it gives rise to the nasolacrimal duct. The 8 mm long duct empties into the inferior meatus, after passing through a bony canal.

NASOLACRIMAL DUCT OBSTRUCTION

Clinical Presentation and Evaluation

Within the first 2 to 3 weeks of life, as the baseline lacrimation increases, cases of nasolacrimal duct obstruction (NLDO) usually become evident. The parents will report that one or both eyes appear moist and that tears overflow and stream down the cheek. Chronic or intermittent infections of the upper drainage system cause mucopurulent material to appear on the surface of the eye. The eyelids and eyelashes may become perpetually mattered with the crusting exudate (Fig. 3-1). The eyelid and periocular skin often is red and irritated. There may be worsening of the discharge when the child has an upper respiratory illness or temporary improvement when the child is taking antibiotics for another ailment. Usually, the parents, primary care physician, and ophthalmologist will have no trouble recognizing a primary nasolacrimal duct obstruction, although at times, it is misdiagnosed as conjunctivitis. Distinguishing NLDO from congenital glaucoma should not be problem-

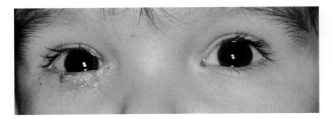

Fig. 3-1   Exudate and crusting secondary to nasolacrimal duct obstruction. See color plate.

Box 3-1   Technique of Lacrimal Sac Massage
1. Place fingertip on the medial canthal region.
2. Apply firm pressure on the sac.
3. Use a short, downward, sliding motion to raise the hydrostatic pressure in the duct and relieve the obstruction.
4. Perform once or more per day.

atic for the ophthalmologist, owing to the frequent presence of mucopurulent discharge in NLDO, as well as the absence of photophobia, corneal clouding, and buphthalmos. Hence, in the office, the ophthalmologist can typically confirm the suspected diagnosis readily; expressing mucopurulent material from the sac is confirmatory and demonstrates to the parents some of the pathologic process. Remember, however, that congenital glaucoma may (rarely) coexist with NLDO.

Fortunately, the visual consequences of NLDO are not severe. There is no evidence to support the fear, which many parents have, that the affected eye will become weaker (amblyopic). The primary consequence of NLDO is the local irritation caused to the patient (and to the parents as well) by the ongoing process. Very rarely, the process may develop into a true dacryocystitis/preseptal cellulitis picture, requiring prompt treatment with systemic antibiotics.

Natural History

Numerous studies have demonstrated what is generally known to most primary care physicians and ophthalmologists: the great majority of cases of NLDO, probably more than 90%, will spontaneously resolve, if given enough time. This natural history provides the context in which the other factors relevant to treatment decision-making are weighed. The timing of definitive treatment, nasolacrimal duct probing and irrigation is indeed controversial, and considerations include the severity of the case and the discomfort of the patient, the general health and age of the patient, and the wishes of the parents.

Treatment

In young patients, those up to about six months of age, it is reasonable to defer probing. Many suggest lacrimal sac "massage" and the use of topical antibiotics (Box 3-1). To perform massage a fingertip is placed on the medial canthal region, and firm pressure is placed on the sac. A short, downward, sliding motion is employed to raise the hydrostatic pressure in the duct, and to relieve the obstruction. This technique is also referred to as

Crigler massage. Massage is performed once or more per day.

Kushner studied the effectiveness of hydrostatic nasolacrimal sac massage compared to simple expression of the sac's contents out of the canaliculi and to observation and found hydrostatic massage significantly more effective than expression or observation. Topical antibiotics are used intermittently to control infections and are believed not to enhance spontaneous resolution of NLDO.

The primary operative goal of a nasolacrimal duct probing and irrigation is to break the membranous *valve of Hasner,* and any other obstructions present, with a probe. Many small variations of our preferred method exist (Box 3-2), and the practitioner will develop his or her own technique.

Probings on awake patients should be done by experienced surgeons, which minimizes the duration of the procedure. Topical anesthesia and secure restraints are used. Confirmation of probe placement and nasolacrimal system irrigation are often omitted.

The decision as to when to perform nasolacrimal duct probing is, in part, related to whether the practitioner prefers to perform probings in the office or in the operating room. Children as old as 6 to 8 months of age can be probed in an office setting. Advocates of this approach argue a number of factors in favor of office probings. First, the patients are not subjected to a general anesthetic as required in older patients. The cost and time expenditure is significantly lower when performed in the office. Some practitioners advocate early in-office probing, before the age of 6 months, because it eliminates the repeated infections that may scar the imperforate valve of Hasner. Such scarring, in theory, reduces the success rate of simple probing. Hence, early probing, besides relieving the patient and family of the problem, may reduce the need for subsequent silicone intubation. On the other hand, early in-office probing is traumatic to the patient, offers less control to the surgeon, and may largely be unnecessary, since many of the patients will have spontaneous resolution anyway. Katowitz and Welsh found that initial probings performed before age 13 months were more likely to be curative than those done later. There is general agreement that

Box 3-2   Technique of Nasolacrimal Duct Probing and Irrigation

- The surgeon sits at the head of the bed.
- Good illumination and, if required, magnification is used to examine the eyelids and puncta.
- A lubricated punctum dilator is introduced into the upper punctum and rotated 90 degrees toward the canaliculus.
  - Temporal traction on the upper eyelid is essential.
- The dilator is gently twisted in the fingertips as it is advanced.
  - This is done for a few seconds to allow the elastic punctum to fully expand.
- The punctal dilator is removed.
- A size 0-Bowman probe is introduced into the punctum.
- The eyelid is, again, pulled laterally, and the probe is turned into and advanced the length of the canaliculus.
  - *Most mistakes are made during this seemingly simple step.*
  - If the canaliculus is not straightened and made taut by lateral eyelid traction, it will kink as the probe is passed. This will result in tissue being dragged into the lacrimal sac or the creation of a false passage to the sac.
  - A clean pass will encounter minimal resistance and will allow the tip of the probe to palpably strike the lacrimal bone medial to the lacrimal sac.
- Gently tapping the tip of the probe against the firm medial wall of the sac will confirm its proper placement.
- Once proper placement is confirmed, eyelid traction may be released.
- The probe is then rotated downward into the duct.
  - Again, repeatedly tap the bony wall to ensure that no mucosa is engaged and dragged along with the tip.

- The probe should be kept on the horizontal plane as it is turned, taking care not to raise the trailing end of the probe, which makes it more difficult to properly enter the duct.
- As the probe is advanced forward, a discrete membrane or membranes will often be encountered.
  - By breaking through them, the surgeon can be confident that the problem is likely to be solved.
  - Other times, only minimal resistance is felt.
- Most practitioners, the authors included, will then confirm that the tip of the probe is truly in the nasal cavity.
- A nasal speculum is used to visualize the lower turbinate.
- A second, larger probe or a Freer elevator is guided below the turbinate, into the inferior meatus, keeping to the medial aspect of the nose.
  - You should be able to feel "metal on metal" contact as confirmation of proper placement.
  - Viewing with the nasal speculum also provides an opportunity to determine whether the turbinate is tightly opposed to the nasal septum, perhaps contributing to or causing the obstruction. If such a situation is found, we do not hesitate to infracture the turbinate with an elevator, a safe and easy maneuver.
- The probe is then removed and irrigation is performed.
- Balanced saline stained with fluorescein is gently injected into the lacrimal sac with a blunt cannula.
- Recovery of the solution from the nose with a suction cannula demonstrates that the system is patent.

cases which have not spontaneously resolved by age 12 or 13 months should be treated with probing and irrigation. In summary, in the United States, the approach to treatment of NLDO varies widely. We have performed probings in both fashions and, in most circumstances, prefer the control that is present in anesthetized patients. Although no scientific data on this point exist, we are concerned about the possibility of psychologically traumatizing babies who undergo awake probings.

Following one or two failed probings, silicone intubation of the nasolacrimal system is typically performed. It is also indicated in children older than 18 to 24 months because simple probing and irrigation typically fails in these patients. Some surgeons will place tubes even at the first probing if a bony stenosis is encountered. Also, simple probing and irrigation has a high failure rate in patients with craniofacial disorders; primary placement of silicone tubes is suggested in these patients (Box 3-3).

Box 3-3   Nasolacrimal Duct Obstruction: Instances in Which Simple Probing and Irrigation Is Likely to Fail

Older children
Congenital anomalies of the mid-face
Craniosynostosis
Down syndrome
Trauma

Once placed, these flexible stents are left in for 3 to 6 months. Improvement may be seen shortly after they are inserted but may be delayed until after removal. The implant used by most surgeons today consists of a moderately flexible stainless steel wire probe bonded to ei-

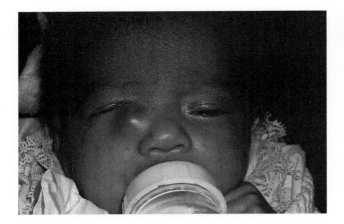

Fig. 3-2   Infected dacryocystocele. See color plate.

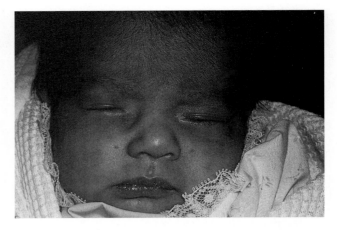

Fig. 3-3   Same patient as Fig. 3-2 immediately following probing of the nasolacrimal duct. See color plate.

ther end of a thin silicone tube. Within the tube is a silk suture. The nasolacrimal system first is cannulated from one punctum, with the wire passed in the usual fashion. The wire probe, which has at its tip a small ball, is retrieved through the nose with a Crawford hook and pulled through. The process is repeated with the remaining end through the other punctum. The wire probes are cut off and discarded, and the ends of the tubes are tied together. This leaves a small loop of tubing in the medial corner of the eye, spanning the upper and lower puncta. Many variations to secure the tubing in the nose have been described. Most strip off the silicone and tie the ends of the bare suture; others knot the silicone tubing without stripping. Regardless of the particular method employed, it is most important to tie the tubing so that no tension is placed on the puncta and canaliculi.

The most difficult step of silicone intubation is often the retrieval of the wire probes with the hook, typically a blind maneuver. This is made easier if you start by packing the nose with phenylephrine to shrink the mucous membranes and have a good understanding of the anatomy of the nose. The proper location to retrieve the wire is inferior and medial in the nose.

CONGENITAL DACRYOCYSTOCELE

The congenital dacryocystocele, also referred to as a dacryocele, mucocele, amniotocele, and lacrimal sac cyst, appears as a blue, cyst-like mass below the medial canthal tendon in a newborn. This uncommon condition is distinct from the usual NLDO and is managed differently. Dacryocystoceles occur when the nasolacrimal sac and duct become distended with fluid. A lower duct obstruction, combined with a functional upper blockage at the valve of Rosenmuller, trap mucoid material and

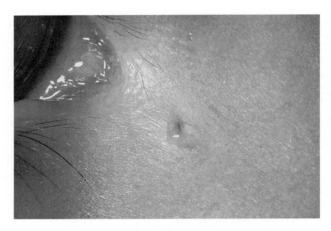

Fig. 3-4   An anomalous punctum, producing a tear.

create a tense, mass-like enlargement of the sac, which frequently becomes secondarily infected. Progression to infection, abscess formation, and preseptal cellulitis may occur rapidly; therefore these patients must be followed closely.

Various approaches to management have been suggested. A small percentage will spontaneously decompress and resolve permanently. Others will resolve with digital massage of the lacrimal sac and the use of topical antibiotics, and this is now usually suggested as the first management step. Probing of the nasolacrimal system, if no infection is present, is safe and very often effective. However, repeated probings may be required. Typically, within a few days to weeks, if the swelling has not resolved, secondary infection (dacryocystitis, cellulitis) will ensue (Figs. 3-2 and 3-3). Probing and systemic antibiotics are then indicated. External incision and drainage are to be avoided as skin fistulas may result. The differential diagnosis of dacryocystoceles includes meningoencephaloceles, hemangiomas, and dermoid cysts.

OTHER ANOMALIES OF THE NASOLACRIMAL DRAINAGE SYSTEM

Rarely, the lacrimal puncta fail to form. Careful inspection will show a small dimple or membrane in the region where the punctum should lie, and a safety pin can be used to create an opening into the canaliculus, which is then probed. Another uncommon anomaly is the external fistula of the lacrimal sac, a congenital epithelial tract from the lacrimal sac to the overlying skin (Fig. 3-4). Production of tears from such an orifice implies an obstruction of the lower system, which should be cleared before treatment of the fistula is undertaken.

LACRIMAL GLAND DISORDERS

Congenital absence of aqueous tear production, or severe hyposecretion, is referred to as alacrima. Very rarely, the lacrimal gland fails to form, but more often, the gland is present but secretes insufficiently. In Riley-Day syndrome (familial dysautonomia), a systemic condition affecting Ashkenazi Jews, there is decreased lacrimation and widespread autonomic dysfunction.

Alacrima may occur in association with orbital and ocular developmental disorders, ectodermal aplasia, and as an isolated condition. Affected patients have a viscous tear film, punctate epithelial keratitis, and photophobia. No tearing occurs in response to psychogenic stimuli, such as emotional crying.

Ectopic lacrimal gland tissue may be found in the eyelids, conjunctiva, cornea, uvea, and orbit. Such tissue may become cystic or neoplastic.

SUGGESTED READINGS

Baker JD: Treatment of congenital nasolacrimal system obstruction, *J Pediatr Ophthalmol Strabismus* 22(1):34-35, 1985.

Cassady JV: Developmental anatomy of nasolacrimal duct, *Arch Ophthalmol* 47:141-158, 1952.

Crawford JS, Pashby RC: Lacrimal system disorders, *Int Ophthal Clin* 24(1):39-53, 1984.

Crawford JS: Intubation of the lacrimal system, *Ophthal Plast Reconstr Surg* 5(4):261-265, 1989.

Goldberg MF, Payne JW, Brunt PW: Ophthalmologic studies of familial dysautonomia: the Riley-Day syndrome, *Arch Ophthalmol* 80:732-743, 1968.

Katowitz JA, Welsh MG: Timing of initial probing and irrigation in congenital nasolacrimal duct obstruction, *Ophthalmology* 94(6):698-705, 1987.

Keith CG, Boldt DW: Congenital absence of the lacrimal gland, *Am J Ophthalmol* 102(6): 800-801, 1986.

Kushner BJ: Congenital nasolacrimal system obstruction, *Arch Ophthalmol* 100:597-600, 1982.

MacEwen CJ, Young JDH: Epiphora during the first year of life, *Eye* 5:596-600, 1991.

Mansour AM, Cheng KP, Mumma JV, et al: Congenital dacryocele, *Ophthalmology* 98(11):1744-1751, 1991.

Nelson LB, Calhoun JH, Menduke H: Medical management of congenital nasolacrimal duct obstruction, *Ophthalmology* 92(9):1187-1190, 1985.

Paul TO, Shepherd R: Congenital nasolacrimal duct obstruction: natural history and the timing of optimal intervention, *J Pediatr Ophthalmol Strabismus* 31:362-367, 1994.

Petersen RA, Robb RM: The natural course of congenital obstruction of the nasolacrimal duct, *J Pediatr Ophthalmol Strabismus* 15(4):246-250, 1978.

Ratliff CD, Meyer DR: Silicone intubation without intranasal fixation for treatment of congenital nasolacrimal duct obstruction, *Am J Ophthalmol* 118:781-785, 1994.

Robb RM: Probing and irrigation for congenital nasolacrimal duct obstruction, *Arch Ophthalmol* 104:378-379, 1986.

Rush A, Leone Jr CR: Ectopic lacrimal gland cyst of the orbit, *Am J Ophthalmol* 92:198-201, 1981.

Scott WE, Fabre JA, Ossoinig KC: Congenital mucocele of the lacrimal sac, *Arch Ophthalmol* 97:1656-1658, 1979.

Welham RAN, Bergin DJ: Congenital lacrimal fistulas, *Arch Ophthalmol* 103:545-548, 1985.

Wesley RE: Inferior turbinate fracture in the treatment of congenital nasolacrimal duct obstruction and congenital nasolacrimal duct anomaly, *Ophthalmic Surg* 16(6)368-371, 1985.

Proptosis and Orbital Disease

In this chapter the important conditions of the pediatric orbit are covered. Preseptal and orbital cellulitis are not unique to children, but the spectrum of causative organisms differs, as does the differential diagnosis. Clinicians must be familiar with the diagnosis and treatment of the common orbital tumors, which are covered in the following discussion. Finally, the more common congenital craniofacial disorders are reviewed.

INFECTIONS AND INFLAMMATIONS

Preseptal and orbital cellulitis are covered together because of their similar etiologies and frequent coincidence. Both are more common in children than in adults and more common in the winter months.

Preseptal Cellulitis

Preseptal or periorbital cellulitis is by definition an infection of the eyelids and soft tissue structures anterior to the orbital septum. The septum is a thin fascial structure that extends from the orbital rims to the tarsus inferiorly and the levator aponeurosis superiorly. Anterior infections may pass through this imperfect barrier to involve the orbit. Preseptal cellulitis is a fairly common condition in children. Historical information, physical findings and, in some cases, radiologic findings help in defining the etiology and extent of the process. Clinically, there may be mild to very severe eyelid edema and erythema, but systemic signs are usually mild (Fig. 4-1). The ocular motility and pupil reactions are normal. Preseptal cellulitis in the absence of skin trauma or infection is presumably secondary to upper respiratory or sinus infection. Thus the most common organism causing preseptal cellulitis in children is *Streptococcus pneumoniae*. Cases secondary to abrasions, lacerations, impetigo, herpes simplex, insect bites, and hordeola involve different organisms, most often *Staphylococcus aureus* and *Streptococcus pyogenes*.

Evaluation and treatment of preseptal cellulitis depends on a number of factors listed in Box 4-1.

Although there are no firm rules, in general, the younger the patient and the more severe the case, the more likely we are to obtain laboratory tests and initiate inpatient treatment. If there is drainage from a skin infection, a swab for Gram's stain and culture is obtained. A complete blood count may be obtained, and in the more severe cases, blood cultures. Eyelid or brow trauma may result in abscess formation requiring incisional drainage. In cases without skin infection or trauma, some have advocated obtaining pharyngeal swabs for culture, but

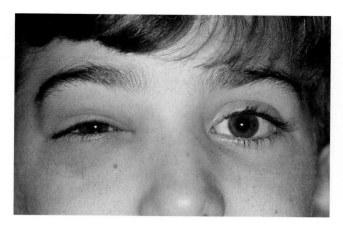

Fig. 4-1   Preseptal cellulitis, right eye. There is mild erythema and edema of the upper and lower eyelids. There is no proptosis and the vision is normal. See color plate.

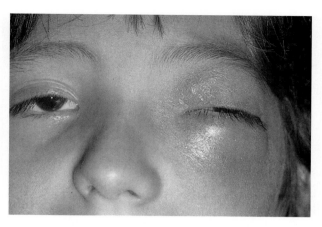

Fig. 4-2   Orbital cellulitis, left eye. Note the proptosis. Impaired ocular motility was also present. See color plate. (Courtesy Dr. Kenneth W. Wright.)

Box 4-1   Factors to Consider in the Evaluation and Treatment of Preseptal Cellulitis

Age of the patient
Severity of the condition, including associated
    systemic findings
Certainty with which the physician can distinguish
    preseptal cellulitis from orbital cellulitis
Family social situation

---

we have found that this rarely changes our antibiotic choice. Systemic evaluation should include assessment of the child's general state to determine if there is fever, signs of meningitis, and so on. The presence of preauricular and submandibular adenopathy should be sought. Very young children and babies are often cared for in concert with the pediatrician or primary care physician. When eyelid swelling is very severe, imaging is indicated. In such instances we usually obtain a computed tomography (CT) scan of the orbits to assess the paranasal sinuses, posterior extension into the orbit, and the presence of subperiosteal or orbital abscesses.

Which antibiotic to choose depends in part on the presumed source of the cellulitis. When skin organisms (staphylococcus and streptococcus species, and beta-hemolytic streptococcus) are suspected, mild cases may be treated with dicloxacillin, cefaclor, or amoxicillin-clavulanate potassium (Augmentin). Severe cases requiring hospitalization may be initially treated with nafcillin (or vancomycin, if the patient is allergic to penicillin) and gentamicin.

Infections associated with upper respiratory infections differ in etiology depending on the patient's age,

with *Staphylococcus aureus* and *Streptococcus pneumoniae* predominant in neonates. In older children, *Streptococcus pneumoniae*, non-typable *Haemophilus influenzae* and *Moraxella catarrhalis* are the important pathogens. It is important to note that *H. influenzae* type b infections, which occur secondary to bacteremia, are now quite rare because of the widespread use of an effective vaccine. Consequently, if there is no skin source evident, coexisting sinus disease is now to be expected. Effective oral agents include cephalosporins (cefaclor, cephalexin), newer macrolides (clarithromycin), and amoxicillin-clavulanate potassium (Augmentin.) Severe cases of preseptal cellulitis may require intravenous antibiotics as in orbital cellulitis (see the following discussion).

Orbital Cellulitis

Orbital cellulitis refers to an infectious process posterior to the orbital septum that affects the orbital contents. Thus the common manifestations are pain, particularly with eye movement, proptosis of the globe, impairment of the pupillary reactions, and limited ocular motility. As in preseptal cellulitis, eyelid edema and erythema are common (Fig. 4-2). Orbital cellulitis is a serious medical emergency that can damage the optic nerve and even progress intracranially through the valveless orbital veins. Bacteremia and sepsis is more common in small children than in adults. Meningitis occurs in 1.9% of all cases of orbital cellulitis.

In children, orbital cellulitis commonly occurs as a result of bacterial infection of an adjacent paranasal sinus, particularly the ethmoids. The lamina papyracea comprising the medial orbital wall is thin and contains neurovascular foramina and thus provides little mechanical resistance to the contiguous spread of infection. However, since the periosteum is loosely adherent here,

---

Box 4-2   Clinical Signs of Mucormycosis in Patients at Risk

Red eye
Orbital or preseptal cellulitis
Proptosis
Pain
Ophthalmoplegia
Visual loss

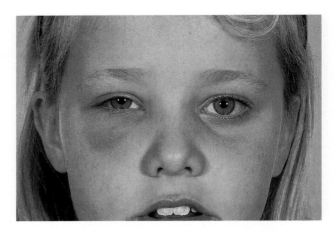

Fig. 4-3   A 12-year-old girl with left orbital pseudotumor. Note the lateral conjunctival injection and lower eyelid erythema. There was pain with eye movement. See color plate. (Courtesy Gregory Kosmorsky, Cleveland Clinic Foundation.)

the infection may be partially contained, forming a subperiosteal abscess. This must be specifically looked for when viewing a CT scan and appears as a dome-shaped elevation of the periosteum of the medial orbital wall. The abscess and adjacent ethmoid sinuses are opacified by purulent material. Infants may develop orbital cellulitis secondary to dacryocystitis.

Mixed flora infections are common (Staphylococcus, Streptococcus) with or without anaerobes. Recommended drugs for initial treatment include ticarcillin-clavulanate (Timentin), cefuroxime, cefotaxime, or ceftriaxone. Ceftriaxone has the advantage of crossing the blood-brain barrier, but may not adequately cover gram-positive infections. Clindamycin may be added if anaerobic infection is suspected. The presence of an abscess usually requires surgical intervention. However, early orbital and subperiosteal abscesses may respond to antibiotics alone. Obviously, such patients require careful monitoring in the hospital since surgery may become necessary.

Immunocompromised patients are susceptible to orbital infections resulting from aspergillosis and mucormycosis. Aspergillus is ubiquitous and causes two distinct patterns of disease. Infectious orbital cellulitis from aspergillosis, seen in immunocompromised patients, produces a rapidly progressive proptosis, with limited ocular motility, chemosis, fever, malaise, and other related symptoms. Aspergillus causes a necrotizing vasculitis and invades the orbit and cranium from the paranasal sinuses. Death can occur from overwhelming systemic or intracranial disease, despite treatment with amphotericin B and surgical debridement. Patients who are otherwise healthy, particularly those who live in warm, humid climates, may develop allergic fungal sinusitis. In this condition, chronic colonization of the paranasal sinuses causes a syndrome of nasal congestion and postnasal drip, with recurrent episodes of superimposed infection. In advanced cases, orbital invasion and proptosis can occur. This condition is treated surgically.

Mucormycosis is an often fatal fungal infection of the pharynx, paranasal sinuses, orbit, and intracranial cavity caused by members of the genera *Absidia, Rhizopus,* and *Mucor.* Affected patients are almost always immunocompromised, most often from diabetes with ketoacidosis, hematologic malignancies, or chronic alcoholism. These organisms invade blood vessels, causing thrombosis and tissue necrosis. Hence, little bleeding is encountered during biopsy or debridement of affected tissue. The clinician must consider this diagnosis early in patients at risk exhibiting certain conditions (Box 4-2).

An orbital apex syndrome is characteristic. Initial evaluation should include examination of the oropharynx and nasopharynx, with biopsy of necrotic tissue if encountered, as well as imaging with CT or magnetic resonance imaging (MRI). Aggressive treatment is required to avoid death and includes wide excision and high-dose amphotericin B.

Orbital Pseudotumor

Orbital pseudotumor is an idiopathic, noninfectious inflammatory condition of the orbit that affects all ages. In children, it may resemble cellulitis in that there is an abrupt onset of proptosis, with pain that worsens with eye movement (Fig. 4-3). However, unlike cellulitis, pseudotumor is often bilateral. Systemic findings such as malaise, fever, anorexia, headache, nausea, and vomiting may be present. Iritis may be present and even a prominent feature. Extraocular muscle involvement may restrict ocular motility and cause binocular diplopia and, in severe cases, visual loss resulting from optic neuropathy may occur.

To establish the diagnosis of orbital pseudotumor, cellulitis, and orbital and ocular neoplasms must be ruled out. Graves' disease does occur in children but is quite rare. Microbiologic studies are obtained as necessary; imaging with CT is recommended. This helps in the evaluation by identifying discrete masses and bony erosion suggestive of neoplastic processes and indicators of infection such as sinusitis. The CT appearance of pseudotumor includes some fairly characteristic features such as inhomogeneous fat opacification and a "ragged" appearance of the extraocular muscles. There may be a prominent myositic component, with enlargement of the muscle insertions. Enlargement of rectus muscle insertions is common in pseudotumor and uncommon in thyroid ophthalmopathy. In some patients, a scleritis-type picture may predominate, with scleral thickening and adjacent radiolucency or echolucency, indicating edema. Lacrimal gland enlargement also is common in pseudotumor.

The decision to obtain a biopsy must be made on a case-by-case basis. If the clinical presentation and CT scan are strongly suggestive of orbital pseudotumor, we usually do not perform a biopsy. However, in atypical cases or in recurrent cases, a biopsy should be performed to rule out infectious, neoplasms, or granulomatous inflammations. Treatment consists of relatively large doses of systemic corticosteroids. This provides rapid, significant relief, within 1 to 2 days; such a response is so characteristic that it supports the diagnosis. An overview of the causes and characteristics of proptosis in childhood is given in Box 4-3.

NEOPLASTIC DISORDERS

Capillary Hemangioma

Periocular capillary hemangiomas are common benign tumors of childhood that often affect the eyelids, orbit, and face (Fig. 4-4). They are the most common eyelid and orbital tumors of infancy and childhood. Most appear within the first 3 to 6 months of life, although congenital hemangiomas occasionally occur. Untreated, the natural history is characterized by an early, rapid enlargement over the first 6 to 18 months of life, followed by a period of relatively stable size. Gradual spontaneous resolution typically occurs over the course of the subsequent years, resulting in a crepe paper appearance of the skin. Superficial capillary hemangiomas appear as sharply delineated, red, elevated masses that do not blanch with pressure. They are painless and have a firm sponginess. Subdermal and deeper tumors may appear deep red, purple, or blue. In tumors affecting the eyelids, inspection of the palpebral conjunctiva is important and may allow confirmation of the diagnosis. Microscopically, the tumor displays abundant endothelial cells with narrow vascular channels.

Capillary hemangiomas are of great concern to the ophthalmologist because of their potential to cause amblyopia. Tumors involving the eyelids may cause ptosis and subsequent deprivation amblyopia; or the mass may

---

Box 4-3   Etiology and Features of Proptosis in Childhood

ACUTE PROPTOSIS

Orbital Cellulitis

Bacterial: Fever, malaise, pain, ptosis, chemosis, ophthalmoplegia, sinusitis

Fungal: Immune deficiency, pain, ophthalmoplegia, ptosis, optic neuropathy, pharyngeal eschar

Hemorrhage

Traumatic: Sudden onset, ecchymosis, subconjunctival blood, elevated IOP, orbital fractures

Associated with lymphangioma: Conjunctival channels, eyelid ecchymoses, enlarged orbit indicating long-standing tumor

Neoplasm

Rhabdomyosarcoma: Axial proptosis with downward and outward displacement common, average age 8 years, ptosis/eyelid mass

Neuroblastoma: Age ½ to 3 years common, often bilateral, periorbital ecchymoses, Horner's syndrome, opsoclonus, abdominal or neck mass palpable

Leukemia: "Chloroma," often bilateral, intraocular and optic nerve more commonly involved

Inflammatory

Orbital pseudotumor: Often bilateral, pain, eyelid edema, ophthalmoplegia, iritis, disc edema

Dermoid cyst (ruptured): Eyelid erythema, tenderness, fullness over lacrimal fossa

Vascular

Carotid-cavernous fistula: Usually traumatic, "corkscrew" episcleral veins, ophthalmoplegia, globe pulsations, glaucoma

CHRONIC PROPTOSIS

Neoplastic

Optic glioma: 10% to 70% will have NF-I, most grow slowly but rapid growth phase possible, RAPD, disc pallor

Neurofibroma: NF-I, globe displacement, S-shaped lid deformity, glaucoma common

Dermoid tumor: Superolateral mass, axial and nonaxial displacement, bony expansion

Lymphangioma: Orbital enlargement, more common in females, increased proptosis with URIs, no spontaneous regression

Hemangioma: Enlargement in first 6 months followed by regression, eyelid involvement, amblyopia, strabismus

Fibrous dysplasia: Orbital and skull deformity, teenage years, ocular motility disturbance, optic neuropathy

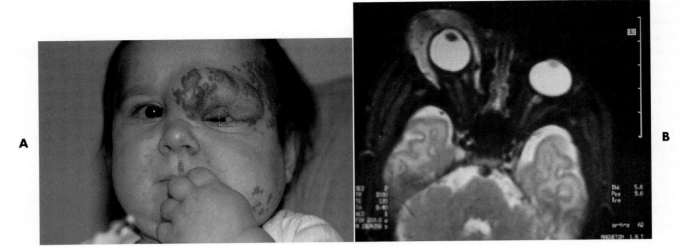

Fig. 4-4   A, Capillary hemangioma involving superficial and orbital structures. **B,** T2-weighted MRI depicts medial and lateral orbital involvement. See color plate. (Courtesy Jill Foster, Cleveland Clinic Foundation.)

warp the cornea, inducing significant astigmatism and subsequent meridional amblyopia. Finally, orbital hemangiomas may interfere with ocular motility, leading to strabismic amblyopia.

Evaluation of a patient with a periocular capillary hemangioma should, therefore, have as its foremost goal the assessment of visual function and the determination of whether or not amblyopia is present. Retinoscopy should be performed and repeated at frequent intervals if there is a risk of induced astigmatism. We do not hesitate to prescribe glasses even to small babies, who have about 1.5 D of astigmatism or more. The presence of a compensatory face turn in the setting of childhood ptosis should not be viewed as signifying that there is no amblyopia. We found that almost 50% of such patients did, indeed, have amblyopia. We use fixation preference and, when needed, the vertical prism test to determine ocular dominance. Glasses should be updated as often as required. The usual principles of amblyopia management are applied.

The diagnosis of superficial lesions can usually be made clinically, but in orbital lesions, imaging is usually obtained to assist in the diagnosis and guide treatment. MRI is the most useful tool in such cases, but B-scan ultrasonography can help to differentiate it from lymphangioma and cavernous hemangioma. Capillary hemangiomas appear as fairly solid tumors; whereas, lymphangiomas often have large echolucent fluid-filled spaces. Cavernous hemangiomas are usually intraconal and encapsulated. The primary entity in the differential diagnosis is lymphangioma. Overall, capillary hemangiomas are significantly more common than lymphangiomas, but lymphangiomas are frequently misdiagnosed as hemangiomas.

The *Kasabach-Merrit syndrome* consists of thrombocytopenia resulting from platelet entrapment within a large hemangioma. Ophthalmologists and anesthesiologists should also remember that, rarely, a subglottic hemangioma may coexist with a periorbital capillary hemangioma.

Consideration of treatment is indicated for the reasons indicated in the earlier discussion, ptosis and amblyopia, as well as for disfiguring or cosmetically objectionable lesions. The most commonly utilized treatment is the intralesional injection of corticosteroids. Treatment early in the first year of life, when the tumor is in the rapid growth phase, is more effective than later treatment. Usually equal volumes of the short-acting steroid, triamcinolone (Kenalog, 40 mg/ml) and the depot preparation betamethasone sodium phosphate (Celestone, 6 mg/ml) are combined and injected from the same syringe. A small gauge needle (27 or 30) is used, and multiple very small aliquots of the mixture are injected into the tumor under very low pressure. This last point is of critical importance since a known complication of treatment is retinal arterial thrombosis, which is thought to be caused by retrograde flow of the particulate-containing steroid mixture into the ocular circulation via the ophthalmic artery. Pulling back on the plunger before injecting is probably also advisable to make sure the tip is not in a large vascular channel. Generally, no more than 2 ml are injected during a given treatment. Additional complications of intralesional corticosteroid treatment include skin depigmentation and atrophy and, rarely, transient growth retardation caused by systemic absorption. At least some effect is obtained from most treatments within 1 to 2 weeks, but it may be variable, ranging from rapid and significant shrinkage to a slowing down of a growing tumor. Multiple treatments may be needed, but even these may have systemic side effects such as causing growth retardation.

Systemic steroids are effective in inducing regression of capillary hemangiomas (perhaps less effective than local treatment) but are less frequently used because of their propensity to cause growth retardation. Systemic interferon alfa 2a and 2b have been shown to be partially effective but are not yet widely used in the United States. Capillary hemangiomas are quite radiosensitive, especially when in their rapid growth phase, but irradiation is rarely used in this country because of possible secondary effects on the growing orbit.

Lymphangiomas

Lymphangiomas are orbital tumors that are frequently mistaken for capillary hemangiomas. They are, of course, quite different in their composition, natural history, and response to treatment so proper diagnosis is imperative. Lymphangiomas consist of vascular elements and dilated lymphatic spaces, as well as lymphoid tissue aggregates, all of which infiltrate the usual orbital tissue. These pathologic features explain the common clinical phenomena observed with this tumor. Spontaneous regression, as seen with capillary hemangiomas, does not occur. Spontaneous hemorrhage or hemorrhage brought on by minor trauma is extremely common, as the fragile blood vessels bleed into the lymphatic spaces. As the blood breaks down, "chocolate cysts" develop, which are essentially a diagnostic feature of lymphangiomas (Fig. 4-5). Bleeding may be sudden, massive, and quite difficult to contain. Another clinical characteristic is that the resident lymphoid tissue may grow during systemic infections, resulting in a temporary enlargement of the tumor.

Treatment of lymphangiomas can be very frustrating for the patient, as well as the physician. Large tumors are cosmetically objectionable and may cause severe proptosis with visual loss. Unfortunately, they cannot be surgically cured because of their infiltrative nature. When surgery is undertaken, it is usually to debulk the tumor and to drain blood. These cases are challenging, since care must be taken to minimize damage to orbital structures such as extraocular muscles while accomplishing the goals of the operation. Severe hemorrhage may accompany or follow surgery. Thus the decision to operate must be made with caution.

Optic Pathway Gliomas

Primary astrocytomas of the optic nerves, chiasm, and tracts are collectively referred to as optic pathway gliomas. These are generally slow growing, pilocytic astro-

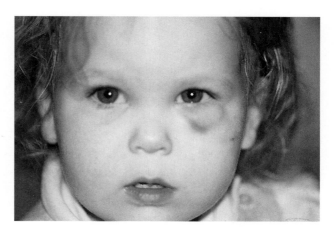

Fig. 4-5   Lymphangioma of left orbit. Note ecchymosis that occurred spontaneously. See color plate.

cytomas that are common but not restricted to patients with neurofibromatosis type I (NF-I). Magnetic resonance imaging allows fairly certain noninvasive diagnosis, once an orbital process is suspected. Therefore, over the past decade, the main issues concerning these tumors have evolved to include treatment of optic pathway gliomas and screening of asymptomatic NF-I patients.

Optic pathway gliomas may involve one or both nerves, tracts, or the chiasm. Orbital involvement causes a slowly progressive and painless axial proptosis, with variable effect on ocular motility. Because of the young age of the patients usually involved, the patients are generally visually asymptomatic. The mean age of presentation is 9 years, but gliomas can be discovered at any age. There is no sex predilection. The visual loss may lead to a sensory strabismus, which may be the presenting sign. However, early tumors may cause no visual loss. The optic nerve in cases of orbital gliomas may be pale or swollen, and a relative afferent pupillary defect may be detectable. Associated choroidal folds may be present because of the mass effect of the tumor. Currently, many gliomas are identified during an initial evaluation for NF-I, either upon examination or by imaging.

Optic pathway gliomas diffusely infiltrate the resident neural structures, causing a progressive, fusiform, or nodular enlargement. The astrocytes comprising the tumor are spindle-shaped or hair-like, the latter appearance giving rise to the term *pilocytic*. Rosenthal fibers, which are elongated foci of eosinophilic, degenerated cell processes, may be seen. Other characteristic histopathologic findings include focal calcification and microcystic degeneration. In NF-I associated cases, commonly there is an associated arachnoidal gliomatosis, which may lead to confusion with optic nerve sheath meningiomas in terms of imaging.

CT shows an enlarged optic nerve and enlargement of the optic canal if the tumor extends sufficiently posteri-

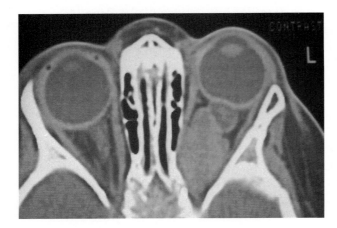

Fig. 4-6   Axial CT scan displaying a left optic nerve glioma with fusiform enlargement and cyst formation.

orly (Fig. 4-6). MRI is the optimum method to determine the nature and extent of optic pathway gliomas that appear isointense on T1-weighted images and isointense or highly intense on proton and T2-weighted images. MRI also depicts chiasmal and tract involvement nicely, as well as diencephalic extension and the benign high signal intensity nodules often seen in NF-I.

Fifteen percent of patients with NF-I will develop an optic pathway glioma. On the other hand, the reported incidence of NF-I among all patients with optic pathway glioma has ranged from 10% to 70%. Gliomas in NF-I patients tend to arise earlier than in those without (5 years versus 12 years) and are more likely to be bilateral or multifocal. Whether or not and when to perform screening MRIs on patients with NF-I are hotly debated topics, since asymptomatic patients may harbor the tumor.

The natural history of optic pathway gliomas is unpredictable; therefore treatment considerations are particularly difficult. Most demonstrate slow growth over years. However, a rapid growth phase may develop; thus patients with optic pathway gliomas must be followed indefinitely. Many authorities believe that the tumors in NF-I tend to have a more indolent course, with better preservation of vision than isolated tumors. Further complicating management is the fact that bilateral and multifocal tumors are common in NF-I. In anterior, unilateral cases, monitoring (clinical examination, visual field testing, MR imaging, VEPs) is done largely to make sure the chiasm does not become threatened, which would eliminate the chance for a surgical cure. The factors that must be taken into account when considering the surgical excision of an optic nerve glioma include the level of vision in the eye, the degree of proptosis, and how far the tumor extends posteriorly. Obviously, these issues require detailed and frank discussions with the patient's family, as well as the input of the neurosurgeon and radiologist. Chemotherapy and radiation therapy may be indicated in certain instances, particularly with chiasmal and diencephalic involvement, but obtaining a cure is difficult, and the side effects of these treatments are severe.

Rhabdomyosarcoma

Although rare, this is the most common malignant orbital tumor of childhood. Its usual presentation is that of a rapidly growing mass in the superonasal orbit, causing proptosis and displacement of the globe (Fig. 4-7). Ptosis is common, and in some cases, eyelid involvement may predominate. The average age of occurrence is 7 to 8 years, but any age may be affected, including newborns. Rhabdomyosarcomas are thought to arise from embryonic tissue rests, not from the extraocular muscles. The main clinical differential diagnoses include the causes of rapidly expanding orbital masses (Box 4-4). Once suspected, urgent imaging with CT or MRI is performed, followed by diagnostic biopsy.

It is important to try to classify the tumor into one of the four histologic varieties that occur for prognostic reasons, and electron microscopy is often used toward this end. The embryonal form is most common, comprising about 75% of cases. These are composed of poorly differentiated myoblasts. Next in frequency is the alveolar form (15%), which is differentiated from embryonal tumors by the presence of septae. It carries the worst prognosis of all the varieties. Pleomorphic rhabdomyosarcomas show the most differentiation, with cells containing cross-striations but rare mitoses. They have the best prognosis but are least common. The botryoid form refers to subconjunctival tumors that grossly assume a grape-like appearance.

Significant improvement in survival has occurred in the past 20 years, largely resulting from a move away from surgical treatment, to the use of systemic chemotherapeutic agents combined with external beam radiation. In tumors confined to the orbit, the 3-year survival rate is about 90% but significantly worse with extraorbital (intracranial, sinus) extension. Common metastatic sites are lungs, brain, and lymph nodes.

Plexiform Neurofibroma

Plexiform neurofibromas occur as part of the syndrome of NF-I. These are diffusely infiltrating tumors, composed of Schwann's cells and endoneural fibroblasts, surrounded by perineural sheaths. In the orbit, they present in childhood as a slowly growing mass causing proptosis and globe displacement. Eyelid involvement is common, leading to the classic S-shaped lid deformity, or the "bag of worms" picture (Fig. 4-8). Important associated

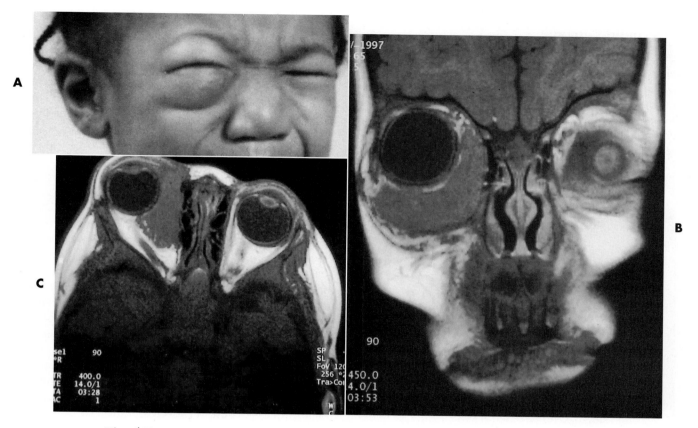

Fig. 4-7 **A,** A one-year-old patient with rhabdomyosarcoma, which presented with eyelid swelling. **B,** Coronal MRI showing large inferonasal tumor. **C,** Axial MRI showing proptosis and displacement of the optic nerve and globe. See color plate.

Box 4-4 Causes of Rapidly Expanding Orbital Masses

Rhabdomyosarcoma
Cellulitis
Pseudotumor
Lymphangioma
Ruptured dermoid cyst
Neuroblastoma
Lymphoma

---

findings in affected patients include congenital or juvenile glaucoma and sphenoid wing dysplasia; the latter may cause proptosis and globe pulsations in synchrony with the heartbeat.

Like lymphangiomas, plexiform neurofibromas pose extremely difficult surgical problems because they infiltrate the normal tissue so extensively. Multiple surgeries may be required over the course of an affected patient's life. The hideous facial deformity that plexiform neurofibromas can cause is well known.

Neuroblastoma

Neuroblastoma is a childhood malignancy that may arise anywhere in the post-ganglionic sympathetic chain, but arises most commonly from the abdomen. Hematologic metastases to the orbit are not uncommon, producing rapidly progressive proptosis, often with characteristic periorbital ecchymosis (Fig. 4-9). When the diagnosis is suspected, support may be obtained by palpation of the neck and abdomen for masses. Horner's syndrome may also be present if the tumor involves the ascending sympathetic chain in the neck or the lung apex. The initial work-up involves imaging, often including the abdomen and chest, and testing the urine for catecholamine metabolites. Do not rely on the catecholamine levels to rule out neuroblastoma because their production by the tumor may vary. The differential diagnosis, in addition to the previously mentioned causes of rapidly progressive proptosis in children, includes child abuse.

Dermoid Tumor

Orbital dermoid tumors or cysts are congenital masses that occur in the eyelids or orbit. They are painless, slow-growing cystic lesions with walls containing dermal appendages such as sebaceous glands and hair follicles. These elements produce the cyst's contents (cholesterol, keratin, sebum, hair). When anterior and palpable, they are often firm and rubbery. Symptoms, such as propto-

sis, depend on the location within the orbit; commonly, they are found adjacent to or attached to bone at suture lines, which is consistent with the theory that they arise from trapped embryonic ectoderm (Fig. 4-10). Bony erosion does occur because of sustained pressure. Dermoid tumors may spontaneously rupture, causing a severe inflammatory reaction. Thus, when a surgeon removes an unruptured dermoid, the goal is *in toto* excision without liberating the contents into the orbit.

LANGERHANS' CELL HISTIOCYTOSIS (HISTIOCYTOSIS X)

The rubric Langerhans' cell histiocytosis refers to a spectrum of nonneoplastic disorders with variable clinical manifestations. The common feature is the presence of a proliferation of Langerhans' cells, a type of tissue macrophage that, among other characteristics, contains Birbeck granules. Histiocytosis X was the general term used before the cells in question were determined to be Langerhans' cells. Eosinophilic granuloma, Hand-Schüller-Christian disease, and Letterer-Siwe disease are old designations that describe various clinical presentations of what is now understood to be a common pathologic process. These terms create artificial distinctions and so are becoming outmoded but still persist in the clinical vernacular.

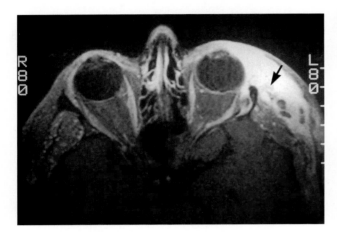

Fig. 4-8 Axial MRI of a plexiform neurofibroma involving the left eyelid and anterior orbit. (Courtesy Dr. Barrett Haik.)

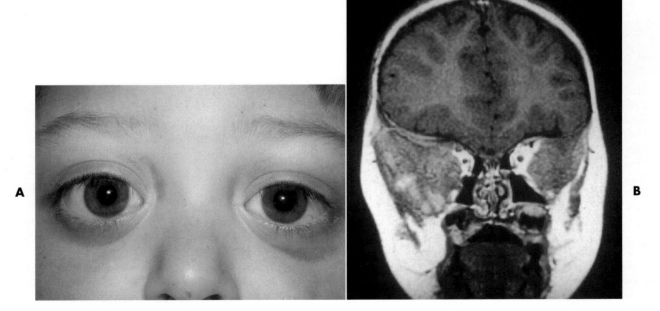

Fig. 4-9 Bilateral metastatic neuroblastoma to orbit. **A,** Clinical presentation with right proptosis and left lower eyelid ecchymosis. **B,** Coronal MRI showing bilateral orbital masses. (Courtesy Dr. Barrett Haik.)

Overall, these are uncommon entities, but they do affect the orbit and may present there. Orbital involvement is characteristic of what was referred to as eosinophilic granuloma, in which a slow-growing mass or masses involving the bone in a child cause proptosis, ptosis, pain, and tenderness. The skull, ribs, and long bones may also be affected. These soft lesions expand and break through bone, causing the lytic and bony defects seen with CT or MRI. Treatment is often successful with excision, local radiation, or systemic corticosteroids. A more aggressive and widespread variety, often affecting the skull with multiple lesions, was previously called Hand-Schüller-Christian disease. The disseminated and most dangerous form of the disease (Letterer-Siwe disease) affects multiple visceral organs and is treated with systemic chemotherapy.

Juvenile xanthogranuloma (JXG) is caused by a proliferation of non-Langerhans' histiocytes and is covered in Chapter 11.

FIBROUS DYSPLASIA

Fibrous dysplasia of bone is another condition that often affects the orbit and so is of interest to the ophthalmologist. This is an idiopathic, slowly progressive

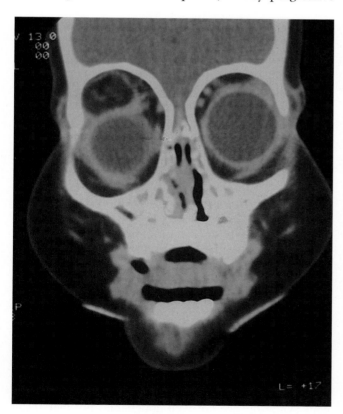

Fig. 4-10 Orbital dermoid, coronal CT scan. Note downward displacement of globe.

proliferation of abnormal bone that expands and distorts the normal orbital architecture. Onset before age 10 with progression through adolescence and early adulthood is typical. Most often there is unilateral proptosis and globe displacement; other findings such as motility disturbance, optic nerve compression, and pain may occur to a variable degree, depending on the location of the abnormal bone. The orbit and skull may become extremely distorted, resulting in significant disfigurement (Fig. 4-11). *Albright's syndrome* affects girls and consists of polyostotic fibrous dysplasia, abnormal skin pigmentation, and premature menarche.

Plain films and CT scans can effectively demonstrate the characteristic hyperostosis with both lytic and sclerotic areas. Cases that are predominantly sclerotic may be difficult to distinguish from meningiomas. Histologically, there is a proliferation of benign spindle cells along with islands of woven bone. Treatment is surgical and is often done in concert with a neurosurgeon; multiple surgeries may be required.

CRANIOFACIAL DISORDERS

Crouzon and Apert's Syndromes

These are rare, autosomal-dominant conditions caused by premature closure of cranial sutures (craniosynostosis). Crouzon and Apert's syndromes become evident in the first few years of life and are felt primarily to involve the coronal suture. The prominent facial features include a steep forehead, maxillary hypoplasia (resulting in a flat appearance), telecanthus, and proptosis (Fig. 4-12). The orbits are characteristically shallow, resulting in eyelid retraction, corneal exposure, and a tendency toward globe prolapse. This can be so severe as to threaten the globe. Strabismus occurs frequently, typically with a V pattern. Structurally abnormal orbits, and abnormally positioned extraocular muscle insertions may promote the development of strabismus. Strabismic and anisometropic amblyopia occur often. Optic atrophy is also common and may result from papilledema, or optic nerve compression or traction. These conditions differ in a number of ways. In Apert's syndrome there is syndactyly of the hands and feet (Fig. 4-13). Structural brain abnormalities and mental retardation are common. Also the proptosis may be less severe than in Crouzon syndrome. Mutations responsible for both syndromes have been found on chromosome 10.

Optic nerve edema or progressive optic atrophy may signal increased intracranial pressure, which may require neurosurgical intervention (shunting). Extensive facial reconstruction is often required and may involve advancement of the orbital walls to increase their volume. Strabismus surgery is usually reserved until after

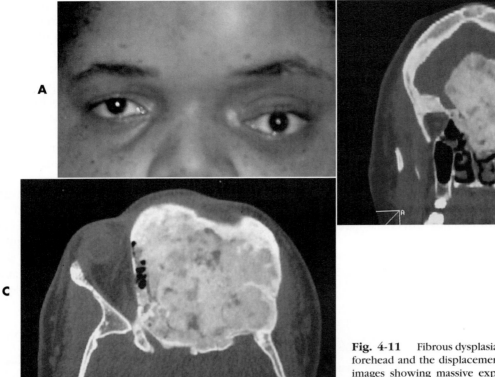

Fig. 4-11   Fibrous dysplasia. **A,** Note the deformity of the left forehead and the displacement of the left globe. **B,** and **C,** CT images showing massive expansion of the bones around the orbit. The fibrous tissue shows characteristic areas of differing densities. See color plate.

orbital surgery and has as its main goal ocular alignment in primary and down gaze. The presence of abnormal extraocular muscle insertions may complicate the surgery.

Goldenhar Syndrome (Oculoauriculovertebral spectrum)

Goldenhar's syndrome is a sporadic, heterogenous spectrum of congenital defects primarily affecting the face, eyes, and ears. Goldenhar's initial 1952 description included mandibular hypoplasia, preauricular appendages, and epibulbar dermoid tumors. Subsequently, it has become evident that this triad of findings is actually a portion of a larger syndrome that can variably involve the heart, lungs, kidneys, cervical vertebral column, and central nervous system (CNS). Thus in many cases the designation, *oculoauriculovertebral* spectrum or *facial microsomia* are more precise terms.

The clinical findings are extremely variable in severity. Marked facial asymmetry, "facial microsomia," is very common, particularly involving the mandible and condyle on one side. The ears are often involved, ranging from anotia to the presence of a small pretragal tag. The ears may be downwardly displaced and malformed, and often there is hearing loss. Cervical spine malformations, such as *Klippel-Feil syndrome,* scoliosis, and spina bifida are present in about 55% of cases. CNS anomalies (e.g., hydrocephalus) are found in as many as 15% of cases and heart, lung, or kidney malformations in up to half.

The globe and ocular adnexa are frequently involved. Probably the most important entity for the ophthalmologist is the *epibulbar dermoid.* These are white, smooth tumors usually found at or near the inferotemporal limbus. They may impinge on the cornea to cause astigmatism or deeply invade the globe, creating the well-known hazard of globe penetration, should excision be attempted. Sometimes, surgery is undertaken because of an adjacent corneal delle or for cosmetic reasons; in such instances, shaving the mass to flatten it is usually more advisable than complete excision. It is important that the parents understand that the result will not be a normal appearing cornea, as the residual tumor remains opaque. Other common findings include ptosis and narrowing of the palpebral fissures, upper eyelid colobomas, conjunctival dermolipomas, amblyopia, and strabismus, including Duane's syndrome. Since conjunctival dermolipomas may extend quite far posteriorly, complete excision is usually not performed. The cause or causes of Goldenhar's syndrome are not well understood but may result from a disturbance in neural crest cell migration. The risk to a future sibling of an affected patient is about 2% to 3%.

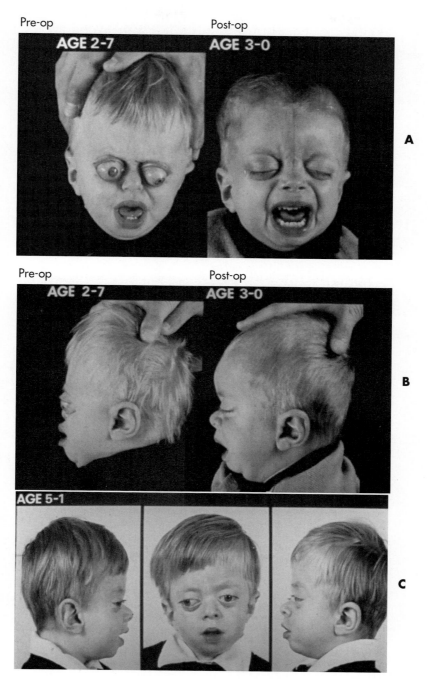

Fig. 4-12   Crouzon syndrome, preoperative and postoperative views. **A,** Before surgery there is globe luxation. Following craniofacial reconstructive surgery, the eyelids adequately cover the globes. **B,** Note the preoperative appearance of midfacial hypoplasia and increased vertical dimension of the skull. Both are improved postoperatively. **C,** At age 5 years, there is no corneal exposure. However, an exotropia requiring surgery is present.

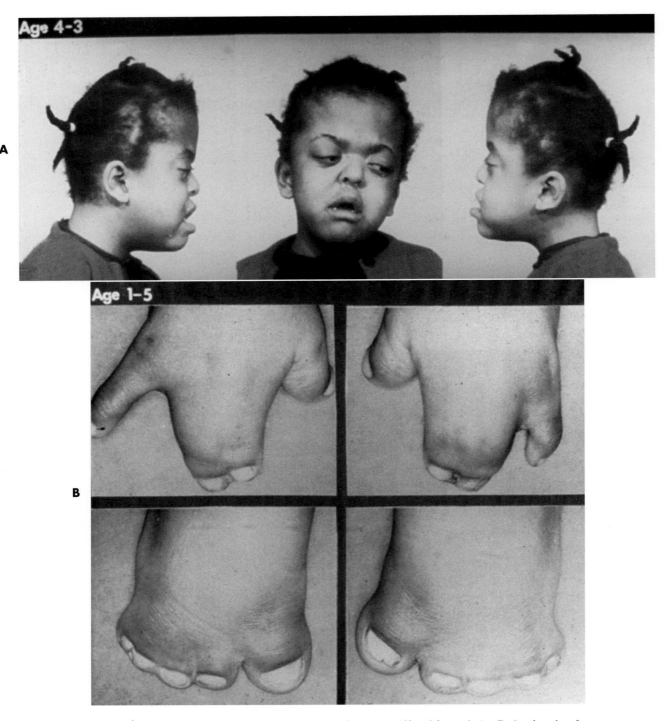

Fig. 4-13   Apert's syndrome. **A,** Facial views showing midfacial hypoplasia. **B,** Syndactyly of hands and feet.

Treacher Collins Syndrome (Mandibulofacial Dysostosis)

Treacher Collins syndrome is an autosomal-dominant clefting syndrome characterized by symmetric malar and mandibular hypoplasia, antimongoloid slant of the palpebral fissures, and lateral colobomas of the lower eyelids. Other common features include cleft palate, micrognathia, macrostomia, and hypoplasia of the zygoma (Fig. 4-14). The responsible gene locus is on chromosome 5q31.3-q33.3. Box 4-5 summarizes the clinical features of the more common craniofacial disorders with ophthalmic manifestations.

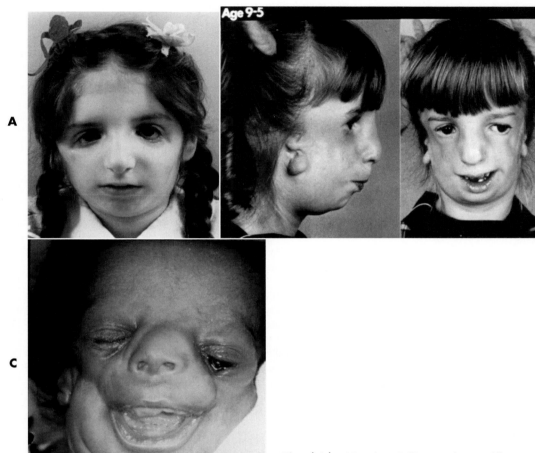

Fig. 4-14   Treacher Collins syndrome. Three patients with different degrees of severity of Treacher Collins syndrome. Note the eyelid deformity, microtia, and midfacial hypoplasia.

Box 4-5   Features of Common Craniofacial Disorders of Ophthalmic Importance

CROUZON SYNDROME

Autosomal dominant, severe proptosis, shallow orbits, optic atrophy, V-pattern strabismus, midfacial hypoplasia

APERT'S SYNDROME

Syndactyly, mental retardation, shallow orbits, proptosis, hypertelorism, downward slanting palpebral fissures, V-pattern strabismus

GOLDENHAR'S SYNDROME

Sporadic occurrence, variable phenotypic expression, facial asymmetry, epibulbar dermoid, conjunctival lipodermoid, upper eyelid coloboma, strabismus (comitant and Duane's retraction syndrome), ear malformations and displacement, spina bifida, scoliosis, heart, lung, and kidney malformations

TREACHER COLLINS SYNDROME

Lower eyelid coloboma, antimongoloid slant of palpebral fissures, canthal dystopia, malar hypoplasia, hypoplastic jaw, poor dentition, nasolacrimal duct obstruction, limbal and orbital dermoids

◤ **MAJOR POINTS** ◢

Preseptal cellulitis subsequent to skin trauma is most often caused by *Staphylococcus aureus* and *Streptococcus pyogenes.*

Preseptal cellulitis associated with sinusitis is most commonly caused by *Streptococcus pneumoniae.*

The main clinical findings in orbital cellulitis are pain, proptosis, decreased ocular motility, and pupil dysfunction.

Computed tomography scanning in suspected orbital cellulitis is mandatory to define the extent of the process and whether or not an abscess is present.

Pediatric orbital pseudotumor is often bilateral and accompanied by malaise, fever, and anorexia.

Capillary hemangiomas may cause deprivation, meridional, or strabismic amblyopia.

Complications of intralesional steroid injections for capillary hemangiomas include retinal artery thrombosis, skin depigmentation and atrophy, and growth retardation.

Lymphangiomas are frequently misdiagnosed as hemangiomas; one important way that they differ is that lymphangiomas do not spontaneously regress.

Optic pathway gliomas occur in about 15% of patients with NF-I.

Most optic pathway gliomas grow slowly, but unpredictable rapid growth can occur.

Rhabdomyosarcoma is the most common orbital malignancy in children and has an average age of occurrence of 7 to 8 years.

Rhabdomyosarcoma is treated with chemotherapy and external beam radiation, and has a 90% 3-year survival rate if it is limited to the orbit.

Neuroblastoma commonly metastasizes to the orbits and may be bilateral.

Langerhans' cell histiocytoses are composed of Langerhans' cells, a tissue macrophage with Birbeck granules.

Fibrous dysplasia may cause unilateral proptosis, globe displacement, ocular motility disturbances, optic nerve compression, and pain.

Crouzon and Apert's syndromes are autosomal-dominant and caused by premature closure of cranial sutures (craniosynostosis).

SUGGESTED READINGS

Barone SR, Aiuto LT: Periorbital and orbital cellulitis in the *Haemophilus influenzae* vaccine era, *J Pediatr Ophthalmol Strabismus* 34:293-296, 1997.

Chen YR, Fairholm D: Fronto-orbital-sphenoidal fibrous dysplasia, *Ann Plast Surg* 15:190-203, 1985.

Hemmer KM, Marsh JL, Milder B: Orbital lymphangioma, *Plastic Reconstr Surg* 82:340-343, 1988.

Lewis RA, Gerson LP, Axelson KA, et al: von Recklinghausen neurofibromatosis: II. incidence of optic gliomata, *Ophthalmology* 91:929-935, 1984.

Mills RP, Kartash JM: Orbital wall thickness and spread of infection from the paranasal sinuses, *Clin Otolaryngol* 10: 209-216, 1985.

Moore RT: Fibrous dysplasia of the orbit, *Survey Ophthalmol* 13:321-334, 1969.

Mottow LW, Jakobiec FA: Idiopathic inflammatory orbital pseudotumor in childhood, *Arch Ophthalmol* 96:1410-1417, 1978.

Noel LP, Clarke WN, MacDonald N: Clinical management of orbital cellulitis in children, *Can J Ophthalmol* 25:11-16, 1990.

Rodary C, Gehan EA, Flamert F, et al: Parognostic factors in 951 nonmetastatic rhabdomyosarcoma in children: a report from the International Rhabdomyosarcoma Workshop, *Med Pediatr Oncol* 19:89-95, 1991.

Rubin SE, Rubin LG, Zito J, et al: Medical management of orbital subperiosteal abscess in children, *J Pediatr Ophthalmol Strabismus* 26:21-27, 1989.

Shields JA, Bakewell B, Augsberger JJ, et al: Space occupying orbital diseases in children, *Ophthalmology* 93:379-384, 1986.

Wharam M, Beltangady M, Hays D, et al: Localized orbital rhabdomyosarcoma: an interim report of the Intergroup Rhabdomyosarcoma Study Committee, *Ophthalmology* 94(3): 251-254, 1987.

Wright JE, McNab AA, McDonald WI: Optic nerve glioma and the management of optic nerve tumours in the young, *Br J Ophthalmol* 73:967-974, 1989.

Pediatric Conjunctival Disease

In this chapter, we will cover conjunctivitis in the newborn and older children, as well as reviewing conjunctival nevi in the pediatric population. Although the list of possible causes of conjunctivitis in a newborn is short, the ophthalmologist must have a good working knowledge because decisive action may be required. As in adults, there are more causes of conjunctivitis in older children, requiring attention to historical clues and physical findings to establish the correct diagnosis.

OPHTHALMIA NEONATORUM

Conjunctivitis in the newborn is caused by only a few organisms and chemical irritants. The etiology is usually not difficult to establish on the basis of the clinical appearance and basic laboratory testing. The time of onset of the conjunctivitis usually provides an important clue to the causative agent, with chemical conjunctivitis occurring in the first day of life, gonococcal conjunctivitis at approximately age 2 to 4 days, and chlamydial conjunctivitis at age 4 to 10 days. Since gonococcal in-

fection can be rapidly progressive and destructive, the first goal of the clinician should be to rule out this organism, or at least initiate antibiotic treatment while definitive diagnosis is pending. Box 5-1 gives the causes of ophthalmia neonatorum, along with suggested treatments.

Chemical Conjunctivitis

Topical disinfectants are used routinely in newborns as prophylaxis against infection. Previously, the standard agent used was silver nitrate (*Credé prophylaxis*), which was fairly effective against gonococcal infection. However, it is not useful in preventing chlamydial infections; thus its use is decreasing. Conjunctivitis following the instillation of silver nitrate drops is common, occurring in about 90% of cases. It occurs within the first 24 hours after use, and is characterized by bilateral, mild eyelid edema, bulbar conjunctival injection, and a clear, watery discharge. Spontaneous recovery occurs within a few days. As tetracycline and erythromycin ointment are replacing silver nitrate, this form of conjunctivitis is becoming much less common in the United States. Dilute povidone-iodine solution has been shown to be effective against the common infectious agents, and its use is increasing.

Gonococcal Conjunctivitis

Infection caused by *Neisseria gonorrhea* is rare in the United States (0.3 cases per 1000 live births) because of effective prophylaxis, but it must be considered and ruled out because of its dangerous potential.

Transmission occurs via the birth canal. The conjunctivitis is severe and purulent, with chemosis and eyelid edema (Fig. 5-1). A serosanguinous discharge may be present. Onset may be earlier than the typical 48 hours of age if there has been premature rupture of the amniotic membranes. *N. gonorrhea* is one of the few organisms that has the ability to invade the intact corneal epithelium (remember the others: *Corynebacterium diphtheriae, Listeria,* and *Haemophilus aegyptius*). Therefore the conjunctivitis can rapidly progress to keratitis, corneal ulceration, and even corneal perforation. If suspected, a Gram's stain should be immediately performed on the discharge to demonstrate the typical gram-negative intracellular diplococci. Growth on Thayer-Martin culture media will confirm the diagnosis.

Treatment primarily consists of the prompt administration of systemic ceftriaxone (IV, 30 to 50 mg/kg/day in divided doses) or penicillin G (50,000 units/kg every 12 hours for 7 days). Many practitioners, including the authors, prefer ceftriaxone because of the increasing prevalence of penicillinase producing *N. gonorrhea*. Although it seems likely that a single intramuscular dose of ceftriaxone may be curative, as shown in adults, this has

yet to be proven in children. Topical erythromycin ointment is also used, as well as frequent topical saline irrigation to remove the purulent material.

Chlamydial Conjunctivitis

Chlamydial conjunctivitis is probably the most common type of infectious neonatal conjunctivitis in developed countries. It usually appears somewhat later than gonococcal infection, at age 4 to 7 days, and has a milder, more indolent course. However, there may be severe lid swelling and even pseudomembrane formation (Fig. 5-2). Giemsa-stained conjunctival swabbings show intracytoplasmic basophilic inclusion bodies, and confirmation can be made with fluorescent antibody staining. Treatment consists of topical erythromycin ointment and oral erythromycin (30 to 50 mg/kg/day in four divided doses) for 2 weeks to treat concomitant (presumptive or proven) pneumonitis. The parents, even if asymptomatic, also should be treated.

Herpetic Conjunctivitis

Neonatal conjunctivitis as a result of Herpes simplex occurs somewhat later than the previously reviewed causes, usually 1 to 2 weeks postpartum. Transmission is also by way of the birth canal during delivery; therefore most cases are caused by HSV2. Neonatal herpetic infections are often generalized, involving the central nervous system, liver, and lungs. Typically, there is a serous discharge with conjunctival injection and geographic keratitis (Fig. 5-3). Cataracts and retinochoroiditis also may be present. Gram's stain of the conjunctival smear shows multinucleated giant cells, and the Papanicolaou stain shows typical intranuclear inclusion bodies. Viral cultures are confirmatory but may take 7 to 10 days

---

Box 5-1   Etiologies and Treatments of Ophthalmia Neonatorum

Chemical
Conservative measures

Gonorrhea
Systemic antibiotics, topical erythromycin, saline
irrigation

Chlamydia
Oral and topical erythromycin

Herpes
Topical and systemic antivirals

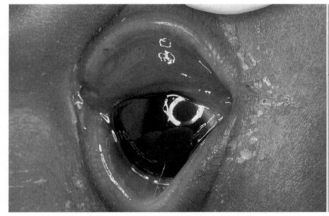 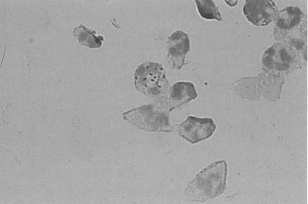

A   B

Fig. 5-1 *Neisseria gonorrhea* neonatal conjunctivitis. **A,** The patient had purulent discharge, conjunctival edema and injection, and punctate keratopathy. **B,** Conjunctival swab showing polymorphonuclear leukocytes with intracellular gram-negative diplococci.

to become positive. Initial treatment consists of a topical antiviral agent such as trifluorothymidine, as well as systemic acyclovir. As in adults, secondary bacterial infections may occur.

PEDIATRIC CONJUNCTIVITIS

Bacterial Conjunctivitis

The manifestations of bacterial conjunctivitis in children are often nonspecific, making it challenging to differentiate such cases from conjunctivitis caused by other agents, such as viruses. Bacterial conjunctivitis is not rare, but is probably over-diagnosed, particularly by physicians other than ophthalmologists. A common scenario is a patient being referred after an ineffective course of topical antibiotics, and in these cases the correct diagnosis is usually an allergic or viral condition. Alternatively, viral conjunctivitis is assumed, but antibiotics are given as an "extra" measure of safety. Nevertheless, it is important to know about the common pathogens responsible for pediatric bacterial conjunctivitis: *Haemophilus, Streptococcus, Pneumococcus,* and *Staphylococcus* (Box 5-2). In addition to the typical purulent exudate, bacterial infections tend to cause acute bulbar and tarsal conjunctivitis, often with a tarsal papillary reaction, although follicles may be present. The conjunctivitis caused by Moraxella tends to be subacute and causes an angular conjunctivitis. One study in which cultures of 99 children with acute conjunctivitis were obtained found about 50% of cases caused by bacteria (*Haemophilus influenzae* and *Streptococcus pneumoniae*), 20% by adenovirus, and 30% culture negative.

Haemophilus influenzae infection may be distinctive since it usually causes a hemorrhagic conjunctivitis (Fig. 5-4). Small, subcutaneous hemorrhages of the eyelids may also be present, imparting them with a violaceous

hue. Thus it is possible to mistake this conjunctivitis for bruising from trauma, as well as viral conjunctivitis. Otitis media commonly occurs with this conjunctivitis; therefore examination of the ears may provide an important clue, as well as disclosing another problem requiring treatment. Untyped *H. influenzae* continues to be important because it is not covered by the *H. influenzae* vaccination. In theory, the best antibiotic choice for haemophilus would be trimethoprim-polymixin B, but a study by Lohr, et al, showed topical gentamicin and sulfacetamide also to be associated with high rates of clinical improvement or cure.

Chlamydial Conjunctivitis

The Chlamydiaceae are obligate intracellular organisms responsible for trachoma (serotypes A-C), inclusion conjunctivitis and urethritis and cervicitis (serotypes D-K) and lymphogranuloma venereum (serotypes L1, L2, and L3). Inclusion conjunctivitis is spread by sexual contact and thus may be seen in sexually abused children and adolescents. There may be an acute mucopurulent infection or a more indolent, chronic conjunctivitis. Characteristically, large tarsal conjunctival follicles are present, and a peripheral keratitis is often also present (Fig. 5-5). Confirmation of the diagnosis can be made by direct fluorescent antibody staining or culture. Treatment with tetracycline, doxycycline, or erythromycin is usually curative and should be given to the patient's sexual partners as well.

Viral Conjunctivitis

The clinical profile and features of viral conjunctivitis in children are similar to those in adults. Adenovirus serotypes 8 and 19 are responsible for epidemic keratoconjunctivitis (EKC) and serotypes 3 and 7 for pharyngocon-

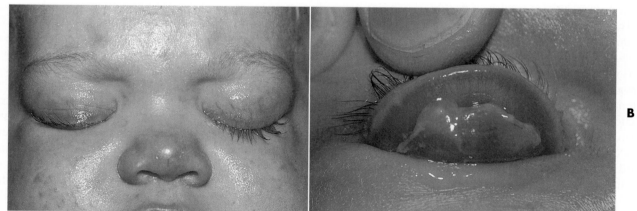

A **B**

Fig. 5-2 Neonatal chlamydia conjunctivitis in a 10-day-old infant. **A,** Bilateral lid swelling. **B,** Superior tarsal conjunctival pseudomembrane.

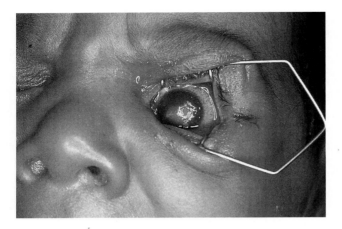

Fig. 5-3   Herpes simplex keratitis with secondary strepto-coccal infection in a 5-week-old infant. Note geographic corneal infiltrate.

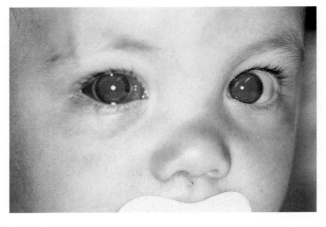

Fig. 5-4   *Haemophilus influenzae* conjunctivitis. Note hemor-rhagic conjunctivitis, lid swelling, and violaceous hue of the eyelid skin. See color plate.

Box 5-2   Bacterial Causes of Pediatric Conjunctivitis
Haemophilus influenzae *Streptococcus pneumoniae* *Staphylococcus* *Pneumococcus* *Moraxella lacunata* *Chlamydia trachomatis* *Bartonella henselae* (agent of cat scratch disease)

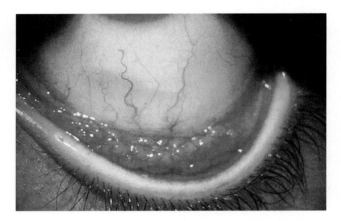

Fig. 5-5   Numerous large follicles of tarsal conjunctiva caused by chlamydial conjunctivitis.

junctival fever. Other adenoviral serotypes may cause conjunctivitis (Box 5-3). These highly contagious infec-tions occur in association with systemic viral infections and cause an acute follicular reaction, often bilateral, with watery discharge, hyperemia, chemosis, itching, superficial keratitis, and preauricular adenopathy (Fig. 5-6). Cases with prominent conjunctival hemorrhage (acute hemorrhagic conjunctivitis) are often caused by the picornavirus, enterovirus type 70.

The follicular conjunctivitis seen in association with molluscum contagiosum can be cured by treating the eyelid lesions (see Chapter 2).

Conjunctivitis resulting from primary herpes simplex (usually type 1) infection is an acute, follicular process, often with a profuse watery discharge. The presence of eyelid and eyelid margin ulcers and vesicles, periocular dermatitis, stomatitis, preauricular adenopathy, and cor-neal involvement usually make this diagnosis straightfor-ward. Topical antiviral treatment with trifluorothymidine or vidarabine ointment should be prescribed.

Hay Fever Conjunctivitis

Hay fever conjunctivitis (seasonal allergic conjunctivi-tis) is a relatively benign but irritating seasonal condition characterized by conjunctival injection, chemosis, and *itching*. Itching is so characteristic that the diagnosis should rarely be made in its absence. Exacerbations come on in the spring when increased airborne pollen, molds, dust, and dander cause an IgE-mediated reaction with subsequent mast cell degranulation. Concomitant rhinitis is typical. Although the diagnosis is not usually difficult to make, conjunctival scrapings may show rare eosinophils; this is notable because scrapings from nor-mal persons have no eosinophils.

Avoiding the offending allergen is often recommended but usually difficult. Treatment with topical antihis-tamine-vasoconstrictor combinations is often effective. Levocabastine (Livostin) is a potent topical antihistamine that provides good symptom relief. Topical NSAIDs such as ketorolac (Acular) are surprisingly effective in re-lieving itching in some patients. The mast cell stabiliz-ers, lodoxamide tromethamine (Alomide) and cromolyn (Opticrom), prevent the release of histamine and leuko-trienes. These agents are very safe but do not become effective for at least 1 week. Topical corticosteroids

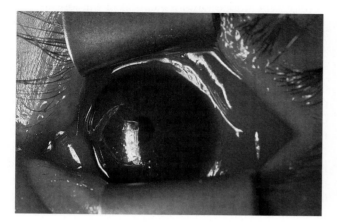

Fig. 5-6   Epidemic keratoconjunctivitis in a 3 year old. Note the hemorrhagic conjunctivitis, chemosis, and punctate keratitis.

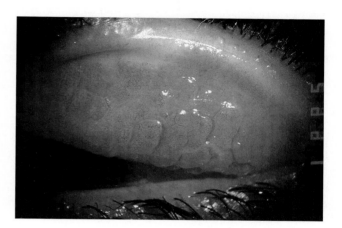

Fig. 5-7   Vernal conjunctivitis with giant "cobblestone" papillae of superior tarsal conjunctiva.

are the most effective drugs, but, because of their side effects and the availability of many good alternatives, should only be used in rare cases and for limited courses.

Atopic Keratoconjunctivitis

Atopy refers to an IgE-mediated clinical syndrome that affects the respiratory tract, skin, and eyes. Atopic individuals have an increased sensitivity to certain allergens and often have asthma, urticaria, and hay fever. A family history of these disorders is often present. Atopic keratoconjunctivitis (AKC) is a chronic bilateral condition that occurs in association with 15% to 40% of patients with atopic dermatitis, particularly in those with eyelid involvement. The prevalence of atopic dermatitis in the general population is 3%. AKC can begin in childhood but more often comes on in the later teens or early adulthood. Bilateral ocular itching is the primary symptom, along with blurred vision and photophobia. The tarsal conjunctiva develops a papillary hypertrophy, with an associated stringy, ropy discharge. The eyelids may be swollen, indurated and scaly, with an irregular margin. Complications of AKC are listed in Box 5-4.

Types I and IV hypersensitivity reactions are thought to be involved in the etiology of AKC. Increased serum and tear levels of IgE are present during exacerbations. Treatment aimed at reducing the inflammation and the

symptoms it causes may consist of multiple agents, in addition to allergen avoidance. Systemic antihistamines, and topical antihistamine-vasoconstrictors, mast cell stabilizers, NSAIDs, and steroids in combination are utilized. If penetrating keratoplasty is required, remember that it carries a relatively high risk of graft failure. In addition, cataract surgery in affected patients is associated with a higher than usual incidence of post-operative retinal detachment.

Vernal Conjunctivitis

Vernal conjunctivitis is a severe allergic process, probably caused by both type I and type IV hypersensitivity reactions, which usually has its onset in childhood. The classic and most common finding is giant papillae of the upper tarsal conjunctiva. These are referred to as cobblestone papillae because of their flattened tops (Fig. 5-7). In the less common limbal form, the conjunctiva near the corneoscleral limbus is predominantly involved. Mixed cases also occur. The limbal vernal variety occurs more often in African Americans than Caucasians. Vernal conjunctivitis is so-named because it often worsens in the spring, but it can occur and be active any time of the year. Males appear to be affected more often than females. The main symptom is itching, as is the case in the other types of allergic conjunctivitis. Accompanying

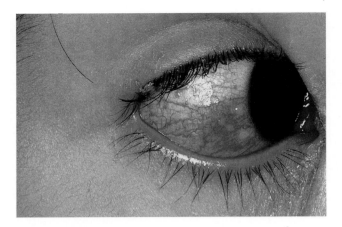

Fig. 5-8 Phlyctenular conjunctivitis. Note the pale nodules temporal to the limbus with conjunctival injection.

this are foreign body sensation, tearing, and photophobia. Other clinical findings include ptosis, resulting from the increased mass of the eyelid; abundant, tenacious, ropy conjunctival discharge; punctate epitheliopathy; and shield ulcers of the cornea. Thus this condition is often a keratoconjunctivitis. In the limbal form, large papillae with Horner-Trantas dots form at the limbus. Conjunctival scrapings in both types reveal more than three to four eosinophils per high-powered field.

Of the variety of agents available for ocular allergy, the most important in vernal conjunctivitis are, by far, the mast cell stabilizers (lodoxamide, cromolyn). Prolonged use may be required to keep the process in check. In addition to starting one of these agents, quicker control of the inflammation and symptom relief can be obtained with topical corticosteroids. Short, infrequent courses of relatively high doses are recommended. Vasoconstrictor-antihistamine preparations also may be useful, and the application of cold compresses usually provides some relief of the itching.

Phlyctenular Keratoconjunctivitis

Phlyctenular keratoconjunctivitis presents with pink to pale-gray inflammatory nodules, usually near the limbus, with associated vascular injection and mild to moderate ocular irritation (Fig. 5-8). Although the details regarding pathophysiology are not well established, phlyctenulosis is felt to be a hypersensitivity reaction to a variety of infectious organisms. Conjunctival involvement causes episodes of mild tearing and irritation. The nodules, typically 1 to 3 mm across, go through a characteristic evolution, with central ulceration, necrosis, and, ultimately, spontaneous resolution, without scarring. The symptoms in corneal involvement may be more severe, and conjunctival vessels often extend across

the cornea to the lesions, which contain lymphocytes, plasma cells, and histiocytes.

In the United States phlyctenulosis most commonly occurs in association with *Staphylococcal aureus* but the first association made was with tuberculosis (skin test reactivity). In regions with a high TB prevalence, phlyctenulosis is most often caused by that agent. Other organisms implicated include *Neisseria gonorrhoeae*, viruses, and chlamydia. In cases caused by presumed staphylococcal hypersensitivity, treatment aimed at improving lid hygiene is usually effective; acutely, topical steroids will induce rapid resolution of the lesions.

Ligneous Conjunctivitis

Ligneous conjunctivitis is a rare, chronic conjunctival disorder that affects children more often than adults. Ligneous means woody, and in the late stages of this condition, there are hypertrophic, nodular, firm, white to red masses replacing the normal superior and inferior tarsal conjunctivae (Fig. 5-9). Chronic tearing and conjunctival injection occur in association with the chronic pseudomembranous conjunctivitis present in early cases. Corneal injury, with punctate keratopathy and secondary infection is the most worrisome complication, but severe cases may cause significant, permanent eyelid deformity. The pain may be significant.

The etiology of this ligneous conjunctivitis is unknown, but proposed theories include a hypersensitivity reaction, an exaggerated inflammatory response following injury, and a viral infection. Microscopically, an amorphous hyaline material (composed largely of immunoglobulins, fibrin, and albumin) with acute and chronic inflammation is found. These findings suggest an aberrant and arrested healing process. Very recent studies have demonstrated plasminogen gene mutations and very low levels of plasminogen in patients with ligneous conjunctivitis. Consequently, decreased levels of plasmin may impair plasmin-mediated fibrinolysis and thus contribute to the pathophysiologic process. Based on this information, patients with ligneous conjunctivitis should be tested for plasminogen activity and antigen level. The ligneous response is not limited to the conjunctiva, having been described in other mucous membranes, including the larynx, vocal cords, trachea, nasopharynx, vagina, gingiva, and tympanic membranes.

Until recently, the main treatments attempted were topical corticosteroids, antibiotics, and hyaluronidase, and generally these were ineffective. Furthermore, simple surgical removal, although quite tempting, usually results in a rapid recurrence. An aggressive, combined surgical and medical approach has been advocated by Holland and Schwartz. Following complete resection of all lesions, frequent doses of acetylcysteine, corticoste-

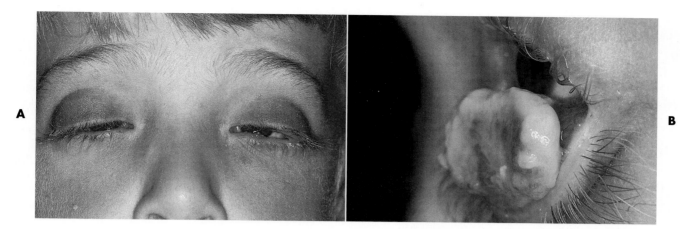

Fig. 5-9   Ligneous conjunctivitis. **A,** Bilateral mechanical ptosis resulting from severe ligneous conjunctivitis. **B,** Large ligneous lesion involving the superior tarsal conjunctiva.

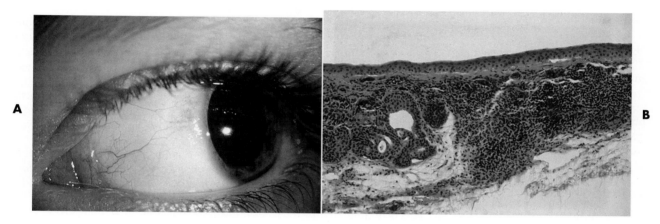

Fig. 5-10   **A,** Lightly pigmented conjunctival nevus of the limbus. Note inclusion cysts. **B,** Histopathologic appearance of nevus from the patient shown in *A.*

roid, alpha-chymotrypsin, and hyaluronidase are started. Topical cyclosporin applications are made to the bed of the lesions, and oral corticosteroids are given. Finally, frequent reexaminations are made and any recurrences are débrided. The relative importance of each of the above medications is not well established, but the introduction of cyclosporin definitely has improved the prognosis in these patients.

CONJUNCTIVAL NEVI

Conjunctival nevi, the most common epibulbar tumors of childhood, may truly be congenital but typically become apparent later. Melanocytes (the melanin-producing cells) and other cells constitute nevi, which are classified depending on their location in relation to the epithelium. All have low malignant potential and move with the epithelium. Conjunctival nevi are well-circumscribed, variably pigmented, and may be flat or elevated (Fig. 5-10). Junctional nevi are confined to the epithelium and appear flat. Compound nevi involve the substantia propria, as well as the epithelium, are often elevated, and often contain inclusion cysts. Subepithelial nevi, less common than the previous two types mentioned, appear flesh-colored to brown, are elevated, and also may contain cysts. Pigmented lesions of the conjunctiva in other locations should arouse greater suspicion. Palpebral conjunctival and forniceal lesions should be biopsied, and recurrent nevi (after excision) also should be studied histopathologically.

Dysplastic nevi occur as part of the dysplastic nevus syndrome (BK mole syndrome), an autosomal dominantly inherited condition in which there are numerous cutaneous nevi and a strong tendency for melanoma formation. Conjunctival nevi may occur in this syndrome, but whether or not there is an increased predisposition is uncertain. Other rare varieties of conjunctival nevi in the pediatric population include Spitz nevi and epithelioid cell nevi.

MAJOR POINTS

Silver nitrate drops cause a mild chemical conjunctivitis in about 90% of cases.

Conjunctivitis caused by *Neisseria gonorrhoeae* is an emergency because of this organism's ability to invade an intact corneal epithelium.

Neonatal conjunctivitis as a result of chlamydia, gonorrhea, and herpes simplex all require systemic therapy.

The common bacterial causes of pediatric conjunctivitis are *Haemophilus, Streptococcus, Pneumococcus,* and *Staphylococcus.*

Haemophilus influenzae often causes a hemorrhagic conjunctivitis.

Chlamydia serotypes A-C cause trachoma; serotypes D-K cause inclusion conjunctivitis.

Epidemic keratoconjunctivitis is most often caused by adenovirus serotypes 8 and 19; serotypes 3 and 7 cause pharyngoconjunctival fever.

Phlyctenules usually occur near the limbus and contain lymphocytes, plasma cells, and histiocytes.

Ligneous conjunctivitis begins as a mild, chronic, pseudomembranous conjunctivitis; nodular masses appear in later stages.

Conjunctival nevi near the limbus have low malignant potential, but pigmented lesions involving the fornix or palpebral conjunctiva should be biopsied.

SUGGESTED READINGS

Abelson MB, Allansmith MR, Friedlaender MH: Effects of topically applied ocular decongestant and antihistamine, *Am J Ophthalmol* 90:254-257, 1980.

Abelson MB, Schaefer K: Conjunctivitis of allergic origin: immunologic mechanisms and current approaches to therapy, *Surv Ophthalmol* 38 (Suppl): 115-132, 1993.

Bateman JB, Pettit TH, Isenberg SJ, et al: Ligneous conjunctivitis: an autosomal recessive disorder, *J Pediatric Ophthalmol Strabismus* 23: 137-140, 1986.

BenEzra D, Pe´er J, Brodsky M, et al: Cyclosporine eyedrops for the treatment of severe vernal keratoconjunctivitis, *Am J Ophthalmol* 101:278-282, 1986.

Foster CS: Evaluation of topical cromolyn sodium in the treatment of vernal keratoconjunctivitis, *Ophthalmology* 95: 194-201, 1988.

Friday GA, Biglan AW, Hiles DA, et al: Treatment of ragweed allergic conjunctivitis with cromolyn sodium 4% ophthalmic solution, *Am J Ophthalmol* 95:169-174, 1983.

Friedlaender MH, Okumoto, M, Kelley J: Diagnosis of allergic conjunctivitis, *Arch Ophthalmol* 102: 1198-1199, 1984.

Gigliotti F, Hendley JO, Morgan J, et al: Efficacy of topical antibiotic therapy in acute conjunctivitis in children, *J Pediatrics* 104: 623-626, 1984.

Gigliotti F, Williams WT, Hayden FG, et al: Etiology of acute conjunctivitis in children, *J Pediatrics* 98: 531-536, 1981.

Grosskreutz C, Smith L: Neonatal conjunctivitis, *Int Ophthalmol Clin* 32: 71-79, 1992.

Haimovici R, Roussel TJ. Treatment of gonococcal conjunctivitis with single-dose intramuscular ceftriaxone, *Am J Ophthalmol* 107: 511-514, 1989.

Harrison JR, English MG, Lee CK, et al: Chlamydia trachomatis infant pneumonitis, *New Engl J Med* 198: 702-708, 1978.

Holland EJ, Chan C, Kuwabra T, et al: Immunohistologic findings and results of treatment with cyclosporine in ligneous conjunctivitis, *Am J Ophthalmol* 107: 160-166, 1989.

Holland EJ, Schwartz GS: Ligneous conjunctivitis. In Krachmer JH, Mannis MJ, Holland E, et al: *Cornea. Cornea and external disease: clinical diagnosis and management,* St. Louis, 1997, Mosby.

Lindquist TD: Ophthalmia neonatorum. In Krachmer JH, Mannis MJ, Holland E, et al: *Cornea. Cornea and external disease: clinical diagnosis and management,* St. Louis, 1997, Mosby.

Lohr JA, Austin RD, Grossman M, et al: Comparison of three topical antimicrobials for acute bacterial conjunctivitis, *Pediatr Infect Dis J* 7: 626-629, 1988.

McConnell JM, Carpenter JD, Jacobs P, et al: Conjunctival melanocytic lesions in children, *Ophthalmology* 96(7): 986-993, 1989.

Schuster V, Mingers A, Seidenspinner S, et al: Homozygous mutations in the plasminogen gene of two unrelated girls with ligneous conjunctivitis, *Blood* 90: 958-966, 1997.

CHAPTER 6

Cornea and Anterior Segment Disease

CLOUDY CORNEA IN INFANCY

STRUCTURAL ANOMALIES OF THE CORNEA
- Megalocornea
- Keratoconus
- Keratoglobus
- Microcornea
- Sclerocornea

ANTERIOR SEGMENT DYSGENESIS
- Posterior Embryotoxon
- Axenfeld-Rieger Syndrome
- Peters' Anomaly

HEREDITARY CORNEAL DYSTROPHIES
- Anterior Dystrophies
- Stromal Dystrophies
- Endothelial Dystrophies

PENETRATING KERATOPLASTY

IRIS ABNORMALITIES
- Aniridia
- Coloboma of the Iris
- CHARGE Association
- Heterochromia Irides
- Brushfield Spots
- Lisch Nodules

The common and important congenital and acquired corneal and anterior segment disorders of childhood are covered in this chapter. The clinician must have a good working knowledge of the causes of corneal clouding in infancy so that an appropriate evaluation can be initiated. This is covered in the first part of this chapter and is followed by a discussion of structural abnormalities, size, and shape of the cornea. A finding, such as microcornea, should evoke a differential diagnosis and trigger a directed examination and further evaluation. This leads to a discussion of the anterior segment dysgeneses. The hereditary corneal dystrophies are covered next, including a discussion of the challenges inherent in penetrating keratoplasty in children. Finally, abnormalities involving the iris, such as aniridia, are covered.

CLOUDY CORNEA IN INFANCY

Table 6-1 is an overview of the main conditions requiring consideration in a neonate or infant with corneal opacity. Infectious causes are among the first that must be ruled out. The time of onset may help distinguish among the possible etiologies of infectious keratitis. Neonatal conjunctivitis resulting from gonococcal infection, which is acquired in the birth canal, comes on within 48 hours after birth, and keratitis and ulceration may follow thereafter. *N. gonorrhoeae* is aggressive and has the ability to penetrate intact corneal epithelium. Abundant purulent discharge, eyelid edema, chemosis, and gram-negative diplococci are the main features. Slit-lamp examination will aid in determining the extent of the keratitis or ulceration. Corneal perforation and endophthalmitis are the most feared complications. Treatment requires the use of topical and systemic antibiotics and frequent topical irrigation.

Herpetic keratitis typically has its onset somewhat later than gonococcal keratitis, at age 4 to 10 days. It is due to herpes simplex II, also transmitted via the birth canal. Most, but not all, of these patients will have periocular skin vesicles. The corneal findings differ somewhat from those in adults; geographic ulceration occurs rather than typical dendrites, and follicles may not appear in these very young patients. Ocular complications include chorioretinitis, vitreitis, optic atrophy, and cataracts. Timely evaluation for the possibility of disseminated herpes is required. The keratitis is treated with topical antiviral medication, as well as systemic acyclovir.

Congenital *rubella* is another infectious entity that may present with corneal clouding in infancy, which may be caused by keratitis or glaucoma. The keratitis clears spontaneously over the course of weeks. Other ocular complications of congenital rubella are microphthalmos, cataract, and pigmentary retinopathy.

Table 6-1 Differential diagnosis of neonatal corneal opacity

Etiology	Age of onset	Corneal signs	Other
Infectious Disease			
Herpes simplex (Type II)	4-10 days	Unilateral corneal ulcer, positive fluorescein staining, often in a geographic configuration	Viral culture for herpes
Rubella	Birth	Diffuse corneal edema, often associated with cataracts	Serology including IgM
Neisseria gonorrhoeae	2-3 days	Diffuse punctate staining with possible corneal ulceration	Gram's stain and culture
Trauma			
Tears in Descemet's membrane	Birth	Vertical corneal striae with edema in the area of breaks in Descemet's membrane	History of forceps delivery, often associated with soft tissue injury of the face
Corneal perforation with amniocentesis	Birth	Local corneal opacity with possible iris synechiae	Amniocentesis; traumatic cataract
Dysgenesis Syndromes			
Peters' anomaly	Birth	Central corneal opacity may extend to the limbus; iridocorneal strands	60% with glaucoma
Sclerocorneal	Birth	Peripheral corneal opacity associated with flattening of the cornea	May be associated with other anterior segment anomalies
Limbal dermoid	Birth	Limbal mass; yellow-white in appearance; also may have hair and follicles	May be isolated or associated with Goldenhar's syndrome
Dystrophies			
Congenital hereditary endothelial dystrophy (CHED)	Birth to several months	Bilateral diffuse corneal edema; corneal thickening; corneal diameters normal	Attenuated or absent endothelium; autosomal dominant
Posterior polymorphous dystrophy (PPMD)	Infrequently at birth to first few years of life	Deep linear opacities and thickening of Descemet's membrane (snail tracks); deep posterior vesicles; corneal edema	Rarely a penetrating keratoplasty is necessary; usually autosomal dominant
Metabolic			
Mucopolysaccharidoses (Hurler's–MPS-I H most severe form)	Unusual at birth, usually first few years of life	Diffuse ground-glass appearance through all layers; bilateral and symmetrical	Urinary glycosaminoglycan autosomal recessive
Mucolipidoses (Type IV)	Early infancy	Anterior and epithelial clouding	Autosomal recessive
Cystinosis (rare)	Rarely birth, usually first year of life	White needle-like crystals within corneal stroma; ground-glass appearance	Renal impairment; systemic crystals also in conjunctiva; autosomal recessive
Tyrosinemia	Neonate	Corneal epithelial deposits	Tyrosine in blood and urine; hyperkeratosis of skin
Congenital Glaucoma			
Congenital glaucoma	Birth to first 6 months	Corneal edema; Haab's striae; Buphthalmos	Increased 10 P; increased optic nerve cupping

Interstitial keratitis secondary to congenital syphilis is not present at birth and usually comes on in early childhood.

Direct ocular trauma from obstetrical forceps may cause Descemet's breaks and subsequent corneal edema. Distinguishing this from congenital glaucoma is usually not difficult. Corneal trauma is suggested by the appropriate history, presence of eyelid and periorbital ecchymoses, unilaterally, and vertically oriented striae. Features of congenital glaucoma include elevated intraocular pressure, buphthalmos, curvilinear striae, and, often, bilaterality.

Anterior segment dysgeneses are present at birth with fixed malformations. *Peters' anomaly* is a sporadic, often bilateral condition in which a central corneal leukoma is present. Varying degrees of other malformations such as iridocorneal strands, cataracts, and corneolenticular apposition may be present. Glaucoma is quite common and may be present at birth. In sclerocornea, scleral tissue extends too far centrally. A preserved island of cornea may be present, or, in complete cases, sclera covers the entire anterior globe. When corneal tissue is present, it is horizontally oval and flat when measured with keratometry. Corneal dermoids, such as those occurring in Goldenhar's syndrome, are elevated, yellow-white limbal masses. They may be bilateral.

The major hereditary corneal stromal dystrophies do not present at birth; but the endothelial disorder, *congenital hereditary endothelial dystrophy* (CHED), may present at birth or shortly thereafter. CHED is a rare, bilateral condition caused by endothelial dysfunction. The opacity involves the entire cornea, which is edematous and bluish in color. The intraocular pressure is normal. *Posterior polymorphous dystrophy* (PPMD) rarely is apparent in infancy. It is an autosomal disorder characterized by band lesions, vesicle-like lesions, and diffuse opacities at the level of Descemet's membrane and the endothelium. Most cases are asymptomatic. *Congenital hereditary stromal dystrophy* (CHSD) is a rare, congenital, bilateral, nonprogressive defect of the corneal stroma. Multiple flake-like opacities are present, without corneal edema.

In most of the metabolic disorders that cause corneal clouding, the opacity is not evident at birth. Mucopolysaccharidosis type IH, Hurler's syndrome, has corneal clouding, optic atrophy, and retinal degeneration as its main features; corneal opacification may be congenital. Cloudiness occurs early in mucolipidosis IV, because of epithelial and anterior stromal involvement. The corneal crystals in cystinosis usually appear at 1 year of age; those in tyrosinemia type II may appear in infancy.

STRUCTURAL ANOMALIES OF THE CORNEA

Megalocornea

Megalocornea is a rare, nonprogressive enlargement of the cornea to 13 mm horizontal diameter or larger, in the absence of glaucoma. Typically, both eyes are affected, and, as most cases are transmitted in an X-linked pattern, 90% of affected patients are male. Clinical examination reveals large, clear corneas, with normal thickness, and increased curvature. With-the-rule astigmatism is common. The key to proper diagnosis is distinguishing isolated megalocornea from buphthalmos in congenital glaucoma. In megalocornea, Haab's striae, corneal clouding, and photophobia are absent, and the

Box 6-1 Conditions Associated with Megalocornea

Aarskog syndrome
Alport's syndrome
Marfan syndrome
Down syndrome
Megalocornea–mental retardation syndrome

remaining structures of the anterior segment are of normal size. Additional ocular changes that may be present include posterior embryotoxon, ectopia lentis et pupillae, mosaic corneal dystrophy, and Krukenberg's spindle. Both glaucoma and cataract may develop at a later time. Associated systemic conditions are listed in Box 6-1. The etiology is not known, but the gene locus is in the region Xq12-q26. The visual prognosis is good.

Keratoconus

Keratoconus is a noninflammatory corneal ectatic disorder that, while typically becoming evident after puberty, may present in childhood or even in early infancy. Childhood cases tend to be mild, but rapid progression can occur in the teenage years and early adulthood. Keratoconus tends to be bilateral and is twice as common in females than males. There is central or paracentral corneal thinning, with early steepening typically occurring inferotemporally. The maximally thinned area is at the apex of the cone, which is usually in the lower half of the cornea. Initially, visual symptoms such as blurred vision, glare, and monocular diplopia result from high degrees of irregular astigmatism and myopia. An early sign of keratoconus is scissoring of the retinoscopic reflex, reflecting the irregular corneal astigmatism. This can be confirmed with photokeratoscopy and mapping of corneal topography. Visible protrusion of the lower eyelid by the cone is referred to as *Munson's sign* and occurs in advanced cases. Other corneal findings are *Fleischer ring*, an epithelial iron ring at the base of the cone; *Vogt's striae*, fine vertical lines in the deep stroma; and, in advanced cases, breaks in Descemet's membrane. Episodes of corneal hydrops occur following Descemet's breaks, as aqueous enters the stroma, resulting in acute corneal edema. There may be residual scarring after the edema clears.

The etiology of keratoconus is not known. Familial cases exist, but most are sporadic. One predisposing factor that appears fairly certain is chronic eye rubbing. This is supported by the fact that atopic keratoconjunctivitis, which often causes rubbing of the eyes, is also a risk factor for keratoconus. Other systemic conditions associated with keratoconus include Ehlers-Danlos syndrome, osteogenesis imperfecta, and Down syndrome. The pathologic changes of the cornea include stromal thinning, breaks in Bowman's layer, scarring of Bowman's layer, and iron staining of the basal epithelium.

Initial treatment involves providing the best optical correction possible. Spectacles are effective in early disease, but rigid contact lenses are more effective in treating irregular astigmatism. Most patients can be satisfactorily managed in this fashion. Acute hydrops may be painful and may dramatically reduce the vision but is not an indication for keratoplasty. Hydrops is managed with cycloplegics for pain control. Occasionally, topical corticosteroids are necessary to reduce inflammation and corneal vascularization. Penetrating keratoplasty is indicated for those with corneal scarring, those in whom glasses and contact lenses do not provide adequate clarity, and those intolerant of contact lenses.

Keratoglobus

Keratoglobus is a rare, bilateral condition that is usually present at birth. This ectatic corneal disorder is characterized by a diffuse thinning of the entire cornea, which appears globular. The corneal diameter is not enlarged, and the remaining structures of the anterior segment are also normal sized. The protruding cornea is very steep as evidenced by high keratometric readings and a very deep anterior chamber. Acute hydrops may occur resulting in corneal edema. Furthermore, the thinness of the cornea makes it susceptible to traumatic rupture. A strong association with Ehlers-Danlos syndrome type IV exists. Shatterproof myopic spectacles provide optical correction, as well as protection from injury.

Microcornea

An eye with an abnormally small cornea, in an otherwise normal-sized globe, is considered to have microcornea. The normal cornea reaches the adult dimension of about 11.75 mm in diameter by age 2 years; diameters of 10 mm or less fall into the microcornea range. *Nanophthalmos* is the correct term if the entire eye is small but structurally normal. If the anterior segment is small but the posterior segment is of normal size, *anterior microphthalmos* is the preferred designation. *Microphthalmos* means the eye is small and disorganized. Hence, after identifying an abnormally small cornea, a thorough evaluation, possibly including ultrasonographic determination of the axial length, is required (Fig. 6-1). Microcornea is an uncommon disorder and may be unilateral or bilateral. It may occur sporadically or may be inherited in an autosomal dominant or (rarely) an autosomal recessive manner.

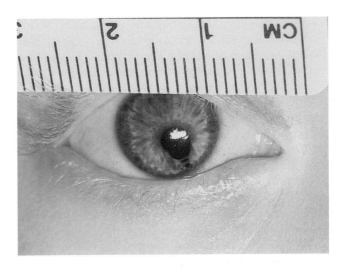

Fig. 6-1   Microphthalmic eye with an iris coloboma.

Good visual potential is possible, depending on the condition of the rest of the globe. The corneas tend to be flat, and, depending on the length of the eye, hyperopic correction is often required. Both angle-closure and open-angle glaucoma occur with greater than usual frequency in these eyes, resulting from the crowding of the anterior segment and, presumably, goniodysgenesis, respectively. The cause of microcornea is not known, but an arrest of corneal development and overgrowth of the tips of the optic cup, impeding corneal growth, have both been hypothesized. Many associated ocular and systemic conditions have been identified, and the most important of these are listed in Box 6-2.

Sclerocornea

Sclerocornea is an uncommon, congenital, nonprogressive condition in which scleral tissue replaces the cornea. In peripheral sclerocornea, central clear corneal tissue is present; diffuse or total sclerocornea affects the entire cornea. The central cornea is flat, with powers between 20 and 40 diopters. The finding of a central corneal curvature that is flatter than the peripheral scleral curvature is felt to be a pathognomonic sign. Since peripheral scleralization and corneal flattening are features of the condition cornea plana, some physicians view these conditions as the same. The abnormal sclera is highly vascularized, and the limbus is poorly developed.

Sclerocornea is usually bilateral and asymmetric, and both autosomal dominant and autosomal recessive transmission has been described. Box 6-3 lists the associated conditions associated with sclerocornea.

Treatment is aimed at providing the best refractive correction possible. Although risky, many cases require penetrating keratoplasty.

Box 6-2 Conditions Associated with Microcornea

OCULAR CONDITIONS

Open-angle glaucoma
Angle-closure glaucoma
Iris colobomas
Cataracts
Microphakia
Retinopathy of prematurity
Persistent hyperplastic primary vitreous
Aniridia

SYSTEMIC CONDITIONS

Ehlers-Danlos syndrome
Marfan syndrome
Alagille syndrome
Hallermann-Streiff syndrome
Norrie's disease
Trisomy 21
Progeria
Rubella
Waardenburg's syndrome
Weill-Marchesani syndrome

Box 6-3 Conditions Associated with Sclerocornea

Hyperopia
Infantile glaucoma
Angle-closure glaucoma
Retinal aplasia
Congenital cataracts
Blue sclerae
Microphthalmos

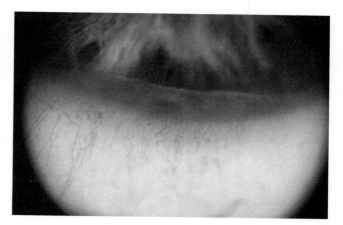

Fig. 6-2 Posterior embryotoxon. (Courtesy of Delmar R. Caldwell, M.D., Tulane University School of Medicine.)

ANTERIOR SEGMENT DYSGENESIS

The anterior segment dysgeneses consist of posterior embryotoxon, Axenfeld-Rieger syndrome, Peters' anomaly, and other disorders. (The term *mesodermal dysgenesis* is obsolete, see the following discussion.) These conditions are examples of neurocristopathies, since there are abnormalities of anterior segment structures derived from neural crest cells.

Posterior Embryotoxon

Posterior embryotoxon is the term for an anteriorly displaced, prominent Schwalbe's line (Fig. 6-2). Usually this line, which marks the peripheral termination of Descemet's membrane, is behind the opaque portion of the anterior limbus and cannot be seen without gonioscopy. However, in up to 15% of normal persons, a fine, white, scalloped ring, on the peripheral inner cornea, is present. It may be complete or discontinuous. Transmission is autosomal dominant. Isolated posterior embryotoxon is a benign condition.

About 90% of patients with *Alagille syndrome* have posterior embryotoxon, often with associated iris strands. Alagille syndrome, or arteriohepatic dysplasia, is an autosomal dominant condition in which too few interlobular bile ducts are present. The result is intrahe-

patic cholestasis in infancy or childhood. Other common features include peripheral pulmonary stenosis, butterfly vertebral arch defects, fundus hypopigmentation, and optic nerve anomalies. Demonstrating the presence of posterior embryotoxon in a young patient with hepatic cholestasis would support a diagnosis of Alagille syndrome rather than other causes of liver disease.

Axenfeld-Rieger Syndrome

The entities referred to as Axenfeld's syndrome and Rieger's syndrome, because of their similarities, are now combined as manifestations of the same condition, as suggested by Shields, et al. In the past, the designation Axenfeld's anomaly referred to an eye with posterior embryotoxon and prominent iris processes, and Axenfeld's syndrome referred to an eye with Axenfeld's anomaly and glaucoma. Rieger's anomaly referred to more severely affected eyes, with iris hypoplasia or atrophy, corectopia, ectropion uveae, and glaucoma. Rieger's syndrome was reserved for cases in which the ocular changes of Rieger's syndrome were accompanied by other various systemic anomalies (see the following discussion). Since the clinical findings are, in practice, dif-

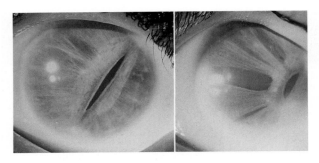

Fig. 6-3   Axenfeld-Rieger anomaly. Note iris atrophy, pseudopolycoria, and corectopia. (Courtesy of Zeynel A. Karcioglu, M.D., New Orleans.)

Box 6-4   Axenfeld-Rieger Syndrome: Differential Diagnosis

Iridocorneal endothelial (ICE) syndrome
Aniridia
Peters' anomaly
Conditions causing anterior segment inflammation with subsequent PAS

---

ficult to cleanly delineate, and because a common genetic problem appears responsible, Axenfeld-Rieger (A-R) syndrome has become the preferred terminology.

Axenfeld-Rieger syndrome is a congenital, bilateral autosomal dominantly inherited condition affecting the structures of the anterior eye and other remote organs. There is no racial or sex predilection, and secondary glaucoma is common, occurring in 50% to 60% of patients. As noted in the previous discussion, great clinical variability exists. The primary ocular findings are posterior embryotoxon, often with iris processes to this anteriorly displaced Schwalbe's line. Iris changes range from mild to severe and include iris atrophy, corectopia, severe hypoplasia, iris hole formation, and ectropion uveae (Fig. 6-3). The morphology of some of these changes is somewhat predictable. In eyes with corectopia, the pupil is drawn toward a large iridocorneal adhesion with iris atrophy and holes seen in the opposite quadrant. The appearance of the iris may change somewhat over the first few years of life, but A-R syndrome is felt to be nonprogressive. The glaucoma is believed to occur as a result of the arrested development of the trabecular meshwork and Schlemm's canal. Most often, its onset is in childhood or early adulthood, but infantile presentations occur.

When the above ocular findings occur in conjunction with certain systemic disorders, Rieger's syndrome is said to be present. The more common systemic abnormalities are dental defects; the teeth may be small (microdontia) or decreased in number. Maxillary hypoplasia, the presence of a broad, flat nose, a thin upper lip with a prominent lower lip, hypertelorism and telecanthus, and redundancy of the periumbilical skin are the other more common anomalies.

Assuming that an adequate examination can be performed, diagnosis of A-R syndrome is usually not difficult, and certain features will distinguish it from other abnormalities. The appearance of the iris in iridocorneal endothelial (ICE) syndrome may resemble that of A-R syndrome, but ICE syndrome is unilateral, and (in Chandler's syndrome) corneal disease is evident. Aniridia does not have the prominent Schwalbe's line and iris processes seen in A-R syndrome. Peters' anomaly typically has a central corneal opacity, although, as discussed in the following section, there is evidence that a common genetic defect is present in Peters' anomaly and A-R syndrome. The differential diagnosis of Axenfield-Rieger syndrome is given in Box 6-4.

The primary management issues in Axenfeld-Rieger syndrome concern the glaucoma. Goniotomies are usually ineffective. Aqueous suppressants are usually tried first, followed by filtering surgery and placement of glaucoma drainage devices.

Peters' Anomaly

Peters' anomaly refers to a collection of congenital disorders of the anterior segment and cornea of which the most prominent feature is corneal opacification. Eighty percent of cases of Peters' anomaly are bilateral, and the condition may be isolated or associated with other ocular or systemic disorders. The common pathologic feature in Peters' anomaly is a zone of absent posterior stroma, Descemet's membrane and endothelium underlying the opacity. Peters' anomaly may be classified into three anatomic groups. Type I Peters' anomaly has only a central corneal opacity or leukoma (Fig. 6-4). Type II also contains a central leukoma, but there are accompanying iris strands that reach across the anterior segment and attach to the edge of the corneal defect. Type III Peters' anomaly contains the above features, with the addition of cataract or adherence of the lens to the cornea. Within each of these anatomic groups, severity of the defects varies widely.

Although autosomal dominant and recessive cases have been reported, most are sporadic, and about 80% are bilateral. Glaucoma is a common and important complication of Peters' anomaly, is present in up to 70% of cases, and is responsible for the majority of blindness in Peters' anomaly. Types I and II tend to be isolated conditions, while type III is often associated with other malformations. The common associated ocular findings are given in Box 6-5.

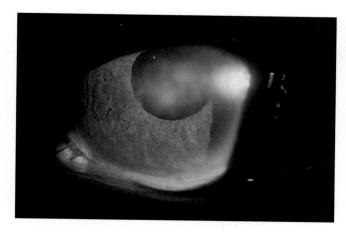

Fig. 6-4   Peters' anomaly, type I, with a posterior corneal defect and leukoma.

The glaucoma may be congenital or juvenile or may develop, following penetrating keratoplasty. As might be expected, deprivation amblyopia is also a common and difficult complication in Peters' anomaly. When systemic disorders are also present, some use the designation "Peters'-plus" syndrome. Recorded malformations include short stature, cleft lip and palate abnormalities, congenital heart defects, genitourinary disorders, and spina bifida.

The etiology of Peters' anomaly remains uncertain, and more than one cause may exist. The entities grouped under the rubric, Peters' anomaly may, in fact, represent diverse mechanisms that yield a similar phenotype. Because of the similarity of some of the manifestations of Peters' anomaly to Axenfeld and Rieger syndrome, Peters' anomaly has been grouped with them as a "mesodermal dysgenesis." The term *mesodermal dysgenesis* is no longer used because the affected tissues derive from neural crest tissue, rather than mesenchyme. There is evidence that at least some cases of Peters' anomaly result from mutations in PAX6. Most cases are sporadic, but autosomal dominant cases exist.

HEREDITARY CORNEAL DYSTROPHIES

Anterior Corneal Dystrophies

Of the three most common anterior corneal dystrophies, Meesmann's dystrophy and Reis-Buckler's dystrophy are common in children. Map-dot-fingerprint dystrophy more often becomes clinically apparent in the third decade.

Meesmann's dystrophy (hereditary juvenile epithelial dystrophy)   Meesmann's dystrophy is a rare bilateral, autosomal dominantly inherited dystrophy. In the first few years of life, innumerable microcysts, visible with direct illumination or retroillumination, appear throughout the corneal epithelium. Affected patients may be asymptomatic or have mild irritation from erosions of the microcysts and photophobia. The vision is either normal or slightly reduced, but many older patients are unaware that they have the condition. Electron microscopy demonstrates filamentary and granular material within the cytoplasm referred to as *peculiar substance*. This material is PAS positive. The cysts contain degenerated epithelial products. Rarely is treatment beyond lubrication required.

Reis-Buckler's dystrophy (dystrophies of Bowman's membrane)   Reis-Buckler's dystrophy is a progressive condition that causes earlier symptoms than Meesmann's dystrophy, typically in the first decade. The nomenclature regarding the dystrophies of Bowman's membrane is evolving, as previous authors have used the designation Reis-Buckler's dystrophy to refer to more than one entity. There appears to be two similar but distinct conditions, referred to by some as corneal dystrophy of Bowman's layer type I (CDB-I or Reis-Buckler's dystrophy) and corneal dystrophy of Bowman's layer type II (CDB-II or Thiel-Behnke dystrophy). Both are bilateral and cause painful corneal erosions. The main early slit-lamp finding is a central, gray-white, reticular, honey-comb-shaped opacity of the anterior stroma and Bowman's membrane (Fig. 6-5). As the condition progresses, the process involves more of the periphery and deep cornea. Repeated erosions lead to subepithelial scarring and irregular astigmatism. Compared to CDB-I, CDB-II tends to disrupt the corneal surface less and disrupt vision later in life. The conditions can also be differentiated with transmission electron microscopy.

Management of these conditions is the same, consisting, first, of treatment of the recurrent erosions. When the opacity significantly impairs vision, phototherapeutic keratectomy (PTK), lamellar keratoplasty or penetrating keratoplasty may be employed. For treatment of recurrent erosions PTK has proven particularly effective.

Map-dot-fingerprint dystrophy   Map-dot-fingerprint dystrophy (*Cogan's microcystic dystrophy*) is the most common dystrophy of the corneal epithelium but typically does not have its onset until patients reach their twenties. It is so named because of the various patterns that can manifest from a defective production of base-

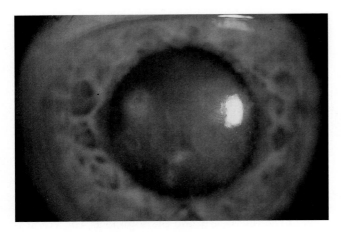

Fig. 6-5 Reis-Buckler's dystrophy. (Courtesy of Delmar R. Caldwell, M.D., Tulane University School of Medicine.)

ment membrane by the basal epithelial cells. Microcysts (the "dots") appear as gray-white oval, round, or irregular opacities in the epithelium. The map figures appear as discrete, irregular, wispy gray lines or bands, which may be multiple. They are composed of abnormal basement membrane within the epithelium. Fingerprint figures appear as regions of multiple, parallel, concentric lines, with normal-appearing regions interspersed. These are best seen with retroillumination. Each of the three patterns may appear in the eye of the affected patient, although the map changes are most common. Map-dot-fingerprint dystrophy may be asymptomatic but often comes to attention because of painful corneal erosions. These occur spontaneously and typically are recurrent. Visual loss is usually not severe and limited to mild blurring secondary to irregular astigmatism.

Stromal Dystrophies

Lattice dystrophy Lattice dystrophy is a dominantly inherited condition in which deposition of *amyloid* occurs in the anterior corneal stroma. Early findings may be visible in childhood, but children rarely are symptomatic. Slit-lamp examination, with direct illumination or retroillumination, reveals the many possible patterns that the depositions display. Early cases show multiple, small, gray opacities. They are subepithelial and round, ovoid, or linear. As they progress, the linear forms come to predominate, taking on a branching or spiculated appearance. Some of the lines may overlap or cross one another, giving rise to the name lattice dystrophy. The intervening areas of clear cornea progressively coalesce, and anterior stromal haze, with a ground-glass appearance, ensues. Amyloid deposition also occurs between Bowman's layer and the epithelium. Therefore recurrent corneal erosions may occur, with consequent pain and scarring.

Two primary types of lattice dystrophy have been described. Type I is limited to the cornea and has the features described above. Type II, also referred to as *Meretoja's syndrome*, is a systemic syndrome, with amyloid deposition in sites other than the eye as well. Type II lattice dystrophy is a condition of older adults. Corneal amyloid deposits may be demonstrated histopathologically with Congo red, PAS, Masson's trichrome, and thioflavin T. Also, dichroism is characteristically seen when viewing through a polarizing filter. The main goal of treatment is to control and treat the erosions. Penetrating keratoplasty is performed in advanced cases with recurrence of the dystrophy more common than in the other stromal dystrophies, occurring in about 50% of cases.

Granular dystrophy The gray-white deposits in the anterior stroma in granular dystrophy may be seen in the first decade, but patients generally do not become symptomatic until the third or fourth decade. The typical opacities, which involve the central portion of the anterior stroma, appear as discrete forms, resembling crumbs or snowflakes. Initially, the intervening stroma remains clear, but the opacities may coalesce in later stages. Erosions are not common, and the main disability results from decreased visual acuity and glare. Inheritance follows an autosomal dominant pattern. *Hyaline deposits* are found through histopathological examination; these stain well with PAS and Masson's trichrome. Penetrating keratoplasty is an effective treatment. More recently, phototherapeutic keratectomy has been shown to be effective in superficial cases.

Avellino corneal dystrophy is felt to be a variant of granular dystrophy; in addition to the typical granular deposits, lattice type I lesions are present, and the patients suffer more from recurrent erosions. Granular, lattice type I, and Avellino dystrophies all appear to result from mutations in the same region of chromosome 5q; they may be different manifestations of a mutation of a single gene.

Macular dystrophy Macular dystrophy differs from the preceding disorders in that its inheritance is autosomal recessive. Also, it is the rarest of the stromal dystrophies, and it is the most severe. The opacities may be visible as early as age 3 years and are composed of intracellular and extracellular *mucopolysaccharide* (glycosaminoglycan) deposits in the stroma. Early changes affect the central cornea, appearing as diffuse superficial clouding. By the second decade of life, the entire corneal stroma becomes involved. There may be formation of guttate, as well as corneal thinning. Recurrent erosions are not a common feature, but visual loss occurs fairly early, requiring penetrating keratoplasty in the second or third decade. On pathological examination, the deposits stain with alcian blue, PAS, colloidal iron, and antibodies to keratin sulfate proteoglycan.

Endothelial Dystrophies

Posterior polymorphous dystrophy (PPMD) Posterior polymorphous dystrophy is a bilateral, autosomal dominantly inherited disease of the corneal endothelium and Descemet's membrane. The condition varies widely in severity and is often discovered as an incidental finding in an asymptomatic adult. However, young children may be affected, with resultant visual loss from corneal clouding. The primary defect in PPMD is the presence of epithelial-like cells admixed with normal-appearing endothelium. The process is thought to represent a metaplasia. These cells display a multilayered configuration, and have microvilli, intermediate fibers, and desmosomes. Additionally, the posterior nonbanded zone of Descemet's membrane is abnormal.

Clinically, three primary patterns of posterior corneal changes may be seen with the slit lamp. Vesicle-like lesions, up to 1 mm in diameter, appear as translucent cysts, and occur singly, in groups, and in linear figures. They are surrounded by a gray halo. Band lesions are horizontal lines with scalloped edges, formed by fused rows of vesicles. Diffuse opacities are 0.5 to 2 mm diameter zones of gray-white lesions. The abnormal cells may migrate across the anterior chamber angle and iris to cause the other important clinical findings in PPMD, broad PAS, and glaucoma. Overall, glaucoma is not a frequent complication, but when it occurs, PAS are usually present. Rarely, corneal edema occurs. Penetrating keratoplasty is indicated when the visual loss is disabling. The prognosis is good in the absence of PAS and glaucoma. The precise gene responsible for PPMD has not yet been determined, but linkage analysis has localized a defect to chromosome 20q11.

Congenital Hereditary Endothelial Dystrophy (CHED) Congenital hereditary endothelial dystrophy is a rare, bilateral dystrophy caused by primary endothelial cell dysfunction. Autosomal dominant and recessive inheritance patterns have been characterized. The usual presentation of the more common, and more severe autosomal recessively inherited form is that of bilateral corneal clouding, present at birth or developing shortly thereafter, with marked corneal thickening but no inflammation (Fig. 6-6). The cornea is gray-blue, with a ground-glass appearance because of diffuse microcystic edema. The intraocular pressure is not elevated, distinguishing this condition from congenital glaucoma, and there is no excessive tearing or photophobia. Typically, the defect is static and isolated. Nystagmus often is present.

Autosomal dominantly inherited cases are much rarer and have a later onset. Typically, these cases come to attention by age 2 years and, in contrast to the early onset cases, may be associated with pain, photophobia, and tearing. Visual loss may be noted, but it occurs too

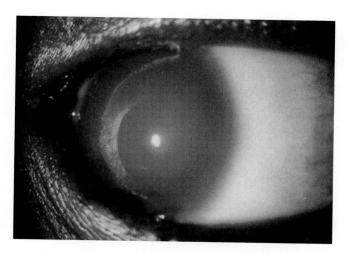

Fig. 6-6 Congenital hereditary endothelial dystrophy. (Courtesy of Delmar R. Caldwell, M.D., Tulane University School of Medicine.)

Box 6-6 **Differential Diagnosis of CHED**
Glaucoma
Metabolic diseases
Forceps injury
Infections
Congenital hereditary stromal dystrophy

late to cause nystagmus. Box 6-6 lists the differential diagnosis of CHED. CHED should be considered a diagnosis of exclusion, since, except for visual loss, no additional complications occur. The primary treatment is penetrating keratoplasty.

PENETRATING KERATOPLASTY

Successful penetrating keratoplasty in children is significantly more difficult than in adults. The surgery is technically challenging, since the graft size may be small and the globes lack rigidity. Post-operative management is hindered by suboptimal examinations in uncooperative patients. Amblyopia typically contributes to the visual impairment and must be vigorously combated. Furthermore, regardless of the ocular condition, all corneal transplants in children pose a high failure risk because of the strong tendency toward immune rejection in young patients, particularly those younger than 1 year of age. Finally, coexisting congenital structural defects and the need to perform other procedures at the time of keratoplasty, such as lensectomy and vitrectomy, add to the risk in these patients. Hence, the decision to perform a cor-

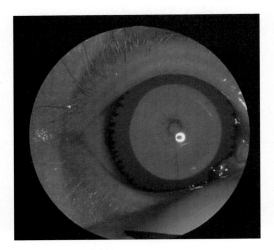

Fig. 6-7   Aniridia. Ciliary processes and the edge of the lens are visible. Note the small anterior polar cataract and persistent pupillary membrane fibers.

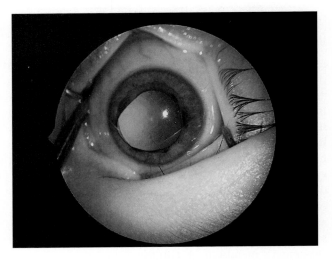

Fig. 6-8   Aniridia. More iris tissue is present in this case than in Fig. 6-7, but there is no iris collarette or pupillary sphincter. (From Traboulsi EL, et al: *Int Pediatr* 5:275-278, 1990.)

neal transplant in a child is made only after careful consideration of many factors beyond the ocular pathology, including the child's social situation (will a responsible caretaker instill frequent eyedrops?); the vision in the fellow eye; and the general medical condition of the child.

The most common conditions requiring penetrating keratoplasty in children include anterior segment dysgenesis, sclerocornea, CHED, glaucoma, trauma, and keratitis. Bilateral Peters' anomaly with dense corneal opacities requires rather urgent care to minimize the effects of deprivation amblyopia. A multicenter, retrospective review of corneal transplants in 108 children younger than 12 years old was reported. At 12 months, 80.2% of the grafts were clear, and 67.4% were clear at 24 months. The most common causes of graft failure were rejection, glaucoma, keratitis or ulceration, and phthisis. However, good visual results are very difficult to achieve because of amblyopia.

IRIS ABNORMALITIES

Aniridia

Aniridia is a rare, surprisingly variable condition named for the lack of iris tissue present in most cases. However, the term *aniridia* is a poor one for two reasons. First, the entire iris is not absent, as the name would imply; careful gonioscopy will usually reveal peripheral hypoplastic tissue, even in the most severe cases. Second, many ocular structures besides the iris are affected. The other common findings in aniridia are cataract, corneal opacification, glaucoma, foveal hypoplasia, optic nerve hypoplasia, and nystagmus.

Iris changes have been considered the hallmark of this condition (Fig. 6-7). Either a rudimentary stump of iris is present, or more iris tissue is present, at times producing a picture resembling a coloboma (Fig. 6-8). Recent work has shown that the iris changes in aniridia may be much more subtle than previously thought. For instance, some affected patients have only corectopia as the main iris finding. Patients with definite aniridia have been described as having round pupils of normal size whose irides have sectors of decreased stromal tissue or absent iris collarettes, as seen with iris fluorescein angiography.

Foveal hypoplasia, another cardinal sign in aniridia, manifests as a decreased or absent foveal reflex. Retinal vessels may pass through the center of the fovea, and the macular pigmentation may be decreased. Angiographically, the foveal avascular zone is reduced or absent. Whereas mild iris changes in the collarette may not be visible in young children, the foveal changes are present from birth and can establish the diagnosis in mild cases. The degree of visual impairment in aniridia is felt to primarily depend on the degree of foveal hypoplasia, and, in certain cases, the presence of optic nerve hypoplasia.

Cataracts, glaucoma, and opacification of the cornea may be progressive, and lead to progressive visual loss. Glaucoma in aniridia is primarily due to progressive angle closure by the rudimentary iris stump. Usually this occurs from age 5 to 15 years. Initially, medical management may be effective, but ultimately, filtering surgery or placement of a glaucoma drainage device is required. Many patients have keratitis, which typically begins peripherally and manifests as cloudiness at the level of Bowman's membrane with anterior stromal neovascularization. The keratitis may progress to involve the central cornea, causing further visual loss. Penetrating keratoplasty is indicated in these patients. There may be overlap between the dominantly inherited form of aniridia and the condition, autosomal dominant keratitis.

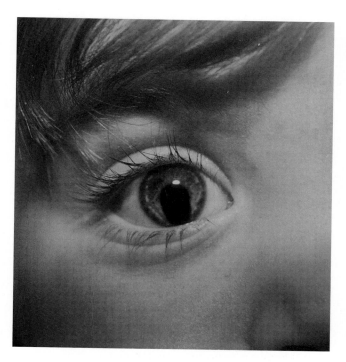

Fig. 6-9 Typical iris coloboma of the right eye.

Aniridia is always bilateral, although one eye may be more severely affected than the other. Photophobia may be a presenting sign.

About two thirds of cases of aniridia are familial, transmitted as an autosomal dominant trait with complete penetrance but variable expressivity. However, remember that some of these cases will be new mutations. Most of the remaining cases are sporadic and nonfamilial. Up to one third of these patients will develop *Wilms' tumor.* The association between sporadic aniridia and Wilms' tumor has been referred to as *Miller syndrome.* The median age of diagnosis of Wilms' tumor in aniridic patients is 3 years. Patients with sporadic aniridia should have abdominal examinations, as well as renal ultrasounds upon diagnosis and at regular intervals thereafter. One suggested ultrasound schedule is every 3 months until age 5 years, followed by every 6 months until age 10, and then yearly until age 16. Some patients with sporadic aniridia also have genitourinary anomalies and mental retardation, forming the *AGR* association. If Wilms' tumor is also present, the acronym *WAGR* may be used.

About 2% of patients with aniridia have *Gillespie's syndrome,* consisting of cerebellar ataxia and mental retardation.

Mutations in the PAX6 gene, on the short arm of chromosome 11, are responsible for familial aniridia. PAX6 is a member of a family of genes that orchestrate organ development. PAX6 is expressed in the neural tube, brain, and eye, and its protein product is felt to be a transcription regulator. PAX6 mutations may also be responsible for at least some cases of Peters' anomaly, congenital cataracts, familial foveal hypoplasia, and autosomal dominant keratitis. Hence, although Peters' anomaly has traditionally been grouped with the anterior segment dysgeneses, Axenfeld-Rieger syndromes, its etiology appears more similar to that of aniridia.

Coloboma of the Iris

Iris colobomas are congenital defects or notches in the iris stroma. Most often, they occur in the inferonasal iris; these are referred to as typical iris colobomas (Fig. 6-9). They form as a result of faulty closure of the embryonic fissure in the fifth week of gestation and are often accompanied by colobomas of the retina and choroid, ciliary body, and optic nerve. Atypical iris colobomas are those present in other areas of the iris. Visual function in eyes with colobomas ranges from normal to profoundly impaired, depending on the structures involved. A very common association with colobomas is microphthalmia, which may be thought of as arising because of low internal pressure in the developing globe, which has not yet become sealed. Most iris colobomas are isolated and sporadic, autosomal dominant, or associated with chromosomal defects. Most isolated iris colobomas do not require treatment.

CHARGE Association

The acronym CHARGE association refers to a set of systemic anomalies which often occur together: Colobomas, Heart defects, Atresia choanae, Retarded growth, Genital hypoplasia, Ear anomalies (and deafness), and, although not specifically designated by a letter in the acronym, mental deficiency. The cause or causes of CHARGE association is unknown. Other systemic syndromes associated with colobomas are listed in Box 6-7, and chromosomal abnormalities associated with colobomas are listed in Box 6-8.

Heterochromia Irides

The list of causes of heterochromia irides is fairly long. The affected iris may be hyperpigmented or hypopigmented compared to the fellow iris. Hyperpigmented causes include melanocytosis (ocular and oculodermal), siderosis, pigmented tumors, congenital iris ectropion (ectropion uveae), and rubeosis. Patients with *melanocytosis* are at increased risk for developing glaucoma and, to a lesser extent, uveal melanoma. (Melanocytosis is covered in Chapter 2.) *Siderosis* causes acquired ocular pigmentation as a result of intraocular iron. This usually occurs because of iron-containing projectiles that lodge in the eye. A green or brown hue is imparted to the iris, and the affected pupil is often larger than the normal

one (iron mydriasis). Progressive pigmentary retinopathy, with visual loss, is seen. *Congenital iris ectropion* is a rare condition in which the posterior pigment epithelium is present on the surface of the iris, creating a dark and glassy smooth surface. Since the posterior pigment epithelium is derived from neural ectoderm and not uvea, the designation *ectropion uveae*, although a widely used term, is a misnomer. Rubeosis iridis may occur in chronic inflammation, following trauma and accompanying intraocular tumors. The first sign of retinoblastoma may be heterochromia resulting from rubeosis.

Hypopigmentation of the iris is seen in Horner's syndrome, Waardenburg's syndrome, Fuchs' heterochromia, and with nonpigmented tumors. In congenital or early-onset Horner's syndrome, the affected eye may fail to develop normal pigmentation because the development of this pigmentation is under sympathetic control. Heterochromia may not be evident in the first 1 to 2 years of life and may not develop at all in naturally blue-eyed patients. In *Waardenburg's syndrome,* both irides may be strikingly hypochromic, or one may be blue and the other normally pigmented. Other features include deafness, a white forelock, and lateral displacement of the medial canthi.

Box 6-8	Coloboma and Chromosomal Abnormalities

Trisomy 13
Triploidy
Cat-eye syndrome
11p⁻
11q⁻
13q⁻
18r
13r
Trisomy 18
Klinefelter's syndrome
Turner's syndrome

Brushfield Spots

Brushfield spots are focal condensations of iris stroma surrounded by areas of hypoplasia and are seen in 38% to 90% of blue-eyed patients with trisomy 21 (Down syndrome) (Fig. 6-10). Usually they form a ring of spots

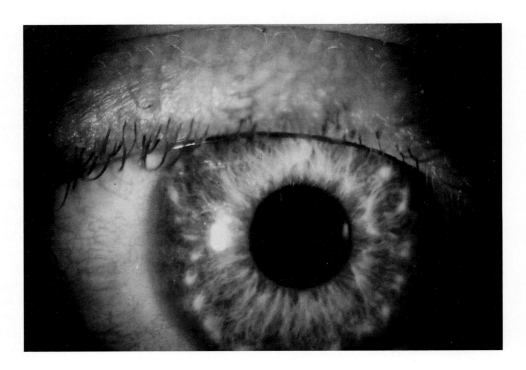

Fig. 6-10 Brushfield spots of trisomy 21. See color plate.

around the pupil, in the mid-iris. They are less easily seen in darker-eyed patients. Similar, although smaller and less distinct findings are seen in normal persons and are referred to as Wolffian nodules.

Lisch Nodules

Lisch nodules occur in neurofibromatosis I and appear as light-tan to brown, flat or dome-shaped, superficial lesions on the iris surface. They are melanocytic hamartomas, not neurofibromas, as the occasional student presumes. Lisch nodules are a highly specific sign

for neurofibromatosis I, although in newborns and young children they are not yet present. About 50% of children with NF-I at age 5 years have Lisch nodules, and about 75% of children at age 15 years have them. Hence, the diagnosis of NF-I is often established in their absence (see Chapter 11).

MAJOR POINTS

The first goal in evaluating an infant with a cloudy cornea is to determine whether or not an infection such as gonorrhea is present.

The major causes of neonatal corneal clouding are infections, glaucoma, trauma, Peters' anomaly, and corneal dystrophies.

Rapid progression of keratoconus may occur in the teenage years.

Acute hydrops, although it may be accompanied by pain and visual loss, is managed conservatively with hypertonic saline drops or ointment, cycloplegics, and patching or bandage contact lenses.

Nanophthalmos is defined as an eye that is structurally normal but small.

In eyes with sclerocornea the cornea is flatter than usual.

Although posterior embryotoxon is a common normal finding, its presence in children with hepatic cholestasis suggests the diagnosis of Alagille syndrome.

Glaucoma occurs in 50% to 60% of patients with Axenfeld-Rieger syndrome, with the usual presentation in childhood or early adulthood.

Approximately 80% of cases of Peters' anomaly are bilateral, and most occur sporadically.

Reis-Buckler's dystrophy comes on in childhood with bilateral, painful, corneal erosions.

Macular dystrophy is a rare autosomal recessive stromal dystrophy that may present in early childhood.

Posterior polymorphous dystropy is autosomal dominantly inherited, varies significantly in severity from case to case, and often is associated with glaucoma.

Autosomal recessive cases of congenital hereditary endothelial dystrophy present at birth or in infancy, whereas autosomal dominantly inherited cases present later.

About two thirds of the cases of aniridia have autosomal dominant inheritance. Of the remaining sporadic cases, up to one third will develop Wilms' tumor.

SUGGESTED READINGS

Angell LK, Robb RM, Berson FG: Visual prognosis in patients with ruptures in Descemet's membrane due to forceps injuries, *Arch Ophthalmol* 99:2137-2139, 1981.

Beauchamp GR, Knepper PA: Role of the neural crest in anterior segment development and disease, *J Pediatr Ophthalmol Strabismus* 21:209-214, 1984.

Brooks AMV, Grant G, Gillies WE: Differentiation of posterior polymorphous dystrophy from other posterior corneal opacities by specular microscopy, *Ophthalmology* 96:1639-1645, 1989.

Cameron JA: Corneal abnormalities in Ehlers-Danlos syndrome type VI, *Cornea* 12:54-59, 1993.

Dubord PJ, Krachmer JH: Diagnosis of early lattice corneal dystrophy, *Arch Ophthalmol* 100:788-790, 1982.

Folberg R, Stone EM, Sheffield VC, et al: The relationship between granular, lattice type I, and Avellino corneal dystrophies, Arch Ophthalmol 112:1080-1085, 1994.

Hanson IM, Fletcher JM, Jordan T, et al: Mutations at the PAX6 locus are found in heterogeneous anterior segment malformations including Peters' anomaly, *Nat Genet* 6:168-173, 1994.

Héon E, Mathers WD, Alward WLM, et al: Linkage of posterior polymorphous corneal dystrophy to 20q11, *Hum Mol Genet* 4:485-488, 1995.

Hingorani M, Nischal KK, Davies A, et al: Ocular abnormalities in Alagille syndrome, *Ophthalmology* 106:330-337, 1999.

Johnson BL. Ocular pathologic features of arteriohepatic dysplasia (Alagille's syndrome), *Am J Ophthalmol* 110:504-512, 1990.

Jones NP, Postlethwaite RJ, Noble JL: Clearance of corneal crystals in nephropathic cystinosis by topical cysteamine 0.5%, *Br J Ophthalmol* 75:311-312, 1991.

Kaiser-Kupfer MI, Caruso RC, Minkler DS, et al: Long-term ocular manifestations in nephropathic cystinosis, *Arch Ophthalmol* 104:706-711, 1986.

Kivlin JD, Fineman RM, Crandall AS, et al: Peters' anomaly as a consequence of genetic and nongenetic syndromes, *Arch Ophthalmol* 104:61-64, 1986.

Krachmer JH. Posterior polymorphous corneal dystrophy: a disease characterized by epithelial-like endothelial cells which influence management and prognosis, *Tr Am Ophth Soc* LXXXIII:413-475, 1985.

Mackey DA, Buttery RG, Wise GM, et al: Description of x-linked megalocornea with identification of the gene locus, *Arch Ophthalmol* 109:829-833, 1991.

Mackman G, Brightbill FS, Optiz JM: Corneal changes in aniridia, *Am J Ophthalmol* 87:497-502, 1979.

Nelson ME, Talbot JF: Keratoglobus in the Rubinstein-Taybi syndrome, *Br J Ophthalmol* 73:385-387, 1989.

Parmley VC, Stonecipher KG, Rowsey JJ: Peters' anomaly: a review of 26 penetrating keratoplasties in infants, *Ophthalmic Surg* 24:31-35, 1993.

Small KW, Mullen L, Barletta J, et al: Mapping of Reis-Bücklers' corneal dystrophy to chromosome 5q, *Am J Ophthalmol* 121:384-390, 1996.

Steinsapir KD, Lehman E, Ernest JT, et al: Systemic neurocristopathy associated with Rieger's syndrome, *Am J Ophthalmol* 110:437-438, 1990.

Stone EM, Mathers WD, Rosenwasser GOD, et al: Three autosomal dominant corneal dystrophies map to chromosome 5q, *Nat Genet* 6:47-51, 1994.

Sullivan TJ, Clarke MP, Heathcote JG, et al: Multiple congenital contractures (arthrogryposis) in association with Peters' anomaly and chorioretinal colobomata, *J Pediatr Ophthalmol Strabismus* 29:370-373, 1992.

Traboulsi EI, Maumenee IH: Peters' anomaly and associated congenital malformations, *Arch Ophthalmol* 110:1739-1742, 1992.

Tripathi BJ, Tripathi RC: Neural crest origin of human trabecular meshwork and its implications for the pathogenesis of glaucoma, *Am J Ophthalmol* 107:583-590, 1989.

Vaux C, Sheffield L, Keith CG, et al: Evidence that Rieger syndrome maps to 4q25 or 4q27, *J Med Genet* 29:256-258, 1992.

Wells KK, Pulido JS, Judisch GF, et al: Ophthalmic features of Alagille syndrome (arteriohepatic dysplasia), *J Pediatr Ophthalmol Strabismus* 30:130-135, 1993.

Glaucoma

This chapter covers the essential practical and theoretical points in congenital and juvenile glaucoma. Also reviewed are new advances in genetics and medical therapy. Glaucoma occurs in many ocular and systemic syndromes. The essential glaucoma-associated conditions with which every ophthalmologist should be familiar are presented in the last part of this chapter.

CONGENITAL GLAUCOMA

Clinical Features

Congenital or infantile glaucoma affects children in the first few years of life, causing the classic findings of buphthalmos (enlargement of the eye), corneal edema, corneal striae, and myopia. In the isolated, primary form of congenital glaucoma, characteristic abnormalities of the angle impair aqueous drainage and lead to the predictable sequelae of pressure elevation in the immature eye.

The incidence of congenital glaucoma in the United States is about 1:10,000 live births. Most cases appear to occur sporadically, but a certain percentage is likely inherited in an autosomal recessive manner. This is supported by the fact that in Saudi Arabia, where consanguineous pairings are relatively common, the estimated incidence is 1:2,500.

Congenital glaucoma may be evident at birth or develop soon thereafter. At least 60% of cases are diagnosed before 6 months of age and 80% by 1 year of age. Males are affected more often than females, at a 3 to 2 ratio, a finding that thus far has not been well explained. About 75% of patients have bilateral involvement, although the onset may be sequential rather than simultaneous. Severe cases will not pose a serious diagnostic challenge to the ophthalmologist. However, inexperienced clinicians may incorrectly diagnose conjunctivitis and delay correct diagnosis. Alternatively, mild cases, without the usual findings of tearing, photophobia, and corneal edema, may not come to attention until the child is somewhat older. Bilaterally symmetrical cases with buphthalmos may fail to be recognized because of the absence of a normal eye for comparison.

Box 7-1   Gonioscopic Findings in Primary Congenital Glaucoma

Flat insertion of peripheral iris
Anterior insertion of peripheral iris
  into TM
Absent or rudimentary scleral spur
Absence of a true angle recess
Iris processes (not a constant feature)

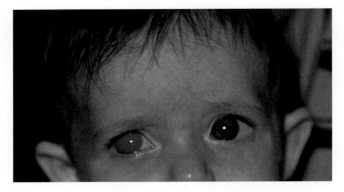

Fig. 7-1   Corneal edema in infantile glaucoma. See color plate.

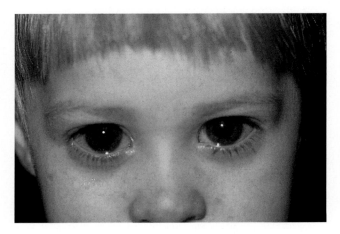

Fig. 7-2   Patient with congenital glaucoma who presented with epiphora, photophobia, and megalocornea. See color plate.

Knowledge of the anatomy and gonioscopic appearance of the angle in congenital glaucoma is essential. In congenital glaucoma, the peripheral iris is flat and inserts anteriorly, without a normal recess, into the trabecular meshwork. The scleral spur may be absent or rudimentary. Iris processes are often, but not always, present. Finally, a fine, glistening, wispy structure, covering the angle, may appear to be present. This is what has been referred to as *Barkan's membrane* (see the following discussion). The gonioscopic findings in primary congenital glaucoma are listed in Box 7-1.

The primitive drainage angle becomes visible at 12 to 15 weeks gestation. The trabecular meshwork is felt to be derived from neural crest tissue, and Schlemm's canal is believed to be derived from mesoderm. Beginning at about 15 weeks gestation, trabecular anlage form, with a separation of the anterior mesenchyme into corneoscleral and iridociliary regions, and a deepening of the angle recess. This is followed by further differentiation into ciliary muscles, the folding of the neural ectoderm into ciliary processes, and formation of Schlemm's canal. Then, according to Anderson, the ciliary body and iris root begin to migrate posteriorly, resulting from differential growth of these tissues. This exposes the trabecular meshwork and gives rise to the normal-appearing angle. In primary congenital glaucoma, this posterior migration fails to occur. In addition, the trabecular beams are thickened and compacted. The result is a decreased facility of aqueous outflow, increased intraocular pressure, and the spectrum of characteristic changes seen in congenital glaucoma.

The pathologic changes in congenital glaucoma are readily explained by the elasticity of the infant eye. However, it must be remembered that findings may be mild or develop later than expected. The infant globe, both sclera and cornea, is more elastic than the mature globe and becomes distended when subjected to excessive pressure. The buphthalmic eye is thinned and, therefore the sclera may appear blue because of the increased visibility of the uvea. In general, buphthalmos and megalocornea only occur in children younger than 3 years of age. Increased corneal diameter is a cardinal sign of congenital glaucoma. Normal term newborns' corneal diameters average 10 mm, and at 1 year, the normal corneal diameter is 11 mm. An adult-size cornea, 11.6 mm, is reached by 2 years of age. A corneal diameter of 12 mm or more at 1 year old is considered abnormal *(megalocornea)*. Progressive axial myopia may also occur in cases of elevated IOP before 3 years of age and sometimes in older children. Astigmatism and anisometropia are also common. Progressive corneal enlargement causes breaks in Descemet's membrane, with subsequent corneal edema resulting from aqueous influx (Fig. 7-1). Corneal clouding and bullous keratopathy lead to photophobia, blepharospasm, and tearing (Fig. 7-2).

Descemet's breaks in glaucoma are referred to as *Haab's striae* (Fig. 7-3). These occur because of the relative inelasticity of the membrane and appear as curvilinear, often horizontal, lines, which often can be seen without the aid of magnification because of their length and scrolled edges. In contrast, traumatic breaks in Descemet's membrane are more often linear and vertical. In such cases, the cornea is not enlarged, and other evidence of the trauma, such as eyelid ecchymoses and edema, is often present. Haab's striae and secondary

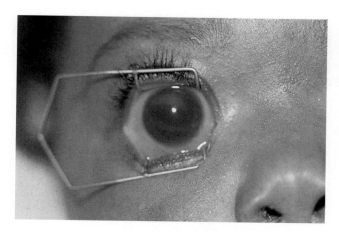

Fig. 7-3   Congenital glaucoma with Haab's striae and corneal stroma scarring. See color plate.

scarring may limit the visual acuity. Amblyopia is common in congenital glaucoma and is due to corneal opacity (edema and scarring), irregular astigmatism, anisometropia, and strabismus.

Knowledge of the optic nerve changes in congenital glaucoma is essential. Glaucomatous nerves usually show cupping, whereas nerves of normal infants seldom are cupped. The glaucomatous cups are central in the disc, round, deep, and surrounded by healthy-appearing neural tissue. Asymmetric optic nerve cupping should also raise the physician's suspicion for the presence of glaucoma. Since the lamina cribrosa, like the other structures of the immature globe, is elastic, part or all of the cupping may be caused by posterior bowing of the lamina. Hence, reducing the intraocular pressure, particularly in younger patients, often lessens the cupping. Also, keep in mind that not all cupping in childhood is glaucomatous. For example, children with periventricular leukomalacia often have a peculiar type of optic nerve hypoplasia characterized by normal-sized discs with large cups.

Advanced and uncontrolled cases of congenital glaucoma may cause keratitis and corneal scarring, lens subluxation resulting from stretched and broken zonules, and phthisis. In summary, the primary factors responsible for visual loss in congenital glaucoma are optic nerve damage, corneal opacities and irregularities, and amblyopia. Box 7-2 summarizes the main clinical findings in congenital glaucoma, and Box 7-3 lists the primary factors responsible for visual loss in congenital glaucoma.

Intraocular Pressure

A measurement of elevated intraocular pressure is only one aspect of the comprehensive evaluation of a patient with congenital glaucoma. Much has been written about intraocular pressure (IOP) measurement in babies with suspected glaucoma. It is true that in some (but not many), a good measurement can be made during sleep or feeding. Measurements can be attempted in crying patients, but elevated readings may be unreliable. Jaafar and Kazi advocate the use of oral chloral hydrate if sedation is required and the use of a dose of 100 mg/kg for the first 10 kg of body weight, plus an additional 50 mg/kg thereafter. This is a higher dose than recommended by the manufacturer but appears necessary to achieve the required level of sedation. Ketamine can elevate the IOP and is not appropriate for office use. Other general anesthetics will lower the IOP; thus the reading should be made as soon as possible after induction. The authors' preference is to use an instrument such as the Perkins tonometer, which we find most reliable, but many routinely use electronic devices such as the Tonopen. We no longer use the Schiøtz tonometer. Remember that normal IOPs of children younger than 3 to 4 years of age are significantly lower than IOPs of adults. For example, Pensiero, et al., found the average pressure to be 9.59 +/−2.3 mm Hg in newborns and 12.58 +/−1.46 mm Hg in children aged 2 to 3 years.

Treatment

For the most part, congenital glaucoma is a surgical disease. It is remarkable that cures can be obtained even with a single procedure. This is possible because the basic abnormality is a limited, localized dysgenesis of the

---

Box 7-4 Differential Diagnosis of the Common Signs in Congenital Glaucoma

ENLARGED GLOBE STRUCTURES

Axial myopia
Primary megalocornea (usually X-linked recessive)

CORNEAL FINDINGS

Sclerocornea
Congenital hereditary endothelial dystrophy—this
   is the most difficult to differentiate
Keratitis
Storage disease (mucopolysaccharidosis)
Cystinosis
Tyrosinemia
Birth trauma
Posterior polymorphous dystrophy

EPIPHORA

Nasolacrimal duct obstruction

Box 7-5 EUA for Suspected Congenital Glaucoma: Checklist

Scan quickly to check adnexa
Measure IOP
Measure corneal diameters
Slit-lamp examination: Haab's striae
Gonioscopy
Ophthalmoscopy with disc photo or drawing
Retinoscopy
Be prepared to perform surgery if necessary

Remember: A good magnified view of the optic nerve,
   even through small pupils, is possible by using the
   Koeppe lens and the direct ophthalmoscope.

---

superficial angle structures, and trabeculotomy and goniotomy both overcome this anatomic problem. Early surgery provides the best chance of favorable results, so once the diagnosis is confirmed, surgery should be performed expediently. If the diagnosis is uncertain, an examination under anesthesia (EUA) should be performed. The elements of an EUA for such a patient are listed in Box 7-5.

Short courses of pressure-lowering medications are useful in a number of ways. First, corneal clearing can be obtained before examination under anesthesia and surgery. Second, until surgery is performed, the lower pressures obtained with medicines lessen optic nerve damage. Finally, medications can be used following surgery for additional pressure lowering. Over the past approximately two decades, the most utilized medications have been timolol, $\frac{1}{4}$% given daily or twice per day, and acetazolamide. New classes of topical agents will certainly be of great use because of their efficacy and minimal side effects. We have found the topical carbonic anhydrase inhibitors, dorzolamide and brinzolamide, quite effective as a first agent or second agent. Also, prostaglandin analogues may be useful and can be administered once daily. Alpha-2 agonists (apraclonidine, brimonidine) can also be helpful as second line therapy.

The primary surgeries for congenital glaucoma are the goniotomy and trabeculotomy. Comparable results have been reported with these two operations, in the range of 75% to 90% success rate with one procedure. Although relatively safe, both of these surgeries require practice to master. As a second or third operation, trabeculectomy, or trabeculectomy combined with trabeculotomy, can be performed. Young patients tend to heal vigorously, but judicious use of antimetabolites can enhance the success rate in these cases.

The *goniotomy*, popularized by Barkan, was designed to incise and open the membrane that he believed covered the trabecular meshwork and prevented aqueous outflow (Fig. 7-4). Even though it has been established that a discrete membrane does not truly exist, the goniotomy remains an appropriate and effective procedure for this type of glaucoma. It requires a clear view of the angle structures. Following pupil constriction with pilocarpine, the eye is stabilized by an assistant. A pair of locking forceps can be used; we usually pass two perilimbal episcleral sutures across from one another and knot them. These provide a secure anchor for the forceps. The angle is visualized with a portable slit-lamp biomicroscope, or with surgical loupes, through a Koeppe-type lens. Excellent illumination is critical. We prefer to maintain the anterior chamber with viscoelastic, but some prefer an irrigating cannula. Through a flat, peripheral corneal stab incision, a goniotomy knife, MVR blade, or similar instrument is introduced 180° from the zone to be treated. The tip of the instrument is carefully advanced across the anterior chamber, and with a deliberate sweeping motion, about 100° of the anterior trabeculae is incised. Both visual and tactile cues are used to judge the correct amount of force to apply. An immediate deepening of the chamber in that region will occur, as the iris falls back to a more normal configuration. A small hyphema frequently results but resolves quickly and without detrimental effect. A suture may or may not be required to close the wound, and subconjunctival antibiotics are given. Complications are rare but include cataract, infection, and large hyphema.

The *trabeculotomy*, or *trabeculotomy ab externo*, is the surgery of choice when the angle structures are obscured from view because of corneal edema; although, as

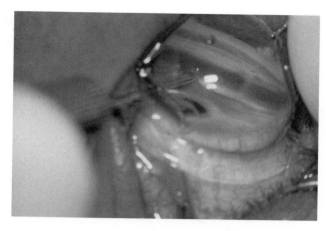

Fig. 7-4 Goniotomy as seen through a Koeppe lens. See color plate.

stated previously, this operation is preferred by some surgeons regardless of the state of the cornea. It creates a communication from the anterior chamber to Schlemm's canal by breaking through from the canal to the anterior chamber. The procedure begins with a limbus-based conjunctival flap to expose the sclera overlying Schlemm's canal. A partial-thickness scleral flap is fashioned, and in its bed, a deeper radial incision transecting Schlemm's canal is made. The canal is located and cannulated with the lower tine of the trabeculotome. Great care must be made so that a false passage is not created. The instrument is then twisted along the axis of the handle, and the tine tears into the anterior chamber. The process is repeated on the other side of the radial incision, the flap is sewn, and the conjunctiva is closed.

The greatest challenge in performing a trabeculotomy can be properly locating Schlemm's canal, particularly in buphthalmic eyes, in which the limbal structures are stretched and enlarged. Premature entry into the anterior chamber will collapse the canal and prevent it from being cannulated. Other complications include hyphema, Descemet's membrane detachment, iridodialysis, and infection.

Trabeculectomy is usually reserved as the third or sometimes second surgery in patients with prior unsuccessful goniotomies or trabeculotomies. Greater success rates in such cases are attributable to the prolonged use of topical corticosteroids, as well as antimetabolites, at the time of surgery. The use of glaucoma valves in uncontrolled cases has increased greatly in recent years. Another surgical option is the combined trabeculotomy-trabeculectomy. This procedure is effective as a first surgery for patients in high-risk ethnic groups, including those from the Middle East and India. Combined trabeculotomy-trabeculectomy may also be performed following failed initial goniotomies.

Anderson reviewed the prognostic factors in congenital glaucoma. The primary characteristic of the more favorable cases was an onset postnatally but before one year of age. Poor prognostic factors were the presence of associated ocular disease; hereditary cases; cases with marked buphthalmos; and cases with prior unsuccessful surgery.

JUVENILE GLAUCOMA

The term *juvenile glaucoma* refers to an open-angle glaucoma that develops from about 3 years of age to early adulthood. Its relatively late onset means gradual, insidious damage can occur before detection.

Linkage analysis of a number of pedigrees has shown a defect in the gene named GLC1A or myocilin on chromosome 1q21-q31. This gene previously was referred to as TIGR (trabecular meshwork induced glucocorticoid response). Mutations of this gene are thought to result in a gene product that hinders aqueous outflow. The affected members display remarkable phenotypic variability in age of onset, severity, and anatomy of the drainage angle. For example, most of the patients in the family from Panama described by Lichter were diagnosed by age 20, but one member was not diagnosed until age 43. Most of them had peak IOPs in their 40s or 50s but in one patient, the highest measured pressure was 23 mm Hg. Some had many iris processes, although others had normal-appearing angles. The commonly shared feature was a poor response to medical and laser treatment. No strong tendency towards myopia was found, but this has been reported in other families. A detailed family history should be obtained when a person in this age group is found to have open-angle glaucoma, and relatives should be screened.

OCULAR AND SYSTEMIC CONDITIONS ASSOCIATED WITH GLAUCOMA

This section covers the important and common ocular and systemic conditions in which glaucoma occurs. It is not intended to be inclusive, since many of these associations are uncommon or concern rare entities. Pediatric glaucoma with associations having known genetic loci are given in Box 7-6.

Aniridia

Glaucoma is common in aniridia but is usually not present at birth. Rather, progressive angle closure develops as the rudimentary iris stump occludes the angle, typically between ages 5 and 15 (Fig. 7-5). The degree of iris changes in aniridia varies, and glaucoma is more likely to develop in severely affected eyes. Satisfactory pressure control can sometimes be initially achieved with

Box 7-6	Conditions and Genetic Loci Associated with Pediatric Glaucoma	
Juvenile open-angle glaucoma	1q21-31
Aniridia	11p13
Posterior polymorphous dystrophy	20q11
Reiger's syndrome	4q25
Lowe syndrome	Xq24-26

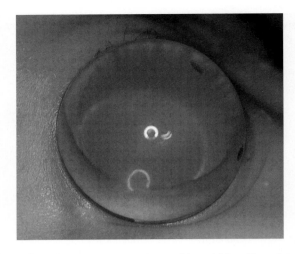

Fig. 7-5 Glaucoma in a patient with aniridia. The view is through a Koeppe lens. Note corneal clouding, ciliary processes, and lens equator.

topical medications, but surgery is eventually required in many patients. Goniotomy and trabeculotomy are often used as initial procedures, but may eventually fail. Trabeculectomy with mitomycin C or glaucoma valve placement may be required in many patients.

Axenfeld-Reiger Syndrome

Since Axenfeld-Reiger syndrome results from abnormal neural crest–derived structures, an association with glaucoma is not surprising (Fig. 7-6). It is present in about half or more of the cases, with a typical onset in childhood to early adulthood. Although the angle structures are abnormal, goniotomy has not proven to be an effective treatment. Instead, aqueous suppressants and trabeculectomy are preferred.

Peters' Anomaly

About 50% to 70% of patients with Peters' anomaly will develop glaucoma, with a usual onset in childhood. Control of the glaucoma before penetrating keratoplasty is desirable. Topical medicines should be tried first, followed by trabeculectomy if needed.

Posterior Polymorphous Dystrophy

Glaucoma occurs in about 13% of patients with posterior polymorphous dystrophy (PPMD), and both open- and closed-angle mechanisms occur. Open-angle glaucoma in PPMD is accompanied by an iris with a high insertion. In closed-angle cases, the drainage angle is covered by the abnormal endothelium characteristic of PPMD, with large, broad-based peripheral anterior synechiae and corectopia. Periodic examinations are required since elevated pressure may develop at any time.

Iridocorneal Endothelial Syndrome

The iridocorneal endothelial syndrome (ICE syndrome) encompasses four entities: essential iris atrophy, Chandler's syndrome, Cogan-Reese syndrome, and iris

nevus syndrome. These conditions are now understood to share the common basic defect of an abnormal corneal endothelium, which produces defective basement membrane. Glaucoma occurs in all varieties because of the drainage angle becoming covered by the abnormal basement membrane and by PAS. Corneal edema, particularly in Chandler's syndrome, may occur without elevated pressures because of deficient endothelial pumping. Some pressure control may be obtained with aqueous suppressants, but the angle closure will often necessitate filtering surgery. Late failure of filtration surgery is common, as a result of endothelialization of the bleb following growth of the membrane into the sclerostomy.

Congenital Ectropion Uveae (Congenital Ectropion of the Iris Pigment Epithelium)

Use of the term *ectropion uveae* to describe the condition in which the iris pigment epithelium turns onto the anterior iris surface, is no longer in favor, because it is now known that the iris pigment epithelium is not uveal tissue. The term *congenital ectropion of the iris pigment epithelium* is more precise. This condition is recognized by the presence of a smooth, pigmented iris surface, without crypts, involving the sphincter and extending to a variable degree to the iris periphery. This is a fairly rare condition, and is unilateral. Glaucoma is extremely common, since many affected eyes have high iris insertions and goniodysgenesis.

Persistent Hyperplastic Primary Vitreous

Secondary glaucoma is a frequent complication of persistent hyperplastic primary vitreous (PHPV), or, as Goldberg has suggested, *persistent fetal vasculature* (PFV).

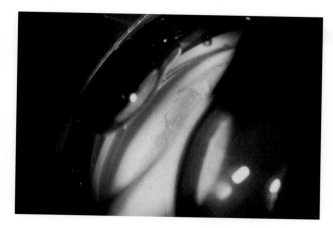

Fig. 7-6   Angle processes in Axenfeld-Rieger syndrome.

Progressive angle closure may result from lens swelling, anterior lens displacement resulting from inward drawn ciliary processes, recurrent hemorrhage, and uveitis. The decision as to whether or not to operate on these eyes must take into account the condition of the entire eye and its visual potential, but in certain instances, simply removing the lens will alleviate the glaucoma.

Retinopathy of Prematurity

Glaucoma has been estimated to occur in 30% of eyes with severe cicatricial ROP. Angle closure caused by contraction of a retrolental fibro-glial mass is the most common mechanism in infants and young children. Other possible causes of angle closure in these patients include inflammation and neovascularization. Additionally, the drainage angles may be developmentally abnormal.

Uveitis

As in adults, glaucoma commonly accompanies uveitis, and in children, the main entities are uveitis associated with juvenile rheumatoid arthritis, other HLA B-27 related iritides, sarcoidosis, and herpetic keratouveitis. The pathophysiologic mechanisms include synechial angle closure, secluded pupil with iris bombé, and neovascular glaucoma. These conditions are covered in Chapter 9.

Nevus of Ota

Nevus of Ota, or oculodermal melanocytosis, is characterized by increased pigmentation of the periocular skin, episclera, and uvea. It is most common in Asians. One study of Thai patients with nevus of Ota found elevated pressure in 10.3%; this included congenital glaucoma, ocular hypertension, open-angle glaucoma, and angle-closure glaucoma.

Ectopia Lentis

Ectopia lentis, whatever the cause, may cause pupillary block glaucoma. In children, the most common cause of ectopia lentis, excluding trauma, is *Marfan syndrome* (lens dislocation present in 80% of cases), but since the lens usually moves upward and out, pupillary block is uncommon. Ectopia lentis occurs in 90% of patients with homocystinuria. The lens tends to move downward, but in about one third of cases, complete dislocation into the anterior chamber or vitreous occurs. Glaucoma, usually a pupillary block mechanism, occurs in about one quarter of such patients. *Weill-Marchesani* syndrome (spherophakia-brachymorphia) is a rare condition in which patients have small, round lenses. Anterior subluxation is a common feature and pupillary block glaucoma occurs in approximately 80% of cases.

Aphakia and Pseudophakia

Chronic glaucoma following cataract extraction has, fortunately, become a smaller problem than it once was. Chrousos, et al, found that 6.1% of their 329 patients undergoing cataract extraction developed glaucoma, when followed for a mean of 5.5 years. Risk factors were leaving residual cortex, performing additional procedures to remove secondary membranes, and the presence of coexisting ocular disease. Almost all of the cases of glaucoma followed needle aspiration, but none came after lensectomy with the Ocutome. We advocate a bimanual technique utilizing a vitrectomy device in which the entire lens is removed before removal of the posterior capsule.

Neoplasms

The most common intraocular neoplasms causing glaucoma in children are medulloepithelioma, retinoblastoma, and juvenile xanthogranuloma. Glaucoma is present in one half of cases of medulloepithelioma at the time of diagnosis. It is also a common presenting sign in retinoblastoma, where forward angle displacement and neovascularization contribute to angle closure. Glaucoma in juvenile xanthogranuloma may occur secondary to spontaneous hyphema characteristic of this disorder.

Hyphemas and Ocular Trauma

Much of the material concerning ocular trauma and glaucoma in adults is applicable to children, but certain differences must be stressed. Most obvious of these is the difficulty obtaining accurate IOPs and performing gonioscopy in these patients. Acute pressure elevations in patients with sickle cell disease and trait can rapidly cause severe optic nerve damage. Furthermore, there is evidence that persons with sickle cell trait carry an increased risk of secondary hemorrhage. Thus the sickle cell status of black children with hyphemas should be determined. Finally, remember that since corneal blood staining can take months to resolve, aggressive actions may be required to avoid permanent loss of vision from amblyopia.

Osteogenesis Imperfecta

Osteogenesis imperfecta, which was classically described by the triad of brittle bones, deafness, and blue sclerae, occurs in about one in 20,000 live births. Open-angle glaucoma may also occur in this condition. Trabeculectomy in these patients may be complicated because of the thin sclera in this disease.

Neurofibromatosis I

Glaucoma is a common and important complication of neurofibromatosis type I, occurring in 50% of cases with an ipsilateral orbital or eyelid neurofibroma (Fig. 7-7). The glaucoma may have its onset in infancy, causing congenital glaucoma with buphthalmos, or it may develop later. Thus patients with orbital neurofibromas must be monitored at regular intervals for life. The causes of glaucoma in NF I include developmentally abnormal drainage angles and angle closure resulting from ciliary body and choroidal neurofibromas. Treatment is individualized, depending on the mechanism.

Sturge-Weber Syndrome

In Sturge-Weber syndrome, intraocular, as well as extraocular, factors probably contribute to the development of glaucoma. Overall, about one third of patients with Sturge-Weber syndrome have increased intraocular pressure; most of these have ipsilateral eyelid, tarsal, and conjunctival involvement (Figs. 7-8 and 7-9). Developmental chamber angle abnormalities, as well as episcleral hemangiomas causing raised episcleral venous pressure, are both cited. In addition, retinal detachment from the intraocular hemangioma may lead to glaucoma. The clinician must remember that in an eye harboring a choroidal hemangioma, intraocular surgery produces a significant risk of choroidal hemorrhage or effusion. Preoperative pressure lowering and creating posterior sclerotomies may reduce these complications.

Glaucoma occasionally occurs in the Klippel-Trénaunay-Weber Syndrome, a sporadic phakomatosis syndrome consisting of large cutaneous port-wine lesions, varicose veins, and soft tissue and bony hypertrophy. Glaucoma is uncommon in von Hippel-Lindau disease, tuberous sclerosis, and Wyburn-Mason's syndrome.

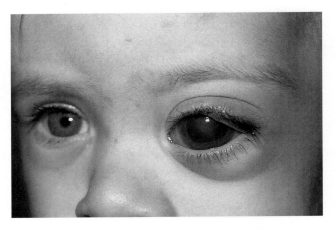

Fig. 7-7   Buphthalmos in a child with neurofibromatosis. An orbital neurofibroma was present.

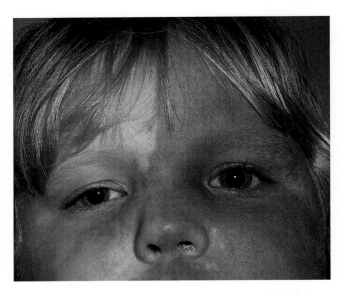

Fig. 7-8   Unilateral glaucoma in a patient with Sturge-Weber syndrome. Note the enlarged size of the left cornea. See color plate.

Congenital Cataracts

Lowe syndrome and *congenital rubella* are the two important conditions in which glaucoma and cataracts may coexist. In Lowe syndrome (oculocerebrorenal syndrome), small lenses with discoid cataracts, congenital glaucoma, and small pupils are typical. The patients have frontal bossing and chubby cheeks. Renal tubular dysfunction leads to metabolic acidosis, secondary hyperparathyroidism, secondary hypophosphatemia, and rickets.

In congenital rubella, cataracts are present in about 30% of patients, and glaucoma is present in about 9% of patients. Thus most babies with congenital rubella do

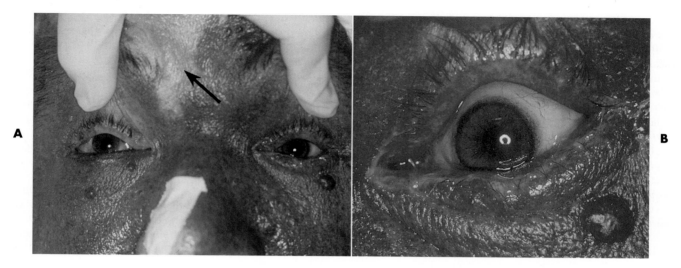

Fig. 7-9   Sturge-Weber syndrome. **A,** This young man has bilateral port wine stains. The *arrow* indicates a region of normal skin. **B,** Magnified view of the same patient's glaucomatous left eye, demonstrating dilated episcleral vessels. See color plate. (Courtesy of Dr. Peter Netland.)

◀ MAJOR POINTS ▶

Congenital glaucoma is bilateral in about 75% of cases.

Eighty percent of cases of congenital glaucoma present by 1 year of age.

The primary causes of visual loss in congenital glaucoma are optic nerve damage, corneal opacity, and amblyopia.

Goniotomy and trabeculotomy both are effective for congenital glaucoma, but the trabeculotomy is preferred when the view of the angle is impaired.

Cases of congenital glaucoma with onset between the immediate postnatal period and 1 year of age have the best prognosis.

A gene responsible for open-angle juvenile glaucoma has been identified on chromosome one.

The glaucoma associated with aniridia is often an angle-closure type that usually occurs in childhood.

In PPMD, periodic examinations are needed because glaucoma can develop anytime during the patient's life.

In patients with nevus of Ota, elevated IOPs and glaucoma are significantly more common than uveal melanomas.

Ectopia lentis frequently causes a pupillary block glaucoma.

In NF I, glaucoma is seen in half of the patients with ipsilateral orbital or eyelid involvement.

Elevated episcleral venous pressures, as well as abnormal aqueous drainage angles, probably contribute to the glaucoma seen in Sturge-Weber syndrome.

not have both cataracts and glaucoma, but rubella should be considered in such cases. However, new cases of rubella have become quite infrequent. The glaucoma may result from inflammation, anomalous drainage angles, or pupillary block. Additional findings of congenital rubella include microphthalmos and retinopathy.

Arthrogryposis Multiplex Congenita

Arthrogryposis multiplex congenita is a heterogeneous congenital condition characterized by multiple joint contractures and skeletal deformities. Rarely, glaucoma may be present, and both congenital and juvenile-onset types have been described.

SUGGESTED READINGS

Anderson DR: Trabeculotomy compared to goniotomy for glaucoma in children, *Ophthalmol* 90:805-806, 1983.

Biglan AW, Hiles DA: The visual results following infantile glaucoma surgery, *J Pediatr Ophthalmol Strabismus* 16:377-381, 1979.

Chrousos GA, Parks MM, O'Neill JF: Incidence of chronic glaucoma, retinal detachment and secondary membrane surgery in pediatric aphakic patients, *Ophthalmology* 91:1238-1241, 1984.

Cibis GW, Tripathi RC, Tripathi BJ: Glaucoma in Sturge-Weber syndrome, *Ophthalmology* 91:1061-1071, 1984.

Debnath SC, Teichmann KD, Salamah K: Trabeculectomy versus trabeculotomy in congenital glaucoma, *Br J Ophthalmol* 73:608-611, 1989.

DeLuise VP, Anderson DR, Primary infantile glaucoma (congenital glaucoma), *Surv Ophthalmol* 28:1-19, 1983.

Hoskins Jr HD, Shaffer RN, Hetherington J: Anatomical classification of the developmental glaucomas, *Arch Ophthalmol* 102:1331-1336, 1984.

Jaafar MS, Kazi GA: Effect of oral chloral hydrate sedation on the intraocular pressure measurement, *J Pediatr Ophthalmol Strabismus* 30:372-376, 1993.

Lichter PR, Richards JE, Boehnke M, et al: Juvenile glaucoma linked to GLC1A in a Panamanian family, *Trans Am Ophthamol Soc* XCIV:335-346, 1996.

Mandal AK, Naduvilath TJ, Jayagandan A: Surgical results of combined trabeculotomy-trabeculectomy for developmental glaucoma, *Ophthalmology* 105:974-982, 1998.

Morin JD, Bryars JH: Causes of loss of vision in congenital glaucoma, *Arch Ophthalmol* 98:1575-1576, 1980.

Nasrullah A, Kerr NC: Sickle cell trait as a risk factor for secondary hemorrhage in children with traumatic hyphema, *Am J Ophthalmol* 123:783-790, 1997.

Netland PA, Wiggs JL, Dreyer EB: Inheritance of glaucoma and genetic counseling of glaucoma patients, *Int Ophthalmol Clin* 33:101-120, 1993.

Pensiero S, Da Pozzo S, Perissutti P, et al: Normal intraocular pressure in children, *J Pediatr Ophthalmol Strabismus* 29: 79-84, 1992.

Richards JE, Lichter PR, Boehnke M, et al: Mapping of a gene for autosomal dominant juvenile-onset open-angle glaucoma to chromosome 1q, *Am J Hum Genet* 54:62-70, 1994.

Schottenstein EM: Peters' anomaly. In Ritch R, Shields MB, Krupin T, editors: *The glaucomas,* ed 2, St Louis, 1996, Mosby.

Seidman, DJ, Nelson LB, Calhoun JH, et al: Signs and symptoms in the presentation of primary infantile glaucoma, *Pediatrics* 77:399-404, 1986.

Sheffield VC, Stone EM, Alward WLM, et al: Genetic linkage of familial open angle glaucoma to chromosome 1q21-q31, *Nat Genet* 4:47-50, 1993.

Shields, MB: Axenfeld-Rieger syndrome: a theory of mechanism and distinctions from the iridocorneal endothelial syndrome, *Trans Am Ophthalmol Soc* LXXXI; 736-784, 1983.

Teekhasaenee C, Ritch R, Rutnin U, et al: Glaucoma in oculodermal melanocytosis, *Ophthalmology* 97:562-570, 1990.

Wiggins Jr RE, Tomey KF: The results of glaucoma surgery in Aniridia, *Arch Ophthalmol* 110:503-505, 1992.

Lens Abnormalities

Lens abnormalities covered in this chapter include lens opacities (cataracts), abnormal lens position, and spherophakia. Despite dramatic improvements in the treatment of infantile cataracts, cataracts continue to be a major cause of decreased vision and blindness in children. By far, the most common cause of a poor visual results after pediatric cataract surgery is irreversible amblyopia. The clinician should be aware of the systemic implications of pediatric cataracts and sublux lenses, since these ocular disorders may be the first presenting sign of important systemic diseases.

PEDIATRIC CATARACTS

Lens Anatomy

An understanding of lens anatomy is necessary to properly classify and describe pediatric cataracts. The crystalline lens consists of a nucleus (embryonic and fetal) and the lens cortex (Fig. 8-1). Embryologically, the *embryonic nucleus* develops first reaching completion by approximately 6 weeks gestation. It is made up of primary lens fibers that come from primitive posterior lens epithelium. On clinical examination, the embryonic nucleus is the central slightly dark core of the lens that is inside the Y sutures. Just peripheral to the embryonic nucleus is the fetal nucleus. The *fetal nucleus* develops from secondary lens fibers from the equatorial anterior epithelial cells. These secondary lens fibers stretch anteriorly and posteriorly around the embryonic nucleus and join to form the anterior and posterior Y sutures. The Y sutures are an important landmark because they identify the extent of the fetal nucleus. Lens material peripheral to the Y sutures is lens cortex, whereas lens material within and including the Y sutures is nuclear. At the slit lamp, the anterior Y suture is oriented up right, and the posterior Y suture is inverted. At birth the fetal and embryonic nuclei make up most of the lens volume. Most of the cortical fibers are produced postnatally from continued metamorphoses of anterior lens epithelium into cortical lens fibers.

The adult lens (over age 35 years) is relatively stiff because of progressive mineralization of the nucleus and cortex. The pediatric lens, however, is soft and pliable. This flexibility allows for a large amplitude of accommodation in children. The soft lens allows for surgical removal by vitrectomy instrumentation, without the need for nuclear delivery or phacoemulsification. Another difference between pediatric and adult cataracts is the pres-

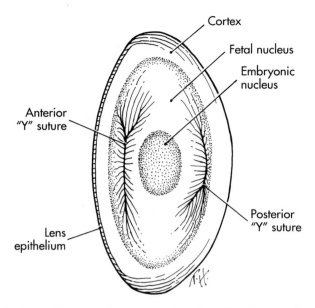

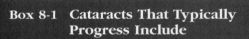

Fig. 8-1   Drawing of a cross-section through a juvenile lens. Note the lens nucleus is that area within the Y sutures. The anterior Y suture is upright while the posterior Y suture is inverted.

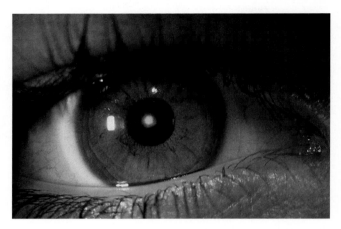

Fig. 8-2   Photograph of anterior polar cataract that is approximately 1.5 mm in diameter, involving the central aspect of the anterior capsule. At the slit lamp, this opacity appears as a fibrosis and scarring of the anterior capsule. This small opacity did not significantly interfere with vision, since visual acuity was 20/25.

Box 8-1   Cataracts That Typically Progress Include

Posterior lenticonus
Persistent hyperplastic primary vitreous (PHPV)
Lamellar
Anterior and posterior subcapsular

---

ence of an attachment between the posterior lens capsule and the anterior vitreous face, called *Wieger's capsulohyaloid ligament.* The capsulohyaloidal ligament represents a remnant of the primary vitreous and provides an attachment between the lens and vitreous. This ligament is why surgical removal of the intact lens by intracapsular lens extraction results in vitreous loss and is dangerous in children and young adults. The capsulohyaloidal ligament dissipates with time and is gone by approximately 40 years of age.

Morphologic Classification of Infantile Cataracts

Documenting the location and morphologic characteristics of a cataract can provide information about the specific type of the cataract, including the onset and the visual prognosis. Making the diagnosis of a specific type of can be difficult. Spread of a cataract to involve multi-

ple lens layers can mask the original location and morphology of the opacity. Cataracts that typically progress are listed in (Box 8-1). Anterior polar and nuclear cataracts tend to be static; however, even these cataracts can occasionally progress. Descriptions of pediatric cataracts should include the location, color, density, shape, and confluence of the opacity. The specific types of cataracts listed in the following discussion are classified according to their morphologic appearance and location.

Anterior Cataracts

Anterior polar cataract   An anterior polar cataract is a small, discrete, white opacity usually less than 3 mm in diameter located on the center of the anterior capsule (Fig. 8-2). They are derived from abnormal separation of the lens vesicle from surface ectoderm during embryonic lens development. One third of anterior polar cataracts are bilateral. The term *anterior polar* refers to the position of the opacity at the anterior pole of the lens. *Persistent pupillary membranes* or iris strands may connect to anterior polar cataracts. Rarely, large areas of the iris can attach to the opacity. The author has managed a rare case where the entire iris was adhered to the anterior polar cataract causing pupillary block glaucoma and iris bombé. Jaafar and Robb found that one third of patients with anterior polar cataracts will have either strabismus, refractive anisometropia, or amblyopia. Close follow-up of patients with anterior polar cataracts is indicated because the opacity may rarely progress.

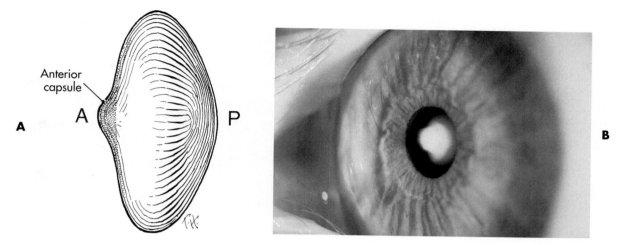

Fig. 8-3 **A,** Drawing of anterior pyramidal cataract. This is a type of anterior polar cataract where the anterior capsule fibrosis forms a pyramid or nipple. **B,** Slit-lamp photograph of anterior pyramidal cataract. Note the white opacity actually protrudes through the pupil into the anterior chamber. The base of the lens opacity was larger than 3 mm and visual acuity was impaired.

Despite these admonitions, anterior polar cataracts are for the most part nonprogressive, usually not visually significant, and in the majority of cases, they can be managed conservatively, without surgery. Anterior polar cataracts occur sporadically in 90% of cases, with less than 10% transmitted in an autosomal dominant fashion.

Anterior pyramidal cataract This is a type of anterior polar cataract that is white, conical in shape, with the apex of the cone projecting into the anterior chamber (Fig. 8-3). The cone is usually 2 to 2.5 mm in diameter, and the base of the cone may be surrounded by cortical opacities. The conical opacity by itself is usually not sufficient to disrupt visual development; however, the surrounding cortical changes can progress, and some cases will require surgery. When operating on these cataracts the surgeon will find the cone opacity to be fibrotic and difficult to fragment and cut with mechanical vitrectomy devices. It may be necessary to deliver the fibrotic cone through a corneal incision. These opacities are usually bilateral, occur sporadically, and are not associated with a specific systemic disease.

Anterior subcapsular cataract This opacity lies immediately beneath the anterior capsule in the anterior lens cortex. Anterior subcapsular cataracts are often idiopathic; however, the clinician must consider the possibility of trauma-induced lens changes or *Alport's syndrome* (hereditary nephritis with hematuria and deafness). Lens changes associated with Alport's syndrome include bilateral anterior subcapsular cataracts and bilateral anterior lenticonus. *Anterior lenticonus* is a thinning and anterior bowing of the anterior capsule. Anterior subcapsular cataracts are usually acquired after birth.

Central Cataracts

When evaluating a cataract located in the central aspect of the lens, it is important to distinguish between an opacity that surrounds the nucleus (cortical lamellar), versus one that truly involves the nucleus (nuclear). The key observation is whether or not the lens material within the Y sutures is involved. Opacities inside and including the Y sutures are nuclear, whereas cataracts peripheral to the Y sutures are cortical.

Nuclear cataract This is an opacity located within the embryonic or fetal nucleus (Fig. 8-4). In general, the presence of a nuclear cataract indicates a congenital onset. Nuclear cataracts tend to be nonprogressive, but can progress to involve adjacent cortical layers. Nuclear cataracts may be unilateral or bilateral, with bilateral cases often associated with autosomal dominant inheritance. Visually significant nuclear cataracts must be operated on early, within the first few weeks of life, to obtain best visual results.

Sutural cataract Sutural cataracts are a type of congenital nuclear cataract with the opacity concentrated along the Y sutures in the area of the fetal nucleus (Figs. 8-5 and 8-6). Sutural cataracts may be progressive and expand into the cortex and central embryonic nucleus. Bilateral sutural cataracts are often associated with an autosomal dominant inheritance pattern, but X-linked recessive cases have also been described.

Lamellar cataract (zonular cataract) This is a whitish cortical opacity that surrounds the lens nucleus, just outside the Y sutures (Fig. 8-7). The cataract develops in layers like an onionskin, with clear zones alternating with white cortical lamella. Because there are zones of

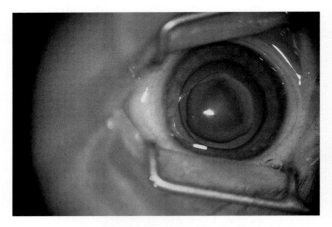

Fig. 8-4   Nuclear cataract in a four-day-old infant. The central opacity involves the nucleus between the Y sutures. See color plate.

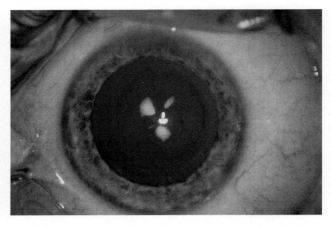

Fig. 8-6   Four year old with bilateral sutural cataracts. Preoperatively visual acuity was 20/80 each eye and postoperatively visual acuity improved to 20/30. Note the white calcific opacities along the Y suture.

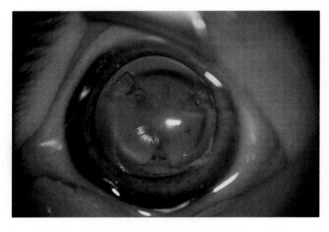

Fig. 8-5   One-week-old infant with sutural cataract. Note that the opacity is within the nucleus and follows the Y sutures. The anterior Y suture is oriented in an upright position. See color plate.

clear and opacified lens cortex, these cataracts are often referred to as *zonular cataracts* since they occupy specific zones. In addition to the circumferential lamellar opacities, spoke-like radial opacities termed *cortical riders* often coexist (see Fig. 8-7, *B*). Lamellar cataracts are developmental with their onset after 4 to 6 months of age. Most lamellar cataracts are progressive and eventually require surgery. Since the lens is relatively clear during the critical period of visual development, lamellar cataracts generally have a good visual prognosis even when surgery is performed in late childhood. The best visual results, however, are obtained by early surgery as soon as the opacity is visually significant. Lamellar cataracts are common, and can be unilateral or bilateral, with bilateral lamellar cataracts frequently inherited as an autosomal dominant trait. Metabolic diseases such as neonatal hypoglycemia and galactosemia can cause bilateral lamellar cataracts.

Posterior Cataracts

Posterior lenticonus and persistent hyperplastic primary vitreous (PHPV) are the two most common causes of a posterior unilateral lens opacity in childhood.

Posterior lenticonus   Posterior lenticonus is a congenital thinning of part of the posterior capsule with posterior bowing of the thinned capsule (Fig. 8-8). In early infancy the lens cortex is relatively clear, but the abnormality of the posterior capsule will distort the light reflex. With time, the posterior cortex becomes opacified, progressing into a posterior subcapsular cataract. Posterior lenticonus is almost always unilateral; it occurs sporadically and often requires surgery. The posterior bowing of the lens capsule may cause myopia and irregular lenticular astigmatism. It is important to monitor visual function in these patients since significant amblyopia can occur even when the lens appears relatively clear. The visual prognosis for posterior lenticonus is generally good even when surgery is performed after the critical period of visual development.

Persistent hyperplastic primary vitreous   Persistent hyperplastic primary vitreous is a disorder related to the persistence and secondary fibrosis of the primitive hyaloid vascular system. A fibrovascular stalk emanates from the optic disc to join the posterior lens capsule (Fig. 8-9, *A*). At the posterior capsule, the stalk fans out to form a white fibrovascular membrane that covers the posterior lens (Fig. 8-9, *B*). This fibrovascular membrane may be quite small, only a few millimeters in diameter (see Mittendorf's dot in the following discussion), or it can extend from the center of the posterior lens capsule to the ciliary processes. If the fibrovascular membrane extends to the ciliary processes, the membrane will produce circumferential traction and pull the ciliary processes towards the center of the pupil (Fig.

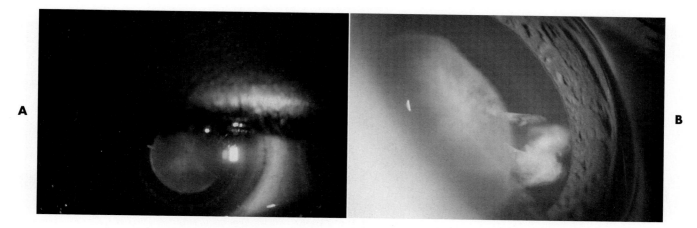

Fig. 8-7   **A,** Ten year old with bilateral lamellar cataracts. At first glance, the opacity appears to be nuclear; however, at slit-lamp examination the opacity surrounds the Y suture. Note the cortical rider or spoke-like opacities just peripheral to the central opacity. **B,** High-magnification slit-lamp photograph of patient with lamellar cataract and cortical riders or spoke opacities. Note the riders or spoked opacities are just peripheral to the central lamellar cataracts. See color plate.

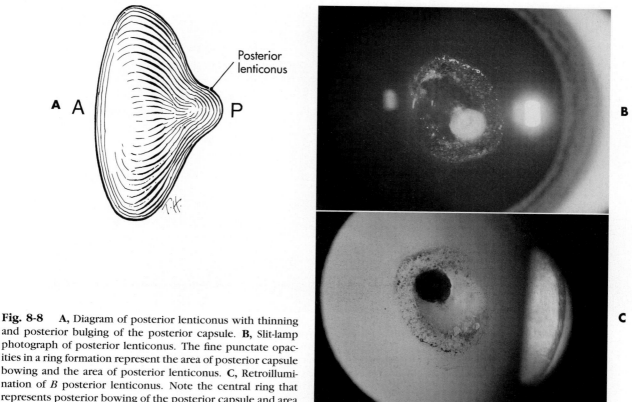

Fig. 8-8   **A,** Diagram of posterior lenticonus with thinning and posterior bulging of the posterior capsule. **B,** Slit-lamp photograph of posterior lenticonus. The fine punctate opacities in a ring formation represent the area of posterior capsule bowing and the area of posterior lenticonus. **C,** Retroillumination of *B* posterior lenticonus. Note the central ring that represents posterior bowing of the posterior capsule and area of posterior lenticonus.

8-9, *C*). Over time the membrane contracts, which pushes the lens iris diaphragm anteriorly, thus shallowing the anterior chamber. If left untreated, angle-closure glaucoma results and eventually over several years the eye will be lost. Recent advancements in surgical techniques have improved the prognosis of PHPV. Intraocular microscissors, intraocular cautery, and vitrectomy instrumentation allow for safe removal of the lens and posterior vascular membrane (Fig. 8-9, *C* and *D*). Optimal treatment is early surgery; however, the visual prognosis is relatively good even when surgery is performed after the critical period of visual development as long as the

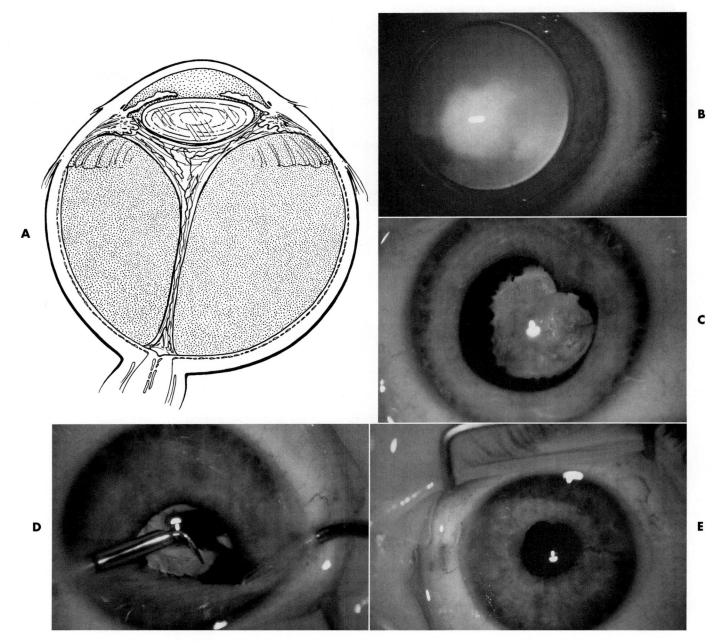

Fig. 8-9   **A,** Drawing showing typical persistent hyperplastic primary vitreous (PHPV) with a fibrovascular stalk emanating from the optic nerve towards the ciliary processes and posterior capsule of the lens. The fibrovascular membrane contracts with time and pulls the ciliary processes centrally, thus pushing the lens iris diaphragm anteriorly, shallowing the anterior chamber. **B,** Photograph of persistent hyperplastic primary vitreous. The central white opacity is a fibrovascular membrane involving the posterior capsule. There is a dark shadow at the 8 o'clock position (inferior nasal) that represents a fibrovascular stalk from the optic nerve to the posterior capsule. **C,** Severe persistent hyperplastic primary vitreous with the posterior fibrovascular membrane pulling the ciliary processes to the center of the pupil. The black pigmented tissue within the pupillary border represents the ciliary processes. Note that the fibrovascular membrane is pinkish in color since there are vessels within the membrane. **D,** Removal of the PHPV membrane requires microsurgical technique using intraocular scissors to segment the fibrovascular membrane, then the membrane is subsequently removed with vitrectomy instrumentation. Intraocular cautery is necessary to provide hemostasis. **E,** Postoperative photograph after removal of PHPV fibrovascular membrane, having used the limbal approach. Note the feeder vessel at the 3 o'clock position was cauterized. See color plate. (Surgery by Dr. Kenneth Wright.)

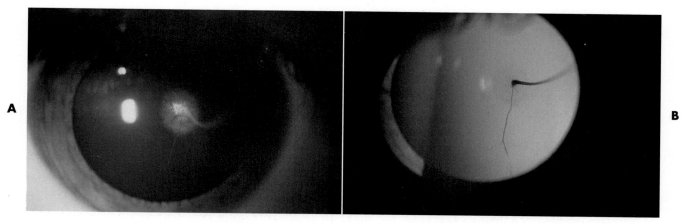

Fig. 8-10   **A,** Slit-lamp photograph of Mittendorf's dot with stalk that emanates from the optic nerve to the lens. **B,** Retroillumination of *A* showing thin fibrovascular stalk that emanates from the optic nerve and connects to the posterior capsule. Note the small vessel coming off the stalk inferiorly.

retina and posterior pole is normal. Karr and Scott reported a patient who underwent surgery at 10 months of age yet achieved 20/50 visual acuity. The authors concur because we reported 4 out of 5 patients with PHPV operated after 10 months obtained vision of 20/60 or better. These good results are probably because even though PHPV is congenital, it is progressive. The opacity may be partial during the first few months of life, which allows visual development to occur. PHPV can be associated with tractional macular detachments and in these instances the visual prognosis is poor. PHPV occurs sporadically, is almost always unilateral, and is typically associated with a small cornea or microphthalmus.

Mittendorf's dot   This is a small congenital white opacity on the posterior capsule, just nasal to the central visual axis (Fig. 8-10, *A*). A small remnant of the hyaloid artery may extend from the optic nerve to the opacity (Fig. 8-10, *B*). Mittendorf's dot occurs sporadically and is found in approximately 2% of normal individuals. Mittendorf's dot with hyaloid artery remnant may represent a very mild form of PHPV. Unlike PHPV, Mittendorf's dot is not progressive and does not interfere with vision.

Posterior subcapsular cataract   This is a cortical opacity just anterior to the posterior capsule. These cataracts are almost always developmental, occurring after birth. Posterior subcapsular cataracts can be associated with Down syndrome, chronic steroid use, blunt trauma, or they may be idiopathic. The most common cause of a unilateral posterior subcapsular cataract in childhood is posterior lenticonus (see the previous discussion). Because of the posterior location, close to the optical nodal point of the eye, posterior subcapsular cataracts tend to be visually significant and often require surgery.

Oil-drop cataract   This is a faint opacity in the central aspect of the posterior lens cortex. On retroillumination this opacity resembles an oil droplet (Fig. 8-11). Oil-drop cataracts have been classically described in association with *galactosemia*. If galactosemia is diagnosed early, dietary restriction of galactose can result in clearing of the cataract.

Diffuse Cataracts

Christmas tree cataract   The Christmas tree cataract has multiple small flecks that, when light is reflected, give the appearance of various colors from the central aspect of the cortex (Fig. 8-12). These cataracts can be associated with myotonic dystrophy, pseudohypoparathyroidism, and hypoparathyroidism.

Cerulean (blue-dot) cataract   These are small, scattered bluish-white opacities throughout the lens cortex (Fig. 8-13). They can be seen with Down syndrome, they can occur during puberty, and they probably represent late-formed cortical fibers that have broken down into granular debris. These opacities lie in the cortex peripheral to the nucleus. They are bilateral, usually nonprogressive, and generally cause minimal visual loss.

Total cataract   Total cataract is an opacity that involves the entire lens so that the inner layers of the lens cannot be visualized. Total cataracts can be associated with Down syndrome, metabolic disorders, autosomal dominant hereditary cataracts, and trauma.

Membranous cataract   This is an end-stage cataract where the lens material has been absorbed and the anterior and posterior capsules are in apposition. Membranous cataracts can be associated with trauma, intrauterine infections (TORCH), or be secondary to anomalous lens development.

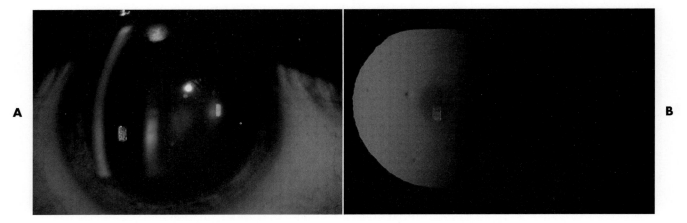

Fig. 8-11   **A,** Slit-lamp photograph of patient with galactosemia and oil-drop cataract. **B,** Retroillumination photograph of *A* showing central oil-drop cataract associated with galactosemia. See color plate.

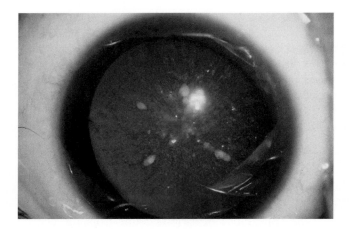

Fig. 8-12   "Christmas tree" cataract with multiple small flecks that reflect multiple colors at the slit lamp. See color plate.

Etiology of Pediatric Cataracts

When considering the etiology of congenital or infantile cataracts, it is helpful to make the distinction between unilateral and bilateral involvement. Box 8-2 contrasts the etiologies of unilateral versus bilateral pediatric cataracts.

Bilateral congenital cataracts   In contrast to unilateral cataracts, bilateral cataracts are often inherited, and may be associated with a systemic disease. The list of associated systemic diseases is long and includes the diseases listed in Box 8-2. Bilateral congenital or infantile cataracts have an identifiable cause or are hereditary in approximately 60% to 70% of cases.

Unilateral congenital cataracts   Most unilateral congenital cataracts are caused by local dysgenesis and, as a rule, are not associated with a systemic disease and are not inherited. Most unilateral pediatric cataracts are of unknown etiology. Box 8-2 lists the types of cataracts associated with ocular dysgenesis. The dysgenesis is not isolated to the lens since unilateral cataracts are often associated with an ipsilateral small cornea. The presence of a unilateral cataract does not rule out the possibility of an associated systemic disease, since diseases such as congenital rubella syndrome can cause unilateral cataracts.

Specific Etiologies

Some of the more common syndromes associated with pediatric cataracts are covered in the following discussion.

Hereditary cataracts   *Autosomal dominant* inheritance pattern is the most common identifiable cause of bilateral infantile cataracts. Approximately 25% of these cases represent a new autosomal dominant mutation. A slit-lamp examination should be performed on the parents of affected children since variable expressivity is a characteristic of autosomal dominantly inherited cataracts. *Autosomal recessive* cataracts are uncommon, and when they occur are often associated with a history of consanguinity. *X-linked* cataracts are rare.

Prematurity   *Transient opacities* have been noted in premature children. They are usually bilateral and appear as vacuoles along the posterior lens suture, but they rarely persist.

Intrauterine infection   Maternally transmitted *intrauterine infections* may result in cataracts. The most common of which may be remembered by the acronym TORCHS, standing for *T*oxoplasmosis, *R*ubella, *C*ytomegalic inclusion disease, *H*erpes simplex, and *S*yphilis. Of these, rubella is most commonly associated with congenital cataracts. The cataracts associated with intrauterine infections are usually dense central opacities and are usually bilateral; however, they may be unilateral. A history of a maternal illness during the pregnancy with a

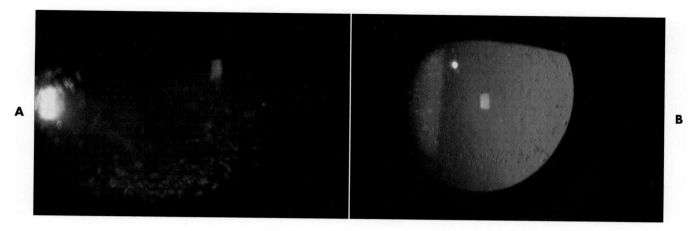

Fig. 8-13 **A,** Cerulean cataract with multiple small cortical opacities with clear zones between the opacities. **B,** Retroillumination of *A* showing multiple fine opacities and relatively clear cortex between the opacities. Visual acuity in this patient was 20/20. See color plate.

rash and fever is suggestive. Elevated infant IgM antibodies against rubella, or serial assays showing increasing IgG titer is indicative of an intrauterine infection.

Rubella cataracts are due to the invasion of the lens by the rubella virus. Rubella cataracts may present with a hazy cornea caused by congenital glaucoma or a keratitis. Wolff found approximately 15% of patients with rubella syndrome had cataracts, with 20% being unilateral (Fig. 8-14). Rubella keratitis will spontaneously resolve in 1 to 2 weeks. Ocular findings include retinopathy (25%), strabismus (20%), microphthalmus (15%), optic atrophy (10%), corneal haze (10%), glaucoma (10%), and phthisis bulbi (2%). Systemic effects include congenital heart defects, hearing loss, and mental retardation. Postoperatively, these eyes are prone to extreme inflammation. The key to good results is complete removal of all lens material and postoperative treatment with topical steroids and mydriatics.

Chromosomal syndromes   There are a number of *chromosomal syndromes* associated with congenital cataracts. These include Down syndrome (trisomy 21), Patau's syndrome (trisomy 13), and Edward's syndrome (trisomy 18).

In *Down syndrome,* the cataract can be present at birth or it can manifest itself in the first years of life. The opacities can be sutural, zonular, or complete. Slit-lamp examination may also reveal Brushfield spots and peripheral iris hypoplasia. For a description of the ocular findings associated with Down syndrome, see Chapter 11.

Patau's syndrome (trisomy 13) is a chromosomal anomaly that profoundly affects development of facial and ocular structures. There is a high incidence of cleft lip and palate, hypotonia, and low birth weight. Ocular findings are listed in Box 8-3. Intraocular cartilage and optic nerve hypoplasia can also been associated with Patau's syndrome.

Trisomy 18 (Edward's syndrome) is associated with microcephaly, micrognathia, low set ears, flexion deformities of the fingers, and club feet and is most common in females. Ocular findings are listed in Box 8-4. They are usually related to the lids and orbits. Other ocular anomalies include corneal opacities, uveal colobomas, microphthalmia, and cataracts.

Metabolic disease   The metabolic causes of pediatric cataracts constitute a diverse group of errors in metabolism. Metabolic disorders usually do not result in truly congenital cataracts since metabolic cataracts develop postnatally.

Galactosemia is a rare cause of congenital cataracts, but should be considered in infants and children who present with unexplained bilateral cataracts. Galactosemia may be caused by a defect of one of three enzymes: galactokinase, galactose-1-phosphate uridyl transferase or uridine diphosphate galactose-epimerase. The disease is inherited as an autosomal recessive trait. The classical early cataract is an oil droplet (see Fig. 8-11), but they can progress to diffuse and lamellar cataracts (Fig. 8-15). The severe form of galactosemia is galactose-1-phosphate uridyl transferase deficiency. Transferase deficiency galactosemia affects multiple organs including the central nervous system, liver, kidney and the lens. It often presents like neonatal sepsis with vomiting, diarrhea, hepatomegaly, jaundice, and lethargy. Patients with galactosemia secondary to galactokinase deficiency present in later childhood usually with cataracts and few systemic signs. Epimerase deficiency galactosemia is a very mild form of the disease, not typically associated with cataracts and there are minimal significant systemic manifestations.

Transferase galactosemic cataracts usually appear during the first few months of life with the onset dependent on the severity of the disease. Removal of milk from the

Box 8-2   Causes of Infantile Cataracts

BILATERAL CATARACTS

1. Idiopathic (60%)
2. Hereditary cataracts (30%), without systemic disease*
    a. Autosomal dominant (most common inheritance pattern)
    b. Autosomal recessive
    c. X-linked
3. Genetic, metabolic, and systemic diseases (5%)
    a. Hallermann-Streiff syndrome
    b. Lowe's oculocerebrorenal syndrome
    c. Smith-Lemli-Opitz syndrome
    d. Galactosemia
    e. Hypoglycemia
    f. Trisomy
        1) Down syndrome
        2) Edward syndrome
        3) Patau's syndrome
    g. Alport syndrome
    h. Myotonic dystrophy
    i. Fabry's disease (ceramide trihexosidase deficiency)
    j. Hypoparathyroidism
    k. Marfan's syndrome
    l. Pseudohypoparathyroidism
    m. Conradi's syndrome
    n. Diabetes mellitus
    o. Peroxisomal disorders
    p. Wilson's disease
4. Maternal infection (3%)
    a. Rubella
    b. Cytomegalovirus
    c. Varicella
    d. Syphilis
    e. Toxoplasmosis
    f. Herpes simplex
5. Ocular abnormalities (2%)
    a. Aniridia
    b. Anterior segment dysgenesis
    c. Microphthalmia
    d. PHPV
    e. Posterior lenticonus

UNILATERAL CATARACTS

1. Idiopathic (80%)
2. Ocular abnormalities (10%)
    a. Posterior lenticonus
    b. Persistent hyperplastic primary vitreous
    c. Anterior segment dysgenesis
    d. Posterior pole tumors
3. Traumatic (10%) (must rule out child abuse)
4. Masked bilateral cataract†
5. Intrauterine infection (rubella)—unusual

*Hereditary cataracts may be congenital or acquired and can occur in older children.
†Asymmetric lens involvement can mimic a unilateral cataract. Be sure to carefully examine the "good eye" to rule out bilateral disease.

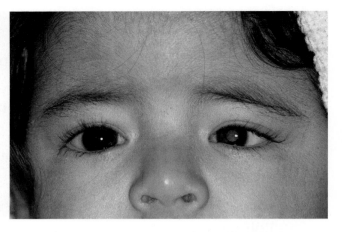

Fig. 8-14   Infant with unilateral congenital cataract secondary to rubella syndrome.

Box 8-3   Ocular Findings of Trisomy 13 (Patau's Syndrome)

Microphthalmia
Uveal colobomas
Hyperplastic vitreous
Retinal dysplasia
Corneal opacities

Box 8-4   Ocular Findings of Trisomy 18 (Edward's Syndrome)

Hypertelorism
Blepharophimosis
Ptosis
Epicanthal folds

diet before 4 months of age will usually result in complete resorption of any lenticular opacities and will prevent the progression of systemic sequelae as well. Urine should be tested for reducing substances 2 hours after a milk feeding in patients with bilateral cataracts of unknown etiology.

Hypoglycemia is a rare cause of congenital cataracts. It is usually seen after a complicated pregnancy. The children are often male and appear small for gestational age. Mental retardation is frequently seen. The cataracts are usually bilateral and of the lamellar type. The diagnosis can be confirmed by low blood glucose levels.

Diabetes mellitus related cataracts are rare in children. However, they have been seen as early as 11 months of age. Slit-lamp examination usually reveals diffuse subcapsular cataracts or snowflake opacities.

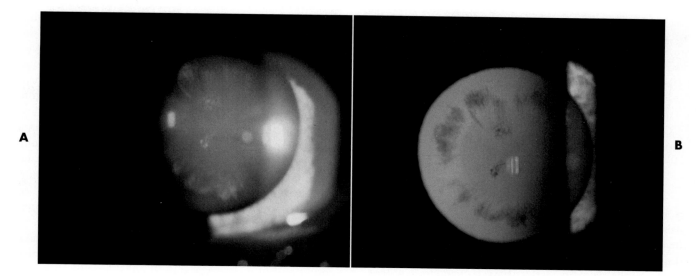

Fig. 8-15 **A,** Cortical cataract associated with galactosemia seen through slit lamp. **B,** Retroillu-mination photograph of *A* showing diffuse cortical cataracts associated with galactosemia. See color plate.

Fabry's disease is a rare X-linked recessive metabolic disease caused by deficient activity of the enzyme alpha-galactosidase. Abnormal storage of glycosphingolipids occurs in the eye, kidneys, central and peripheral nervous system, cardiac muscle, vascular smooth muscle, and vascular endothelium. Symptoms usually begin by 10 years of age as burning sensations or severe pain in the hands, feet, and extremities, as well as unexplained malaise. Punctate dark-red to purple skin lesions develop over the genitalia, thighs, buttocks, and navel (bathing suit area), and are called angiokeratoma corporis diffusum. The disease is generalized and leads to progressive fatigue, hypertension, cerebral aneurysms, cardiomyopathies, myocardial infarction and by age 30 to 40 most patients will have renal failure. Ocular findings include branching posterior spoke-like cataracts, which are pathognomonic of this condition. These cataracts are seen in 50% of patients with Fabry's disease. Other ocular findings include characteristic whorl-like subepithelial corneal opacities, conjunctival and retinal vessel tortuosity, and periorbital or retinal. Since symptoms are so varied and nonspecific in this disease, these patients often see many physicians before a diagnosis is made. The ocular findings are so characteristic that the ophthalmologist may be the first to make the diagnosis. Unfortunately, no specific treatment is known. Female carriers may also manifest a milder form of the disease in later life, including the corneal dystrophy.

Peroxisomal disorders Peroxisomal biogenesis disorders (e.g., in Zellweger syndrome [cerebrohepatorenal syndrome] and rhizomelic chondrodysplasia punctata) have infantile cataracts as a part of the syndrome.

Zellweger syndrome is an autosomal recessive disorder with an incidence of 1:100,000. Clinical findings include a typical facial appearance with a high forehead, epicanthal folds, hypoplastic supraorbital ridges and nasal bridge, micrognathia, and high arched palate. Other findings include hypotonia and hepatic interstitial fibrosis, and renal cortical cysts are also seen. Ocular findings are listed in Box 8-5. Family members who are carriers also possess curvilinear cortical lens opacities. Laboratory evaluation reveals elevated plasma, very long chain fatty acids, and reduced plasmalogen levels.

Rhizomelic chondrodysplasia punctata is the only other peroxisomal disorder that presents with cataracts. It is an autosomal recessive disorder characterized by shortening of the proximal extremities, dermatitis, psychomotor retardation, cataracts, and early death. Infantile cataracts are commonly seen in this condition, and the lens opacities are of the anterior capsular type but posterior lenticonus may also occur. Laboratory evaluation of plasma phytanic acid levels confirms the diagnosis.

Hypoparathyroidism and *pseudohypoparathyroidism* may cause cataracts during childhood. The cataracts associated with this disorder usually consist of multicolor flecks.

Lenticular opacities are found in 15% to 20% of children with *Wilson's disease*. These are posterior subcapsular cataracts made up of copper deposits.

Renal disease *Lowe syndrome* is a rare X-linked recessive disease. It is seen predominantly in Caucasians and Asians. Three major organ systems are affected: the *ocular, cerebral,* and *renal systems*; hence the name oculocerebrorenal syndrome is frequently used to describe this disorder. Children with this disorder have a characteristic facial appearance with frontal bossing and chubby cheeks. The cataracts seen have been described

---

Box 8-5 Ocular Findings of Zellweger Syndrome

Cloudy cornea
Curvilinear cortical cataracts
Retinal abnormalities
Optic nerve pallor
Absent electroretinogram

---

as flattened, central, discoid opacities. They are usually present at birth and often have no demarcation between the nucleus and cortex. Other ocular findings include a frequent association with glaucoma and the presence of miotic pupils. Female carriers have a characteristic lens opacity, but pupillary dilation is often needed to see the cataract. The cataracts in the carriers are punctate, white to gray, and vary in size from one to several millimeters. They may be present in all cortical layers and are considered pathognomonic for the carrier state. Renal tubular dysfunction is seen in early childhood with Lowe syndrome. Renal disease leads to metabolic acidosis, secondary hyperparathyroidism, and secondary hypophosphatemia. This results in severe rickets and demineralization of bone, which further leads to fractures, pain, weakness, hypotonia, and loss of normal motor development. Mental retardation is seen in all patients with this syndrome. A CT scan shows confluent irregular lucencies in cerebral white matter, and an MRI reveals white matter demyelination. The diagnosis is confirmed by identifying amino acids in the urine. Treatment includes early surgery for the cataracts and glaucoma. Patients have a shortened life span and death often occurs in the second decade.

Alport's syndrome is an X-linked dominant disorder that presents as a hemorrhagic nephritis associated with deafness. The most common lens change is the anterior lenticonus (i.e., a central protrusion of the central 3 to 4 mm of the anterior capsule) which is felt by some authors to be seen only with this syndrome. Other lens opacities have been described in association with the syndrome including anterior polar, posterior polar, anterior subcapsular, posterior subcapsular, cortical, and lamellar opacifications. Since anterior lenticonus appears to be specific for Alport's syndrome, it can be used as a noninvasive method of diagnosis, but its absence does not exclude the diagnosis. Laboratory findings include hematuria and proteinuria. Treatment is designed to ward off the complications of renal insufficiency. Anterior lenticonus may result in myopia, which can be corrected with spectacles, but cataract surgery is usually not necessary.

Cataracts associated with drugs Cataracts associated with drugs are usually bilateral. The relationship between systemic corticosteroid treatment and the formation of posterior subcapsular cataracts is well known. The development of cataracts is directly proportional to the dose and duration of corticosteroid treatment. Individual susceptibility also appears to play a role in their formation. Younger subjects tend to develop posterior subcapsular cataracts at lower doses and within a shorter period of time than older subjects. Steroid-induced cataracts have been reported to regress in some patients when the steroids are discontinued. Slit-lamp examination is recommended before institution of chronic systemic steroid treatment and at regular intervals thereafter.

Cataracts and glaucoma Bilateral congenital cataracts associated with congenital glaucoma is a rare condition but it deserves special consideration. The differential diagnosis includes *Lowe syndrome, congenital rubella syndrome, anterior segment dysgenesis,* and *aniridia.*

Systemic Evaluation of Pediatric Cataracts

The systemic evaluation of patients with pediatric cataracts should be based on family history, history of systemic disorders, associated ocular abnormalities, and importantly, whether the cataract is bilateral or unilateral. Box 8-6 shows a summary of the systemic evaluation of patients with bilateral versus unilateral cataracts.

Unilateral pediatric cataracts usually do not require an extensive systemic work-up. A pediatric history and general physical examination, a thorough ocular examination, and serum for TORCH titer is usually all that is needed. A dilated ocular examination is one of the most critical aspects of the work-up. Infants and children are difficult to examine and often require use of a lid speculum and a hand-held slit lamp to obtain a detailed anterior segment examination. First verify that the cataract is in fact unilateral. Assess the morphology of the cataract to establish a specific diagnosis, thus obviating the need for further laboratory studies. Identification of the classical appearance of PHPV or posterior lenticonus provides the diagnosis and no further work-up is needed. Lens position should be examined to rule out the possibility of subluxation. Measure and compare corneal diameters. The iris should also be examined carefully for evidence of iris sphincter tears indicating possible trauma or pseudopolycoria, which would indicate a possible Reiger's syndrome. In older infants and children where unexplained trauma is suspected, the possibility of battered child syndrome should be considered. A dilated indirect ophthalmoscopic fundus examination should be attempted to rule out posterior pole pathology. If the posterior pole and retina cannot be well visualized, then ocular ultrasound is indicated.

In contrast to unilateral cataracts, bilateral cataracts raise the suspicion of an associated systemic disease or inherited pattern. The first aspect of the work-up of a bilateral cataract should be a thorough family history including examination of family members. An infant with a positive family history for autosomal dominant inheritance who is otherwise normal does not need an extensive laboratory work-up. As in the case of unilateral cataracts, bilateral cataracts require a detailed ocular examination including slit-lamp examination and posterior-pole examination. In those cases where there is no clear family history of congenital cataracts, a systemic work-up is indicated. This should include a thorough pediatric examination with developmental assessment, urine for reducing substance after a milk feeding (rule out galactosemia), VDRL, and TORCH titers. In newborns who are suspected of having an intrauterine infection, it is important to obtain IgM titers to avoid confusion with maternal IgG antibodies that cross the placenta. Patients with congenital glaucoma, cataracts, and developmental delay require examination of urine for amino acids to rule out Lowe syndrome. Other laboratory tests and systemic work-up should be pursued in coordination with the pediatric consultants. If dysmorphic features are found or questioned such as presence of midfacial hypoplasia, a dysmorphologist or geneticist should be consulted.

Management of Pediatric Cataracts

Amblyopia and the timing of surgery   Amblyopia is the overwhelming cause of poor vision associated with congenital and infantile cataracts. The first few months of life represent the critical period of visual development, since visual areas in the brain are rapidly developing in response to visual input from the eyes. A unilateral or bilateral blurred retinal image during this critical period will result in irreversible amblyopia. Rodgers, et al, showed that bilateral congenital cataracts that obscure the visual axis will cause irreversible amblyopia and sensory nystagmus unless the retinal images are cleared before 2 months of age. In regards to unilateral congenital cataracts, Birch and Stager suggest operating by 2 months of age. Most authorities agree that visually significant unilateral or bilateral congenital cataracts should be removed and aphakic correction provided as soon as possible, ideally during the first week of life. Very early visual rehabilitation can result in good visual acuity and fusion with stereopsis, even in patients with unilateral congenital cataracts. Newborn nursery screening of every neonate with the red reflex test is essential to identify congenital cataracts before irreversible amblyopia occurs.

It is important to remember that not all congenital cataracts are amblyogenic at birth. Even nuclear cataracts can be partial at birth and later progress to become visually significant. Patients with acquired progressive cataracts have less amblyopia and a much better visual prognosis than patients with cataracts that obscured the visual axis since birth. This is why progressive cataracts such as lamellar cataracts, PHPV, and posterior lenticonus have a relatively good prognosis even when surgery is performed after the critical period of visual development. In general it is difficult to retrospectively determine the onset of a pediatric cataract and to guess the prognosis in regards to amblyopia. One way to estimate the onset is to examine serial baby photographs for a red reflex. Even after examining serial photographs the true onset of the cataract often remains in doubt. It should be pointed out that approximately 40% of older children with unilateral presumed congenital cataracts and 70% with bilateral presumed congenital cataracts will achieve vision of 20/60 or better. Wright's study showed that the best prognosis in older children with unilateral cataracts and straight eyes (no strabismus) PHPV, posterior lenticonus, lamellar cataracts, and bilateral cataracts without nystagmus. Children with bilateral cataracts and sensory nystagmus generally have a poor visual prognosis, but in some cases, even late surgery can reduce the nystagmus and significantly improve visual acuity. Even older children with dense bilateral cataracts and nystagmus may show improvement after cataract surgery.

Is this cataract visually significant? One of the most difficult decisions is when to operate on an infant or preverbal child with a partial cataract. The red reflex, obtained by the direct ophthalmoscope or retinoscope, is the standard method of determining whether an infantile cataract is visually significant. A good rule of thumb is that the central lens opacity must be at least 3 mm to be visually significant. Clinical evaluation should entail examination of monocular and binocular fixation patterns and the ability of the child to pick up small objects in the palm of the hand. The pattern visual evoked potential and preferential looking testing can help in establishing an estimate of visual acuity. Although these tests are useful, the decision of whether or not to operate should be based on the overall clinical picture, rather than an individual test.

In older children who are able to cooperate with optotype acuity testing, the indication for cataract surgery is usually a visual acuity of 20/70 or worse. This is not a hard and fast rule since other factors such as glare and squinting to bright light and progressive loss of stereo acuity are also indications for surgery.

Bilateral patching for congenital cataracts The ideal treatment of a visually significant unilateral or bilateral congenital cataract is immediate removal of the cataract with instantaneous correction of the aphakia. Unfortunately, this ideal is usually not obtainable. Time is required to place the patient on a surgery schedule, obtain medical consultations, and to allow for postoperative recovery before fitting the contact lens. This process of establishing a clear retinal image after cataract surgery can require 3 weeks for unilateral cataracts and longer for bilateral cases. During the critical period of visual development additional time of retinal stimulation with a blurred image can result in irreversible amblyopia.

A method for stopping the amblyogenic effect of a blurred retinal image is to completely eliminate all light in both eyes by bilateral light occlusion or dark rearing. Animal experiments have shown that bilateral light deprivation or dark rearing prolongs the critical period of visual development. Human studies have supported this work, showing that short periods of bilateral light occlusion in neonates will not cause significant amblyopia or visual loss. The length of time bilateral occlusion can be safely given remains unknown. The longest period of bilateral light occlusion reported in humans was 17 days (reported by Wright). This was a 2-week-old infant who

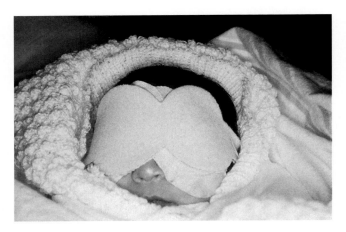

Fig. 8-16   One-month-old infant with bilateral cataracts who is bilaterally patched to prevent the amblyogenic effect of a blurred retinal image. It is important to occlude all light in both eyes symmetrically to avoid pattern distortion amblyopia. Bilateral patching is only a temporary measure and visual rehabilitation should proceed as quickly as possible.

presented with bilateral total hyphemas and vitreous hemorrhages secondary to birth trauma. From these studies, it appears that bilateral patching of a neonate can be safely done for at least 2 weeks.

The author suggests a double occlusive patch over a gauze patch, which is held in place by a Kerlix-type wrap or cloth occluder with Velcro straps (Fig. 8-16). Try to avoid using adhesive tape on the infant's skin since this will cause skin abrasion. Because bilateral patching extends the critical period of visual development, we only patch visually immature infants; those under 4 months of age. Bilateral patching should not be continued longer than 2 weeks unless absolutely necessary, since the effects of long-term total light occlusion have not been well defined in humans. The role of bilateral patching in patients with congenital cataracts remains controversial. Bilateral occlusion does not take the place of immediate surgery and prompt visual rehabilitation. Additionally, bilateral patching is contraindicated in cases of unilateral congenital cataracts if the visual prognosis is poor as in patients with significant macular or optic nerve pathology. It does not make sense to delay visual development of the "good eye" if there is no chance for central vision in the cataractous eye.

Nonsurgical treatment of partial cataracts Not all pediatric cataracts require surgery. Small, partial cataracts of less than 3 mm or pericentral cataracts can be managed by pupillary dilatation with 2½% phenylephrine hydrochloride (Neo-Synephrine) and part-time occlusion therapy of the good eye. If phenylephrine hydrochloride is not sufficient to dilate the pupil, cyclopentolate or Mydriacyl once or twice a day can be added. Daily atropine should be avoided in these patients since prolonged cycloplegia can induce amblyopia. Pupillary dilation is usually reserved for preverbal children (ages 1 year to 6 years) with partial cataracts and borderline amblyopia. These patients should be monitored carefully and, if significant amblyopia persists, cataract extraction should be performed.

Surgical Management

Basic principles In contrast to senile cataracts that have a hard, mineralized nucleus, the lens cortex and nucleus in cataracts of patients under 30 years of age is relatively soft. Pediatric cataracts can therefore be removed by vitrectomy instrumentation that aspirates and cuts both the cortical and nuclear lens material. Phacoemulsification or extracapsular nuclear extraction is not necessary. Intracapsular lens extraction in children is contraindicated since removal of the intact lens causes vitreous traction via *Wieger's capsulohyaloid ligament* and vitreous loss. There is controversy as to the use of an anterior limbal versus a posterior pars plana approach. There are advantages and disadvantages to both methods, but the author prefers the limbal approach. In newborn infants, the pars plana is extremely narrow and almost nonexistent; thus the pars plana incision increases the risk of creating a retinal break. The anterior approach also has the advantage of allowing preservation of the posterior capsule thus facilitating either primary or secondary posterior chamber intraocular lens implantation.

Unlike older adults, posterior capsular opacification occurs in essentially all children who have cataract surgery. Infants can develop capsular opacification very rapidly, literally over days. Because infants are extremely susceptible to amblyopia, even a few days of visual obscuration is significant. Thus infants should have a posterior capsulectomy and anterior vitrectomy as part of the primary procedure. In older cooperative children (usually over 4 years of age) the posterior capsule may be left intact anticipating a YAG laser posterior capsulotomy at some time postoperatively.

Complications of cataract surgery Complications immediately after surgery include acute pupillary block glaucoma, wound leak, iris to the wound, vitreous to the incision, and the rare but devastating complication of endophthalmitis. Postoperative retinal hemorrhages can occur and are probably a result of leaving the eye with a low intraocular pressure at the end surgery. During extubation and at the end of anesthesia, increases in intrathoracic pressure may produce a type of Purtscher's retinopathy. This complication can be prevented by leaving the eye relatively firm at the end of the case. Long-term complications include glaucoma (5% to 10%) and retinal detachment (5% to 10%). The incidence of cystoid macular edema after uncomplicated pediatric cataract surgery is extremely low.

Management of Pediatric Aphakia

The management of pediatric aphakia depends on many factors including the age of the child, the family situation, and the state of the cornea. *Contact lenses* continue to be the treatment of choice for congenital cataracts in infants under 1 year of age. When prescribing aphakic correction, correct for near in infants under 1 year by adding +2.00 to 3.00 diopters to the aphakic correction. For children between 1 to 2 years of age add 1.00 to 1.50 diopters to the aphakic correction. Bifocals are normally prescribed between the ages of 3 to 4 years for bilateral aphakias, but bifocals are not usually prescribed for monocularly aphakic children.

Children with cataracts who are 2 years of age or older should be considered for *intraocular lens* (IOL) implantation. It is important to remember that from birth to 1 year of age there is approximately 10 diopters of lens power reduction because of axial length elongation, but from age 3 years to 8 years there is only a 2 to 3 diopter myopic shift. After 10 years of age the eye is essentially adult size. An eye corrected with an intraocular lens to emmetropia at age 3 years with an IOL will, on the average, have a refractive error of −3.00 as an adult.

Epikeratophakia has been used in the management of pediatric aphakia. The author has also used epikeratophakia in patients with Marfan's syndrome where lensectomy was required to restore vision. Unfortunately, the epikeratophakic grafts are no longer commercially available; however, some eye centers prepare their own grafts.

Aphakic spectacles continue to be useful in children, especially in the treatment of bilateral aphakia. For the most part, aphakic spectacles are reserved for older children with bilateral aphakia. It is important to use a high index of refraction lenses to diminish the weight and size of the aphakic spectacle lenses. Aphakic spectacles are not the treatment of choice for infants since infants do not tolerate spectacles well yet; they require a clear retinal image 100% of the time to stimulate normal visual development.

Secondary intraocular lens implantation for the most part, should be reserved for older children who are contact lens failures, especially those who have at least peripheral binocular fusion. If an older child has strabismus and no binocular function then for all practical purposes the phakic eye is a spare tire eye and a secondary IOL is probably not indicated. If the aphakic eye is needed in future because of loss of the good eye then aphakic spectacles can be prescribed. Dense irreversible amblyopia is a contraindication to secondary lens implantation.

Treatment of Amblyopia

The treatment of amblyopia is based on providing a clear retinal image as soon as possible (ideally first week

Table 8-1 Patching scheme for unilateral congenital cataract (based on visual rehabilitation by 1 month of age)

Months of age	Scheme
0-1 month	no patching
1-2 months	1 to 2 hours/day
2-4 months	2 to 3 hours/day
4-6 months	Up to 50% of waking hours, as indicated by vision assessment
6-12 months	Up to 80% of waking hours, as indicated by vision assessment

of life), then correcting ocular dominance, if present, by patching the "good" eye. In the case of a unilateral congenital cataract, the amount of patching required to promote proper visual development of the aphakic eye depends on the age when the retinal image was cleared. If a unilateral congenital cataract is removed without complication and the contact lens placed in the first week of life, then the initial amblyopia will be mild and part-time patching of an hour or two a day can started after 1 month of age. Table 8-1 gives the suggested patching regimen for a unilateral congenital cataract that is visually rehabilitated before 1 month of age. In contrast, a child who has surgery after 2 months of age will have had a blurred retinal image during the critical period of visual development and will have significant amblyopia. This child requires more extensive patching of at least half the waking hours. Visual acuity assessment by preferential looking or the pattern visual evoked potential is useful in monitoring visual development and modifying the occlusion therapy. Generally, we do not advise patching more than half the waking hours during the first 6 months of life. This conservative approach to patching helps to ensure the normal visual development of the sound eye and allows for the possibility of binocular vision if the cataract was treated early, that is, during the first month of life. Patients with unilateral congenital cataracts will require long-term occlusion therapy. A high percentage of children with unilateral aphakias will show a loss of visual acuity after 2 years of age, so it is important to maintain patching throughout early childhood, usually until 8 or 9 years of age. Parent education about the pathophysiology of amblyopia is critical so the family can understand the treatment strategies and follow through with the rigors of contact lens wear and occlusion therapy.

Prognosis

Monocular infantile cataracts Generally, monocular congenital cataracts have a relatively good prognosis

if surgery and uninterrupted optical correction is provided by 2 months of age. Birch and Stager found that surgery and visual rehabilitation before 2 months of age resulted in a median visual acuity of 20/60, (range 20/800 to 20/30), whereas surgery performed after 2 months produced uniformly poor vision in the range of hand motion to 20/160. Cheng, et al, found similar results could be obtained if cataract surgery was performed by 17 weeks of age. These patients with relatively late cataract surgery, all received full-time occlusion therapy to achieve their good visual results, and all patients developed strabismus. Late visual rehabilitation of patients with truly congenital cataracts necessitates aggressive occlusion therapy and virtually all patients will have strabismus and lack binocular fusion.

Despite the improved visual acuity results in infants receiving early surgery for monocular congenital cataracts, the prognosis for obtaining binocular fusion has been poor. However, binocular fusion is possible if visual rehabilitation is established early. A study by the author showed that of 13 patients with unilateral congenital cataracts who were operated on by 9 weeks of age, 5 showed essentially straight eyes and evidence of motor fusion, whereas 3 demonstrated sensory fusion and stereo acuity by Randot testing. Gregg and Parks reported a case of a patient with unilateral congenital cataract who had 40 second arc stereo acuity and bifoveal fusion. These studies show that binocular fusion is obtainable in patients with unilateral congenital cataracts. Both studies stressed the importance of early visual rehabilitation and limited part-time occlusion therapy during the first few months of life, to enhance binocular visual development.

If a child presents after the critical period of visual development (after 4 to 6 months of age) with a presumed unilateral congenital cataract, should surgery be performed in an attempt to improve vision? Studies by Kushner (1986) and Wright (1992) indicate that some children will show significant visual improvement with late surgery. The author found that of 18 patients operated on between 10 months and 15 years for presumed congenital cataracts, achieved vision of 20/60 or better in approximately 40% of cases. Patients with a relatively good prognosis included those with straight eyes (no strabismus), PHPV, posterior lenticonus, and lamellar cataracts. The relatively good prognosis in patients with PHPV, posterior lenticonus, and lamellar cataracts is probably due to the progressive nature of these lens opacities, with the lens often being clear during early infancy.

Binocular cataracts It has been said that binocular congenital cataracts are less amblyogenic than monocular congenital cataracts. However, this statement is misleading since bilateral congenital cataracts that remain uncorrected past 2 months of age have a poor prog-

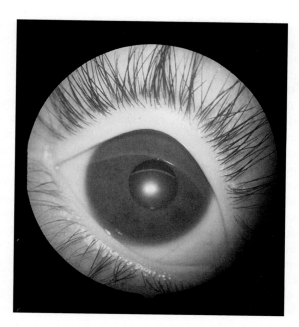

Fig. 8-17   Patient with Marfan's syndrome and an inferiorly sub-luxed lens. Marfan's syndrome is usually associated with a superior temporally dislocated lens; however, the lens position can be variable. See color plate.

nosis, with most patients developing sensory nystagmus. Thus the window of opportunity for bilateral congenital cataracts is similar to that of monocular congenital cataracts, with best results obtained when surgery and visual rehabilitation are instituted before 2 months of age. It is important to note that once sensory nystagmus occurs, the visual prognosis is poor, with most children achieving vision of 20/100 or worse. Since many of these children with bilateral cataracts and sensory nystagmus will be legally blind, it is critical that bilateral cataracts be treated with utmost urgency so that visual rehabilitation occurs early, during the first few weeks of life. In general bilateral cataracts operated on before 2 months of age have an good visual prognosis with approximately 80% achieving vision of 20/50 or better. Unfortunately, not all patients present during early infancy and some patients will present late, with bilateral cataracts and nystagmus. We have found that many of these patients with sensory nystagmus, will show postoperative improvement of the nystagmus and significant visual acuity improvement, with some achieving visual acuity of 20/50 to 20/70. We therefore suggest that cataract surgery should be offered as an option in older patients with significant bilateral cataracts even if nystagmus is present.

SUBLUXATION OF LENS

Subluxation of lens, or ectopia lentis, is displacement of the lens from its normal position in the center of the pupil (Fig. 8-17). This displacement can be partial (sub-

---

Box 8-7   Evaluation of Sublux Lens

I. History
   A. Family: cardiovascular disease, skeletal abnormalities, visual disturbances, mental retardation, early family deaths
   B. Patient: trauma, systemic illness, mental retardation, seizures
II. Complete Eye Examination
   A. Visual acuity
   B. External ocular examination (strabismus)
   C. Anterior segment
     1. Cornea diameter
     2. Anterior chamber depth
     3. Iridocorneal angle
     4. Lens position
     5. Iris configuration (iridodonesis, transillumi-nation, ectopia)
     6. Zonule assessment (phacodonesis)
   D. Retinoscopy/Refraction
     1. Myopia
     2. Astigmatism
   E. Ultrasound
     1. Evaluation of axial length
   F. Keratometry
   G. Posterior segment
     1. Retina (detachment)
III. Laboratory tests
   A. Cardiologist examination
   B. Cardiac ultrasound
   C. Urine for amino acid
   D. X-ray measurements of the hands for possible brachydactyly
   E. Urine for sodium-nitroprusside (homocystinuria screen)

---

luxation) or complete (dislocation), depending on the state of the zonular attachments. Patients with ectopia lentis may present with decreased vision, with monocular diplopia (acquired subluxation), and even pain secondary to pupillary block glaucoma. Ectopia lentis can be idiopathic or may be associated with a systemic or ocular disease. The most common systemic disease associated with bilateral sublux lenses is Marfan's syndrome, which is very important to diagnose because of the life-threatening cardiovascular problems. Refer to Box 8-7 for a guide to the work-up of a patient with ectopia lentis and to Box 8-8 for causes and associated syndromes. In addition to these boxes, specific syndromes commonly associated with ectopia lentis are covered in the following discussion.

Visual loss secondary to ectopia lentis is most commonly caused by anisometropic amblyopia and irregular astigmatism. In some cases the edge of the sublux lens transects the central pupil and distorts the retinal image.

Box 8-8   Causes of Sublux Lens

OCULAR CAUSES

Autosomal dominant
Trauma
Aniridia
Ectopia lentis et pupillae
Idiopathic
Coloboma

SYSTEMIC SYNDROMES

Marfan's syndrome
Homocystinuria
Weill-Marchesani syndrome
Sulfite oxidase deficiency
Hyperlysinemia

In these cases where the edge of the lens prevents clear use of both the phakic or aphakic portions of the pupil lensectomy is required. Recent studies have shown good results with closed eye lensectomy using vitrectomy instrumentation either from a limbal or a pars plana approach. Intracapsular surgery on the other hand is dangerous and associated with a high incidence of retinal detachment.

Ectopia Lentis et Pupillae

Ectopia lentis et pupillae is a rare autosomal recessive disorder characterized by symmetrically displaced pupils and lens. The pupils may be displaced in the same or opposite direction to that of the ectopic lens. The pupils are characteristically oval or slit-shaped, and they frequently dilate poorly. This condition is almost always bilateral. It must be remembered that this disorder involves the entire eye. Other ocular manifestations include persistent pupillary membranes (87%) and iris transillumination (66%). Ectopia lentis et pupillae can be associated with myopia, glaucoma, and retinal detachment may occur.

Marfan's Syndrome

Marfan's syndrome is the most common systemic disease associated with subluxed lens. It is a connective tissue disorder with a prevalence of 4 to 6 per 100,000 people. In most instances it is inherited as an autosomal dominant trait. In approximately 15% of cases no other family member has signs of the syndrome. As in other sporadic dominantly inherited mutations the average paternal age is elevated in these cases. This disorder affects both sexes equally and has no racial or ethnic predilec-

tion. Three major organ systems are predominately affected in Marfan's syndrome: the ocular, skeletal, and cardiovascular systems.

Ocular

Lens Lens subluxation occurs in 80% of patients with Marfan's syndrome. Lens subluxation is thought to occur in utero, hence it is usually visible at the first eye examination *(Maumenee)*. The lens is usually displaced upward and the zonules remain intact permitting normal accommodation. Lens subluxation may also occur inferiorly (Fig. 8-17) or in virtually any location. Amblyopia is often cited as the most common cause of decreased vision in these patients, but lensectomy can restore vision even when performed after the critical period of visual development. Ectopia lentis has been associated with glaucoma in approximately 10% of patients.

Globe Axial length is usually normal and the myopia is lenticular. Retinal detachment can occur and in one study retinal detachment was seen in 9% of phakic eyes.

Cornea The corneal curvature is often flat and the corneal diameter may be increased.

Pupils The pupils are typically small and dilate poorly with mydriatic agents.

Systemic findings

Cardiovascular Cardiovascular complications cause 90% of the early mortality associated with Marfan's syndrome. Aortic weakness leads to dilation of the ascending aorta with subsequent aortic regurgitation and dissecting aortic aneurysm. Echocardiography reveals dilation of the aortic root and is characteristic of this syndrome. Any patient suspected of having Marfan's syndrome must have a cardiologic evaluation and close follow-up.

Skeletal Arachnodactyly (long thin fingers) is the most common skeletal feature in Marfan's syndrome. This phenomenon was seen in 88% of patients with this disorder that were evaluated at Johns Hopkins Hospital. As a rule the upper body segment is much shorter by comparison with the lower body segment. This phenomenon is seen in 76% of patients with Marfan's syndrome. Scoliosis may occur as well. This generally worsens during the adolescent growth spurt and can be a deforming and disabling complication. Pectus excavatum and joint laxity are also seen.

Useful clinical clues to the diagnosis can be elicited via the thumb sign and wrist sign. The thumb sign is considered positive when the thumb projects beyond the ulnar border when making a fist (thumb wrapped under the fingers). The wrist sign is considered positive when the distal phalanges of the first and fifth digit overlap when wrapped around the opposite wrist.

Additional systemic findings Inguinal hernias that tend to recur after surgery and spontaneous pneumothorax have also been reported. Mental deficiency is not a component of this disorder.

Management

Ocular

The presence of a subluxed lens is often compatible with excellent visual acuity. If the subluxation is mild, the patient will view through the phakic portion of the pupil, whereas a patient with a large lens subluxation may achieve the best vision by using aphakic correction and viewing through the aphakic portion of the pupil. In cases where the edge of the lens splits the pupil, a decision must be made regarding the use of the aphakic versus the phakic portion of the pupil versus surgery. A careful refraction with administration of best phakic and aphakic optical correction should be tried. These refractions are difficult and it is often necessary to try many different lenses before the optimum vision is obtained. If the aphakic correction gives the best vision then the entrance pupil can be enlarged by pupillary dilation or application of argon laser to the iris (see laser treatment). If visual acuity fails to improve immediately, amblyopia should be expected and patching therapy of the good eye initiated. Ocular management should be directed toward early optical correction of these patients to prevent amblyopia. In cases where the edge of the lens bisects the pupil, optical distortion by the lens edge may prevent visual acuity improvement despite pupillary dilation, and optical correction of refractive errors. When the edge of the lens interferes with visual rehabilitation, lensectomy should be considered (see lensectomy).

Laser treatment Argon laser spots placed over the iris stroma can cause contraction of the iris thus opening the pupil in the direction of the laser application. If the lens is subluxed superotemporally as with most of the Marfan's lenses, the laser can be applied over the inferonasal iris to draw the pupil down and allowing use of the aphakic space below the lens. YAG laser has been used to break the zonules in order to move the edge of the subluxed lens out of the visual axis. The author has found this technique moves the lens only slightly. The movement is not immediate since the lens will continue to slowly drift for several weeks after laser treatment.

Lensectomy Two indications exist for lens extraction in patients with Marfan's syndrome and sublux lenses in general:

1. Lens positioning where the lens edge bisects the pupil making optical correction of either the aphakic or phakic part of the pupil impossible.
2. Displacement of the lens anteriorly causing secondary glaucoma.

Early studies showed poor results with lensectomy for Marfan's syndrome. In one study, visual acuity was un-altered in 14% of patients undergoing lens extraction and worsened in 18%. Complications included retinal detachment and vitreous loss occurred in 50% of cases. More recent studies with vitrectomy instrumentation have shown that lensectomy can be safely performed of patients with a variety of causes of sublux lens and specifically Marfan's syndrome without increased risks over standard cataract surgery. The safety and surgical outcome of anterior limbal approach versus pars plana approach have been shown to be the same.

Homocystinuria

Homocystinuria is a disease of methionine metabolism. It is due to a deficiency of the enzyme cystathionine synthase. Affected patients have elevated blood levels of homocystine and methionine, and will also have amino aciduria (i.e., homocystine). A screening test for homocystinuria is sodium-nitroprusside for homocystine in the urine. The prevalence of this disorder is 1:200,000 births. Like Marfan's syndrome it affects the ocular, cardiovascular, and skeletal systems.

Ocular The ocular abnormalities do not clearly differentiate homocystinuria from Marfan's syndrome. Ectopia lentis, myopia, retinal detachment, and secondary glaucoma occur in both. McKusick suggested that lenses are most likely to be displaced upwards in Marfan's and downward in homocystinuria. In contradistinction to Marfan's syndrome, the zonules are markedly abnormal; the lens cannot accommodate. In addition, approximately one third of the lenses are eventually completely dislocated into the vitreous or anterior chamber. In Marfan's, the subluxation is relatively stable and complete subluxation rarely occurs. Like Marfan's, dislocation is usually symmetric and occurs in approximately 90% of patients. Anomalies of the iridocorneal angle have not been described in homocystinuria and may be unique to Marfan's.

Systemic/cardiovascular The cardiovascular complications are secondary to thrombosis and occlusion, mainly of medium sized arteries and veins. Cerebrovascular thrombosis, myocardial infarction, pulmonary emboli, intermittent claudication and even death at a relatively young age often result. Anesthesia holds a higher risk for patients with homocystinuria because of the possibility of thromboembolic disease.

Skeletal Arachnodactyly to the degree seen in Marfan's is unusual; however, scoliosis, pectus excavatum, and joint laxity are seen. Hernias have been described with homocystinuria as well. Patients with homocystinuria are often tall with a malar flush and light colored hair. Mental retardation is frequently present with this condition (in contrast to Marfan's), but it is not an invariable manifestation. Infants may fail to thrive and may be developmentally delayed.

Table 8-2 Findings in the Weill-Marchesani syndrome	
Systemic	**Ocular findings**
Brachycephaly	Ectopia lentis
Short build (pyknic)	(down and anterior)
Broad thorax	Spherophakic lens
Brachydactyly	Lenticular myopia
Roentgenologic	Relatively short axial length
brachymetacarpia	Pupillary block glaucoma
Hypoextendable joints	Shallow anterior chamber
Inheritance variable	Angle abnormalities

Management   Ocular management of the sublux lens is the similar to the management of the lens in Marfan's syndrome. Patients with homocystinuria are at increased risk of thromboembolic events especially during anesthesia, thus a more conservative approach is warranted in these patients. At the present time, there is no good satisfactory solution. It is hoped that early dietary manipulation will prevent lens dislocation.

Weill-Marchesani Syndrome (Spherophakia-brachymorphia)

Weill-Marchesani syndrome is a rare disease, with the unclear inheritance pattern. Most cases are thought to be autosomal recessive; however, autosomal dominant cases have been reported. Both sexes are affected equally. Ocular and skeletal abnormalities are characteristic of this disorder.

Ocular   The lens in Weill-Marchesani is microspherophakic being typically small and round. The small steep lens results in lenticular myopia. Subluxation occurs in virtually 100% of cases with over 90% progressing to dislocation by adulthood. On dislocation the lens shifts anteriorly which results in pupillary block glaucoma in approximately 80% of cases. Acute bilateral pupillary block and secondary angle closure after pupillary dilation have been reported as the presenting sign in a patient with previously undiagnosed Weill-Marchesani syndrome. The typical skeletal findings of brachymorphia may be subtle, so suspect Weill-Marchesani syndrome in children who present with unilateral or bilateral angle pupillary block glaucoma. Not infrequently the lens will completely dislocate into the anterior chamber.

Skeletal   Weill-Marchesani syndrome includes systemic findings of brachycephaly, short build, broad thorax, brachydactyl, and hypoextendible joints. In cases where the diagnosis is in question roentgenographic measurements of the hands are helpful. See Table 8-2 for a list of ocular and systemic findings.

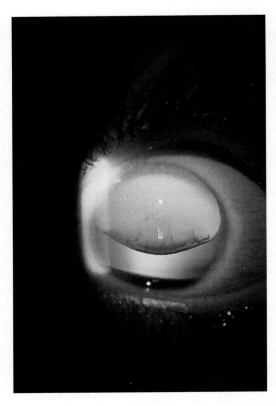

Fig. 8-18   Lens coloboma. Superiorly subluxed lens associated with aniridia. The lens coloboma is inferior. Note the flattened appearance of the inferior margin of the lens where the lens zonules are absent, thus causing a lens coloboma.

Management

Ocular

The major thrust of treatment is to prevent pupillary block glaucoma, which can result in angle closure, and secondary scarring of the angle which in turn causes a chronic glaucoma that is very difficult to treat. The best way to prevent acute pupillary block with angle-closure glaucoma in these patients is controversial. One treatment strategy is to perform a prophylactic laser peripheral iridotomy then keep the patient on miotics to prevent anterior dislocation of the lens. Since the risk of these patients developing angle-closure glaucoma is extremely high (approximately 80%), and the risks of laser peripheral iridectomy is minimal, a prophylactic laser peripheral iridectomy for all patients with Weill-Marchesani syndrome is probably indicated.

Systemic   No specific systemic treatment is required.

Sulfite Oxidase Deficiency

Sulfite oxidase deficiency is an extremely rare metabolic disorder. Sulfite is an important intermediary compound in the metabolic pathway from sulfur amino acids

MAJOR POINTS

The Y sutures are an important landmark since they identify the extent of the fetal nucleus.

Anterior polar cataracts are for the most part nonprogressive, usually not visually significant, and in the majority of cases, they can be managed conservatively, without surgery.

Since the lens is relatively clear during the critical period of visual development, lamellar cataracts generally have a good visual prognosis even when surgery is performed in late childhood.

It is important to monitor visual function in patients with posterior lenticonus as significant amblyopia can occur even when the lens appears relatively clear.

Persistent hyperplastic primary vitreous is a disorder related to the persistence and secondary fibrosis of the primitive hyaloid vascular system.

Most unilateral congenital cataracts are caused by local dysgenesis and, as a rule, are not associated with a systemic disease and are not inherited.

In contrast to unilateral cataracts, bilateral cataracts, raise the suspicion of an associated systemic disease or inherited pattern.

Amblyopia is the overwhelming cause of poor vision associated with congenital and infantile cataracts.

Visually significant unilateral or bilateral congenital cataracts should be removed and aphakic correction provided as soon as possible in the neonatal period, ideally during the first week of life.

In contrast to senile cataracts that have a hard mineralized nucleus, the lens cortex and nucleus in cataracts of patients under 30 years of age is relatively soft.

Children with acquitted cataracts who are older than 2 years of age should be considered for intraocular lens implantation.

The treatment of amblyopia is based on providing a clear retinal image as soon as possible (ideally first week of life), then correcting ocular dominance if present, by patching the "good" eye.

The most common systemic disease associated with bilateral sublux lenses is Marfan's syndrome.

In Weill-Marchesani syndrome subluxation occurs in virtually 100% of cases with pupillary block glaucoma occurring in approximately 80% of cases.

to inorganic sulfate. In sulfite oxidase deficiency, sulfite cannot be converted to sulfate, hence increased amounts of sulfite and its metabolites are excreted in the urine.

Systemic Patients with sulfite oxidase deficiency may present with hemiplegia, progressive choreoathetoid movements, and/or seizures in addition to dislocated lens. The neuropathology reveals atrophic cortical gyri, which is most severe in the parietal area and less marked in the frontal area.

Management Treatment for this condition is limitation of sulfur amino acid ingestion to reduce the production of abnormal metabolites. Unfortunately, although this may limit progression, it will not reverse brain damage. Death usually occurs before 5 years of age.

Spherophakia

Spherophakia is a condition where the lens diameter is relatively small; however, there is increased lens thickness. The lens curvature is quite steep and therefore these patients have lenticular myopia. Spherophakia can occur as an isolated anomaly or be in association with the Weill-Marchesani syndrome.

Lens Coloboma

Lens colobomas are rare and may result from a congenital absence of lens zonules in a localized area. Fig. 8-18 shows a lens coloboma associated with aniridia and absence of inferior lens zonules. A lens coloboma may be considered a type of sublux lens; however, a lens coloboma is displacement of part of the lens, whereas subluxation is displacement of the entire lens.

SUGGESTED READINGS

Behki R, Noel LP, Clarke WN: Limbal lensectomy in the management of ectopia lentis in children, *Arch Ophthalmol* 108:809-811, 1990.

Birch EE, Stager DR: Prevalence of good visual acuity following surgery for congenital unilateral cataract, *Arch Ophthalmol* 106:40-43, 1988.

Cheng KP, Hiles DA, Biglan AW, et al. Management of posterior lenticonus, *J Pediatr Ophthalmol Strabismus* 28(3);143-150, 1991.

Cross HE, Jenson AD: Ocular manifestations in the Marfan syndrome and homocystinuria, *Am J Ophthalmol* 75:405-420, 1973.

Crouch ER Jr, Parks MM: Management of posterior lenticonus complicated by unilateral cataract, *Am J Ophthalmol* 85:503-508, 1978.

Gregg FM, Parks MM: Stereopsis after congenital monocular cataract extraction, *Am J Ophthalmol* 114:314-317, 1992.

Hakin KN, Jacobs M, Rosen P, et al. Management of the subluxed crystalline lens, *Ophthalmology* 99:542-545, 1992.

Hoyt CS: The long-term visual effects of short-term binocular occlusion of at-risk neonates, *Arch Ophthalmol* 98:1967-1970, 1980.

Jaafar MS, Robb RM: Congenital anterior polar cataract: a review of 63 cases, *Ophthalmology* 91(3):249-254, 1984.

Jensen AD, Cross HE, Paton D: Ocular complications in the Weill-Marchesani syndrome, *Am J Ophthalmol* 77:261-269, 1974.

Karr DJ, Scott WE: Visual acuity results following treatment of persistent hyperplastic primary vitreous, *Arch Ophthalmol* 104:662, 1986.

Kushner BJ: Visual results after surgery for monocular juvenile cataracts of undetermined onset, *Am J Ophthalmol* 102: 468-472, 1986.

Maumenee IH: The eye in the Marfan syndrome, *Trans Am Ophthalmol Soc* 69:685-733, 1981.

Parks MM: Visual results in aphakic children, *Am J Ophthalmol* 94:441-449, 1982.

Robb RM, Mayer DL, Moore BD: Results of early treatment of unilateral cataracts, *J Pediatr Ophthalmol Strabismus* 24: 178-181, 1987.

Rogers GL, Tishler CL, Tsou BH, et al: Visual acuities in infants with congenital cataracts operated on before 6 months of age, *Arch Ophthalmol* 99:999-1003, 1981.

Wright KW, Chrousos GA: Weill-Marchesani syndrome with bilateral angle-closure glaucoma, *J Ped Ophthalmol Strab* 22(4):129-132, 1985.

Wright KW, Matusmoto E, Edelman PM: Binocular fusion and stereopsis associated with early surgery for monocular congenital cataracts, *Arch Ophthalmol* 110:1607, 1992.

Wright KW, Christensen LE, Noguchi BA: Results of late surgery for presumed congenital cataracts, *Am J Ophthalmol* 114: 409-415, 1992.

Wright KW, Wehrle MJ, Urrea PT: Bilateral total occlusion during the critical period of visual development, *Arch Ophthalmol* 105:321, 1987.

Pediatric Uveitis

A limited number of clinical entities account for the majority of cases of uveitis in children. Anterior uveitis is usually associated with juvenile rheumatoid arthritis (JRA) or the HLA B27-related spondyloarthropathies; less common, but still important, causes include sarcoidosis and herpetic iridocyclitis. Intermediate uveitis or pars planitis, although most common in young adults, does affect children and is discussed in this chapter. The most common causes of posterior uveitis in children, toxoplasmosis and toxocariasis, are covered in the last section, as well as discussions of Vogt-Koyanagi-Harada syndrome, sympathetic ophthalmia, and cytomegalovirus retinitis.

The above classification scheme, based on anatomic location, is very useful when considering uveitis in children, but analyzing other characteristics (time course, granulomatous versus nongranulomatous inflammation) usually will narrow the differential diagnosis. For example, a granulomatous anterior uveitis is unlikely to be associated with juvenile rheumatoid arthritis and suggests sarcoidosis. Whereas the first episode of isolated, nongranulomatous anterior uveitis in adults often will not trigger an extensive ancillary work-up, chil-

dren in similar circumstances require further systemic evaluation.

ANTERIOR UVEITIS

Juvenile arthritis is a general term that includes the entities juvenile rheumatoid arthritis (JRA) and the HLA B27-related spondyloarthopathies. Of these two categories of arthritis, JRA is much more common, accounting for about 70% of childhood arthritis.

Juvenile Rheumatoid Arthritis

JRA-associated uveitis is typically a bilateral, anterior process that is more common in girls than boys. It may vary greatly in severity and prognosis. Uveitis is sometimes the presenting sign in JRA, but more often it is found when specifically sought in a patient with known JRA. Patients whose disease comes to medical attention because of the ocular involvement may have more severe ocular disease and, possibly, a worse prognosis. Occasionally, the presence of iritis will confirm a diagnosis of possible JRA. Uveitis occurs in 2% to 21% of all patients with JRA, a proportion that will be more or less depending on the specific subtype of arthritis (see the following discussion). A remarkable feature is that the inflammation, although severe at times, often does not induce symptoms of photophobia and pain or external signs such as conjunctival injection. Consequently, significant ocular damage can go undetected; therefore routine screening examinations of JRA patients are required.

The important risk factors for developing ocular involvement in JRA are young age, female gender, the presence of antinuclear antibodies, and the pauciarticular form of arthritis. About 20% of patients with JRA have the systemic form called *Still's disease.* This is characterized by fever, rash, and hepatosplenomegaly; joint in-

Table 9-1 Recommended schedule for ocular examination of patients with JRA	
Type of JRA	**Frequency of screening examination**
Still's disease	Annually
Polyarticular	Every 6 months
Pauciarticular	Every 3 months
Pauciarticular with (+) ANA	Every 2-3 months

Note: Rarely, the onset of uveitis may not occur for a decade or longer after the arthritis begins. Periodic examinations are suggested at least up to the teenage years.

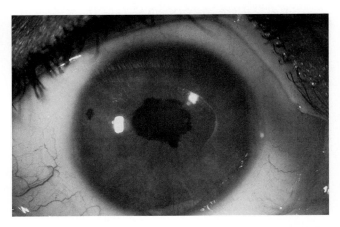

Fig. 9-1 JRA-associated uveitis. Note the presence of posterior synechiae and early band keratopathy.

volvement may be delayed. Patients with Still's disease rarely develop uveitis.

Uveitis is less common with the polyarticular form of JRA, in which patients have involvement of five or more joints, typically the knees, wrists, and ankles within the first 3 months of the disease. Polyarticular JRA, which accounts for 20% of cases of JRA, is further subdivided into rheumatoid factor (RF) positive and RF-negative cases. F-positive patients rarely develop uveitis, whereas 7% to 14% of RF-negative persons develop uveitis. Consequently, screening of asymptomatic RF-negative patients is recommended at 6-month intervals.

Pauciarticular JRA is the most common type of JRA, accounting for 40% to 60% of cases, and is the most likely to be accompanied by uveitis. This form of JRA is defined by the involvement of fewer than five joints in the first 3 months of the illness, regardless of whether or not more joints subsequently become involved. Between 78% and 91% of patients with JRA-associated uveitis have pauciarticular arthritis. Overall, about 20% of patients with pauciarticular JRA develop uveitis. Two varieties of pauciarticular JRA exist. The first variety predominantly involves girls under 5 years of age who have positive ANA tests. About one quarter of such patients develop uveitis, which is typically a chronic iridocyclitis. The second type of pauciarticular JRA affects older boys, 75% of whom are HLA B27 positive. Many of them will have recurrent episodes of acute anterior uveitis.

Clinical findings and sequelae Periodic screening of patients with JRA is performed on a schedule that varies, depending on the particular variety of arthritis (Table 9-1). A careful slit-lamp examination is performed, using a bright, thin beam in a darkened room.

External signs, such as ciliary injection, are usually absent. The most frequent presentation is that of bilateral, nongranulomatous, anterior segment cell and flare. The inflammation may range from rare cells to +4 inflammation. Occasionally, small keratic precipitates may form on the inferior corneal endothelium, a finding that

may aid in the diagnosis, particularly in poorly cooperative patients. Cataracts, particularly posterior subcapsular, occur in up to 42% of patients. Band keratopathy occurs in more than half of patients. Very small white zones at the 3 and 9 o'clock limbus, without involvement of the central cornea, signals early band keratopathy, and thus should be specifically sought. Posterior synechiae may be present at the time the uveitis is recognized (Fig. 9-1). Glaucoma, occurring in 14% to 22% of patients with JRA-associated iritis, is a major problem because it can be quite difficult to control. The glaucoma is caused by progressive-angle closure, steroid response, and other causes. Kanski and Shun-Shin, in 1984, reported that 35% of glaucomatous eyes resulting from JRA-associated uveitis had no light perception at the last examination. This percentage is probably somewhat smaller now, as a result of the use of antimetabolites, which improve the outcomes in filtering surgery, and the effective use of drainage implants in uveitic eyes. A less common, but important, complication is cystoid macular edema because if persistent, permanent macular changes develop. The causes of visual loss in JRA are listed in Box 9-1.

Treatment Successful treatment requires sustained commitment by the patient, his or her family, and the treating physicians. Treatment modifications will be required as the inflammation waxes and wanes. Topical corticosteroids and mydriatic agents are the first-line treatment agents. Despite their inherent risks and side effects, potent steroids with good intraocular penetration, such as prednisolone acetate, must be used. Hourly administration usually will quiet down acute flare-ups, and subsequently the dose can be tapered. Eyes that do not respond adequately may benefit by sub-Tenon's corticosteroid injections. Short-acting topical mydriatics, such as tropicamide, help prevent posterior synechiae formation (but, beware: chronic cycloplegia can cause

Box 9-1   Causes of Visual Loss in JRA

Band keratopathy
Cataract
Glaucoma
Amblyopia
Retinal (cystoid macular edema, macular changes,
    macular hole)
Phthisis bulbi

amblyopia). It is accepted that eyes with aqueous flare, but with no anterior chamber cell, do not require steroid treatment. However, some disagreement exists in the United States as to how aggressive a treatment is required in very mildly inflamed eyes. One approach is to eliminate all cells with frequent administration of drops, while another accepts occasional cells, and treats less vigorously.

More and more use is being made of systemic immunosuppressive agents, methotrexate in particular, to control ocular inflammation and as steroid-sparing agents. Chlorambucil and azathioprine have also been used, but methotrexate appears to be the safest and is becoming more widely used in treatment of childhood arthritis. Obviously, good communication with the rheumatologist is required.

The optimal management of cataracts in JRA is also controversial. Whether or not to operate and whether to implant an intraocular lens or to leave the child aphakic, are the two main issues that must be addressed. Some basic management principles are generally agreed on. In most cases, inflamed eyes should not undergo cataract surgery because a severe postoperative inflammatory reaction is likely. The eye should be quiet for an extended time, 3 months or more, before surgery. Perioperative corticosteroids (systemic, periocular, and topical) should be used in large doses to minimize the inflammatory response. Eyes that have had severe, persistent inflammation are at a greater risk of developing complications that threaten the globe, such as cyclitic membranes, hypotony and phthisis, or glaucoma, following cataract surgery. Currently, most cataracts are managed with lensectomy and anterior vitrectomy, using an automated cutting device. Traditionally, intraocular lenses have not been implanted in uveitic eyes from JRA because of (justified) fears of inciting the same complications listed previously. However, favorable results have been reported in one series utilizing phacoemulsification with placement of a one-piece polymethylmethacrylate lens within the capsule. Long-term data on such eyes are not yet available.

Prognosis Kanski reviewed 103 patients and found that they fell into one of three groups. The first group, comprising about 25% of the cases, had mild disease and did well. The second group, also consisting of about 25% of the cases, had severe and persistent inflammation and often required surgery for cataracts and glaucoma. The third group (50%) had an intermediate severity and course, and the eyes typically responded well to topical corticosteroid treatment. Wolf, et al, reviewed the course of 51 patients with JRA-associated uveitis (the average duration of follow up was 12.7 years) and found that more severe inflammation on presentation correlated with worse visual acuity and more complications. Patients in whom uveitis was the presenting manifestation of JRA were much more likely to have a poor visual outcome than those in which arthritis came first (76% versus 6%).

Sarcoidosis

Clinical features and diagnosis Sarcoidosis is a multisystem disease of unknown origin that causes granulomatous inflammation. The lungs, skin, thoracic lymph nodes, and eyes are the most commonly affected organs. Definitive diagnosis of sarcoidosis is made histopathologically by demonstrating the characteristic noncaseating granulomatous inflammation in the absence of any identifiable inciting agents such as infections or foreign bodies. However, convincing presumptive evidence can be obtained through clinical manifestations and laboratory testing. Although sarcoidosis may manifest in any part of the eye, its discussion is placed here to emphasize the importance of differentiating it from the uveitis seen in JRA and the spondyloarthropathies. Sarcoidosis is not as common in children as in adults but is probably underdiagnosed as a cause of pediatric uveitis.

The demographics of children with sarcoidosis differ somewhat from adults. Among adults in the United States, blacks are affected ten times more often than whites. In contrast, the black to white ratio in children 8 to 15 years of age is 3:1. Whereas adult women are affected 2 to 3 times more often than men, among children the gender ratio appears equal. Sarcoid uveitis in children accounted for less than 1% in Kanski's series (1984).

Sarcoidosis affects children of different ages differently. In children 4 years of age or less, pulmonary involvement is uncommon and the typical patient has joint, eye, and skin involvement (erythema nodosa, rash); skeletal changes, manifested by osteopenia visible on roentgenograms, has an intermediate incidence. In children 4 years of age or older, the lung and hilar lymph nodes are the most commonly affected sites. The inflammation in ocular sarcoidosis can be chronic or recurrent but usually is granulomatous, a feature that distinguishes it from JRA-associated uveitis. Posterior involvement is present in 14% of children with sarcoidosis

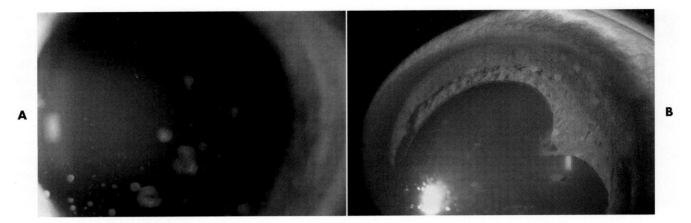

Fig. 9-2   Sarcoidosis, anterior segment findings. **A,** "Mutton-fat" keratic precipitates. **B,** Posterior synechiae with iris nodules. See color plate.

and less than 1% with JRA. The presence of a rash should raise the clinician's suspicion for the presence of sarcoidosis as the cause of uveitis in children.

Anterior segment manifestations of sarcoidosis include an inflammation that is typically chronic and granulomatous, with iris nodules and mutton fat keratic precipitates. Patients with such findings may have only mild symptoms. A smaller percentage of patients may have acute episodes of nongranulomatous anterior uveitis, with pain, photophobia, and injection. Sequelae of the anterior uveitis are anterior and posterior synechiae, secondary glaucoma, cataracts, and band keratopathy (Fig. 9-2). In children, posterior ocular involvement is less common than anterior involvement. Posterior findings include vitreitis, which may form snowball opacities (resembling intermediate uveitis) and papillitis. Retinal periphlebitis is uncommon in children. Other findings include conjunctival granulomas and orbital and lacrimal gland involvement.

Evaluation of a child with suspected ocular sarcoidosis should include a focused physical examination, including inspecting the skin and joints, and a laboratory evaluation. Chest roentgenograms and gallium scans may show evidence of pulmonary and hilar involvement in otherwise asymptomatic patients. The single most valuable blood test is the level of serum angiotensin converting enzyme (ACE). This enzyme is produced by macrophage-derived epithelioid cells that compose the granulomas. The degree of elevation of the angiotensin-converting enzyme is related to the granuloma load in the entire body and correlates with disease activity. One study found elevated ACE levels in 80% of children 8 to 15 years of age at the time sarcoidosis was diagnosed. It should be evident that a normal ACE value does not rule out sarcoidosis as a cause of ocular inflammation. Fur-

thermore, the normal values in children are significantly higher than in adults; thus age appropriate data must be used. Also, ACE levels can be elevated in other conditions such as primary biliary cirrhosis and diabetes mellitus. Serum lysozyme levels can also rise in patients with sarcoidosis. Lysozyme levels are best used in concert with angiotensin converting enzyme levels rather than used alone.

Sites that may be biopsied in children include enlarged lymph nodes, skin affected with a rash or nodules, and conjunctivae, particularly if granulomas are visible.

Treatment   Treatment of acute anterior uveitis caused by sarcoidosis is similar to that caused by other causes, relying on topical and local corticosteroids and cycloplegics. Secondary complications such as glaucoma and cataracts may occur following repeated attacks. Chronic granulomatous panuveitis is a more difficult problem and requires high doses of local and systemic corticosteroids, which are slowly tapered. Obviously, such patients must be managed in concert with the patient's primary care physician since the steroid side effects can be devastating. Cyclosporin and methotrexate may be added to corticosteroids in severe cases, both for improved inflammation control and a steroid-sparing effect. In certain patients, glaucoma and cataracts can present significant management problems. Cataract extraction may be performed with an anterior or pars plana approach, but a significant postoperative inflammatory response should be anticipated. Attempts to mitigate this should be made with a perioperative pulse of large doses of corticosteroids. As in other inflammatory glaucomas, trabeculectomies are more likely to fail in these patients and management must be made on an individualized basis. The natural history of sarcoidosis is variable and unpredictable, but spontaneous remissions occur in some patients.

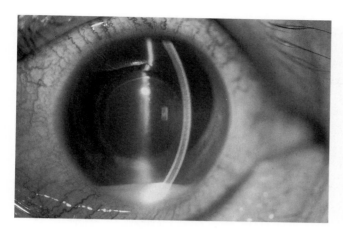

Fig. 9-3   HLA B27-related uveitis. This patient has severe anterior uveitis with hypopyon formation.

Spondyloarthropathies (Uveitis Associated with the HLA B27 Haplotype)

The juvenile spondyloarthopathies, a group of arthritides strongly associated with the HLA B27 haplotype, include ankylosing spondylitis, Reiter's syndrome, psoriatic arthritis, ulcerative colitis, and Crohn's disease. The uveitis associated with these conditions tends to be acute, recurrent, and anterior.

Ankylosing spondylitis   In ankylosing spondylitis (AS), a painful, progressive stiffening of the back occurs. Most patients present with lower back pain resulting from involvement of the sacroiliac joints or lumbosacral spine. A less common presentation is that of a pauciarticular arthritis of the knees, ankles, or heels. Children with ankylosing spondylitis are more often older boys, with a mean age of onset of 11.5 years. Ninety-four percent of children with AS are HLA B27 positive. About one quarter of affected patients develop uveitis. The episodes of iritis in AS may be severe enough to lead to formation of an anterior chamber fibrin membrane or hypopyon, and formation of posterior synechiae is common (Fig. 9-3). Vitreous cells are thought to be a result of spill over from anterior uveitis. The other main ocular manifestation of AS is conjunctivitis. Remember that in patients with suspected ankylosing spondylitis, sacroiliac joint films, rather than lumbar-sacral films should be obtained.

Reiter's syndrome   Reiter's syndrome in classically described as a triad of arthritis, urethritis, and conjunctivitis. Reiter's syndrome may follow episodes of urethritis caused by *Chlamydia* or *Ureaplasma,* but, in children, preceding gram-negative enterocolitis is more common. Both keratitis and iritis may also occur in Reiter's syndrome. The iritis may be acute or chronic and occurs in 3% to 12% of cases.

Psoriatic arthritis   Psoriatic arthritis is an HLA B27-related spondyloarthropathy characterized by the development of psoriasis and arthritis of larger joints, such as the knee. Often, the psoriasis precedes the arthritis, which has a mean onset of 11 to 12 years of age. One study found iridocyclitis in 8% of patients, with a positive ANA being a risk factor for its development.

Crohn's disease and ulcerative colitis   About 5% of patients with inflammatory bowel disease develop uveitis, typically a mild, anterior, nongraulomatous variety. Therefore patients may not be symptomatic when the uveitis is discovered. Episcleritis has also been reported in patients with inflammatory bowel disease. Severe ocular sequelae appear to be uncommon.

Herpetic Iridocyclitis

Anterior uveitis may occur in the context of both herpes simplex, as well as herpes zoster infections. The inflammation may be acute or chronic.

Herpes simplex keratouveitis   Iridocyclitis associated with herpes simplex usually accompanies stromal or disciform keratitis, although, rarely, only epithelial keratitis will be present. Sometimes, no obvious keratitis is present. Whether the uveitis results from active infection or an immune reaction is an unsettled question. Herpetic keratouveitis can cause severe pain, injection, and photophobia. The anterior chamber reaction can range in severity, and keratic precipitates, posterior synechiae, and hypopyons may form. Secondary glaucoma is an important and common complication, especially following repeated episodes of iritis. Transient elevations in IOP, which may occur secondary to trabeculitis, are treated with topical aqueous suppressants. Treatment of the iritis consists of topical antiviral agents (trifluridine, vidarabine), topical corticosteroids (prednisolone acetate, dexamethasone), systemic acyclovir, and cycloplegics. Corticosteroids are the key to suppressing inflammation in herpetic iridocyclitis, although their use may need to be delayed if active epithelial disease is present. Oral acyclovir, in addition to promoting resolution of epithelial disease, may hasten the resolution of iridocyclitis.

Herpes zoster keratouveitis   Reactivation of zoster in the V-I dermatome, causing herpes zoster ophthalmicus, is frequently accompanied by uveitis. When the nasociliary nerve is affected, indicated by involvement of the tip of the nose (*Hutchinson's sign*), uveitis is present in 50% of cases. The inflammation, which usually comes on with keratitis, can be particularly severe. It is thought to be a result of a vasculitis caused by the virus, with resultant vascular occlusion and ischemia. Hence, patchy iris stromal atrophy, sometimes with corectopia, will often be seen following zoster uveitis. The inflammation may be granulomatous or nongranulomatous; common accompanying features are keratic precipitates,

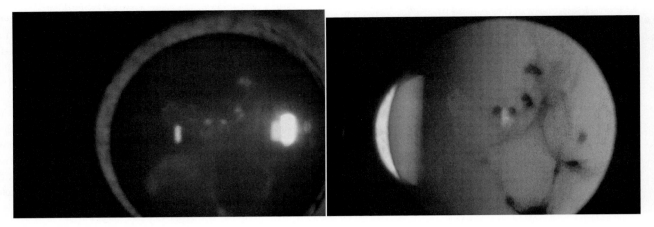

Fig. 9-4 "Snowball" opacities typical of intermediate uveitis.

posterior synechiae, hypopyon, ciliary injection, and photophobia. As in herpes simplex, glaucoma is common and can be difficult to manage. Herpes zoster is uncommon in children; therefore affected children should carefully be evaluated for a predisposing immune deficiency, such as AIDS. Patients who have undergone organ transplantation are also at risk for zoster. Acyclovir is given orally or intravenously, depending on the immune status of the child. Treatment is similar to that described previously for herpes simplex.

INTERMEDIATE UVEITIS

Clinical Features and Evaluation

Intermediate uveitis predominantly affects young adults, but at times it can affect children. The main clinical findings are inflammatory cells and "snowball opacities" in the peripheral vitreous (Fig. 9-4). It is a chronic, painless inflammation, which is bilateral in 80% of patients and curiously involves the inferior eye more than the superior structures. Its etiology is unknown.

The common presenting symptoms are floaters, and, if there is macular edema, metamorphopsia and decreased visual acuity. Pain and photophobia are uncommon. The vitreous and peripheral retinas are the sites most often affected in intermediate uveitis. Vitreous cells are always present in active disease. White or yellow aggregates, usually in the inferior, anterior pars plana, are referred to as snow banks. They are composed of inflammatory cells or masses of fibroglial tissue. In long-standing cases, neovascularization involving the vitreous base and ora serrata is often found. The retina may be involved, showing peripheral periphlebitis and macular edema. Other findings include vitreous hemorrhage, retinal detachment, band keratopathy, and glaucoma.

The clinical course of intermediate uveitis is variable, ranging from a mild and self-limited condition to a chronic and severe one, with blinding complications. The two most common complications of intermediate uveitis are cataracts, occurring in 42% of all cases, and cystoid macular edema (CME), occurring in 28% of cases. Cystoid macular edema and the associated macular degenerative changes are responsible for about three fourths of the cases of eyes with vision worse than 20/40 on long-term follow-up. However, only about 20% of patients with intermediate uveitis lose vision to that level or worse, with long-term follow-up.

Giles studied 60 patients who were diagnosed with intermediate uveitis before age 19. These patients differed from older intermediate uveitis patients in that more than two thirds had marked inflammation at the time of presentation, with photophobia, pain, redness, anterior chamber cell and flare, and keratic precipitates. Seventy percent of his patients had bilateral disease. Laboratory evaluation is generally negative, but obtaining studies to rule out sarcoidosis and Lyme disease is suggested. Conditions associated with intermediate uveitis are listed in Box 9-2.

Treatment Since the inflammation may be chronic and mild, not all patients require treatment on presentation and may be followed. Commonly suggested indications for treatment are given in (Box 9-3). Posterior sub-Tenon's corticosteroids are usually given first; topical steroids are usually not effective. Systemic steroids are a less preferred alternative because of their adverse effects and limited ability to deliver high concentrations into the eye. Multiple periocular injections are frequently needed to control the inflammation, but most eyes can be satisfactorily treated in this fashion. Cryopexy to the peripheral retina and vitreous base generally is used as the next therapeutic step; this reduces or eliminates the neovascularized and diseased tissues that sustain the inflammatory process. If cryopexy fails, vitrectomy may be employed to clear the vitreous of inflammatory debris (which may improve the macular edema) and to treat

Box 9-2   Conditions Associated with Intermediate Uveitis

Sarcoidosis	Intraocular lymphoma
Multiple sclerosis	Whipple's disease
Inflammatory bowel disease	Amyloidosis
Lyme disease	Idiopathic
Toxocariasis	

Box 9-3   Intermediate Uveitis: Treatment Indications

Visual acuity 20/40 or less
Cystoid macular edema
Severe vitreous opacity

secondary complications such as cataract and retinal detachment. Cyclosporin and methotrexate may be useful in severe cases in which the previously mentioned measures are inadequate.

POSTERIOR UVEITIS

Toxoplasmosis

Life cycle Posterior retinochoroiditis caused by toxoplasmosis accounts for 50% or more of cases of posterior uveitis is children. Toxoplasmosis is caused by the protozoan *Toxoplasma gondii,* an obligate intracellular organism for which the cat is the definitive host. Acute infections resemble influenza, with fever, lymphadenopathy, and malaise. In immunocompetent persons, the acute illness is self-limited, and rarely recognized as toxoplasmosis. However, in immunocompromised persons, such as those with AIDS, a life-threatening, multiorgan infection can ensue.

Cats are the definitive hosts of toxoplasmosis and excrete feces containing oocysts. Sheep, swine, and other livestock become infected *via* various vectors. After the animal is infected, the oocysts give rise to tachyzoites, which multiply rapidly and may invade all tissues. The tachyzoites have the ability to form tissue cysts, which, in turn, are transmitted to humans when contaminated, undercooked meats are eaten. Humans can also become infected by eating contaminated feline fecal matter or consuming contaminated produce. The tissue cysts or oocysts invade the human small intestine wall and disseminate throughout the body in the tachyzoite form. The tachyzoites are largely contained by the immune system, but some evolve into tissue cysts in muscle and neural tissue. Rupture of these cysts causes reactivation of the infection.

Except for the self-limited flulike illness, human disease rarely occurs following such an infection. This is remarkable because at least one half of the population in the United States has been infected in such a manner. For unknown reasons, ocular and CNS disease usually does not result from infections acquired postnatally. The patients who develop clinical manifestations of toxoplasmosis, retinochoroiditis in particular, are those whose mothers had a primary infection during pregnancy. Hence, late manifestations of congenital infections cause most of the clinically important sequelae in toxoplasmosis.

Clinical manifestations and diagnosis of ocular toxoplasmosis Active ocular infection presents with painless visual loss or floaters. The characteristic lesion is a round or oval, white region of retinitis. Vitreitis may be limited to the area overlying the retinitis, or the vitreous cavity may be diffusely involved. The "headlight in the fog" appearance refers to the situation in which the retinal findings are partially obscured by the vitreous haze (Fig. 9-5). Very often, the active lesions are characteristically adjacent to areas of inactive scars of healed retinitis. The inflammation often extends into the choroid, producing a retinochoroiditis. Efforts to find healed retinitis should be made during the examination as a means of supporting the diagnosis. Neuroretinitis and retinal vasculitis are less common findings. Sometimes there may be anterior spill over of the inflammatory process with cell and flare, keratic precipitates, and synechiae; such patients may experience photophobia, but the external eye generally appears white and quiet. Signs and symptoms of ocular toxoplasmosis are summarized in Box 9-4, and the severe ocular complications of toxoplasmosis are listed in Box 9-5.

The diagnosis of toxoplasmosis usually can be made clinically, with confirmation provided by laboratory studies. Serologic studies can establish or support the diagnosis; IgG and IgM anti-*T. gondii* antibodies are the most useful. The presence of IgG antibodies indicates that the patient has been infected at some time in the past; therefore toxoplasmosis is a possible etiology. However, such data cannot be used to conclude that a given case of retinochoroiditis is due to toxoplasmosis. First, the prevalence of positive titers in the general population is very high, and high titers can persist for many years following infection. And, second, ocular involvement should not be expected to elevate the serum titers appreciably. Conversely, negative titers may be taken as strong evidence that there is no toxoplasmosis infection, particularly if the test is run on undiluted serum. As mentioned previously, rarely, an acquired infection will cause ocular involvement in an immunocompetent patient. Acute infections can be confirmed by demonstrating rising titers in

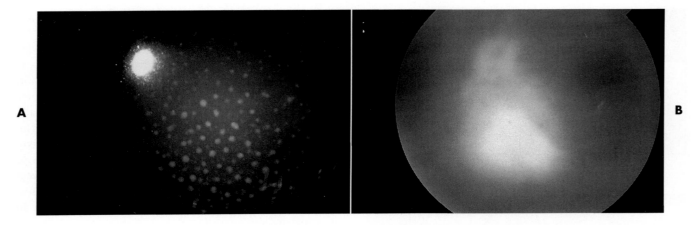

Fig. 9-5   Toxoplasmosis affecting the anterior and posterior segment in one patient. **A,** Keratic precipitates. There is a greater than usual anterior chamber reaction in this case. **B,** Peripapillary retinochoroiditis with vitreitis. See color plate.

Box 9-4   Clinical Features of Ocular Toxoplasmosis

SYMPTOMS

Floaters
Decreased vision

SIGNS

Focal retinochoroiditis
Active lesions adjacent to scars
Vitreitis (headlight in fog appearance)

LESS COMMON SIGNS

Anterior segment inflammation
Retinal vasculitis
Optic nerve inflammation

Box 9-5   Vision Threatening Complications of Toxoplasmosis

Cystoid macular edema
Cataract
Macular infection
Optic nerve involvement
Choroidal neovascularization
Vitreous opacity

Box 9-6   Suggested Indications for Treating Retinochoroiditis Caused by Toxoplasmosis

Lesions within the temporal arcades
Peripapillary lesions
Severe vitreitis
Decreased visual acuity
Persistent lesions

---

serial tests. Antibodies to *T. gondii* can be measured with the Sabin-Feldman dye test (the gold standard), the indirect fluorescent antibody (IFA) test, and the enzyme-linked immunosorbent assay (ELISA). A positive IgM antibody titer suggests, but does not prove, a recently acquired infection because these antibodies can also persist.

Treatment   Most references suggest instituting treatment in the situations indicated in Box 9-6. Such recommendations are based on the fact that the acute episodes of retinochoroiditis are generally self-limited and treatment will not prevent future attacks. Treatment regimens are listed in Box 9-7.

Systemic Congenital Toxoplasmosis

Primary infections acquired during pregnancy pose a significant risk to the developing fetus. Up to 40% of primary maternal infections during pregnancy are transmitted to the fetus. The clinical manifestations of congenital toxoplasmosis are chorioretinitis, intracranial calcifications with hydrocephalus and microcephaly, and hepatosplenomegaly with jaundice. Large, bilateral macular chorioretinal infections are characteristic of congenital toxoplasmosis. The severity varies significantly, with the greatest damage occurring with maternal infections earlier in the pregnancy. The disease is more likely to be transmitted in the latter stages of pregnancy, but with less severe sequelae. Since up to 1% of pregnant women in the United States acquire toxoplasmosis, congenital

Box 9-7 Agents Used in the Treatment of Toxoplasmosis Retinochoroiditis

- Sulfadiazine or triple sulfa
- (Sulfadiazine/sulfamerazine/sulfamethazine) *with* pyrimethamine
  [Folinic acid is given to counteract myelosuppressive effects of pyrimethamine]
  Clindamycin
- Trimethoprim-sulfamethoxazole
- Prednisone [Given concurrently with above regimens]

Note: The listed antibiotics are used in various combinations; the most efficacious regimen has not been determined.

infections are extremely common. Hence, nonimmune women should avoid exposure to cats and cat feces and should not consume undercooked meats during pregnancy.

Toxocariasis

Life cycle Toxocariasis is caused by the dog roundworm, *Toxocara canis,* which passes through the placenta to infect the developing pups. Dogs can also acquire the infection by consuming infected material. Systemic infection in humans may cause a syndrome consisting of fever, cough, malaise, seizures, and eosinophilia referred to as visceral larval migrans (VLM), but most infections do not produce symptoms. The infection is acquired when a child consumes material, typically soil, contaminated with Toxocara eggs. Once in the intestines, the ova mature, and larvae disseminate throughout the body after passing through the intestinal wall. Visceral larval migrans usually occurs in children 6 months to 3 years of age.

Toxocara canis is found throughout the world, and greater than 80% of puppies 2 to 6 months of age harbor the organism. Therefore it is not surprising that Toxocara eggs are found in 10% to 30% of soil samples taken from public playgrounds and parks. The risk factors for developing toxocariasis are exposure to dogs, particularly having puppies in the home, and pica. Ocular toxocariasis is almost never bilateral, a feature that can help differentiate it from retinoblastoma. No good explanation exists to explain the very infrequent coincidence of VLM with ocular involvement. Eighty percent of cases occur in persons 16 years of age or younger.

Clinical features and diagnosis The three primary manifestations of ocular toxocariasis are endophthalmitis, posterior pole granuloma, and peripheral granuloma.
1. *Endophthalmitis.* This presentation is more common in the younger age group (2 to 9 years of age) and

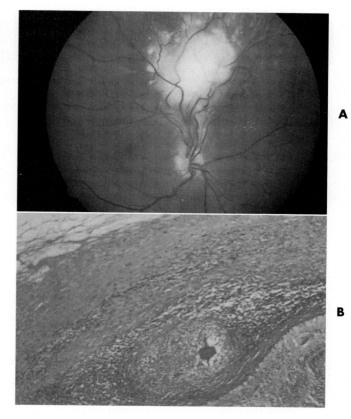

Fig. 9-6 A, Posterior granuloma of toxocariasis. **B,** Histopathology in a case of toxocariasis demonstrating inflammatory response surrounding an encysted nematode. See color plate.

comes to medical attention because of poor vision or leukocoria. A moderate or severe vitreitis exists, sometimes with an associated yellow-white retinal mass. Remarkably, the external eye remains quiet, and discomfort usually is minimal. There may be anterior chamber inflammation, with keratic precipitates, posterior synechiae, hypopyon, and other related symptoms. Severe cases may lead to the formation of a cyclitic membrane.
2. *Posterior pole granuloma.* This form is most often seen in patients 6 to 14 years of age. An elevated, white retinal lesion with overlying vitreitis is typical of this manifestation. The granulomas range in size from one-half disc diameter to four disc diameters and may result in a preretinal fibrotic membrane on resolution.
3. *Peripheral granuloma* (Fig. 9-6). Toxocara inflammatory masses in the peripheral retina tend to affect older patients. Commonly present are traction bands, and radial falciform retinal folds, which extend from the periphery to the macula or optic nerve. Traction bands result from contraction of the peripheral retinal and vitreal inflammatory mass and may cause macular heterotopia. Other, less common clinical findings in-

Table 9-2 Features that may distinguish toxocariasis from retinoblastoma

Clinical finding	Toxocariasis	Retinoblastoma
Average age of onset	7.5 years	Unilateral: 24 mo. Bilateral: 13-15 mo.
Family history	Absent	May be present
Vitreous inflammation	Common	Rare
Vitreous strands	Common	Rare
Calcification	Rare	Common
Bilateral	Very rare	Common

Box 9-8 Systemic Findings in Vogt-Koyanagi-Harada Syndrome

Headache
Meningismus
Hearing loss
Tinnitus
Alopecia
Vitiligo
Poliosis

clude papillitis, anterior segment inflammation, conjunctivitis, and peripheral keratitis.

Echographically, the lesions are solid and highly reflective. Vitreous bands and membranes, traction retinal detachments, and retinal folds may be well visualized with ultrasound.

Histopathologically, there are granulomas with eosinophilic abscesses, with plasma cells, lymphocytes, and fibroblasts. Toxocara larvae may be seen, but multiple sections are often required to find larvae. The other features of the inflammation are sufficiently characteristic to permit a pathologic diagnosis without demonstrating larvae. Other findings in histopathologically examined specimens include retinal detachment, vitreous membranes, and RPE changes.

The differential diagnosis of ocular toxocariasis includes the conditions that cause leukocoria, as well as other ocular inflammations. The important entities are retinoblastoma, Coats' disease, persistent hyperplastic primary vitreous, retinopathy of prematurity, intermediate uveitis, toxoplasmosis, endogenous endophthalmitis, and cataract. Obviously, most worrisome of the previously mentioned is retinoblastoma. Table 9-2 lists features that may differentiate toxocariasis from retinoblastoma. Although most cases of toxocariasis can be diagnosed based on clinical features, often a specific effort to rule out the possibility of retinoblastoma is required.

As stated earlier, the diagnosis of ocular toxocariasis is a clinical one, but laboratory studies can provide supportive evidence. The ELISA test on serum is the most useful; positive results for IgG antibodies at a dilution of 1:8 or greater is very suggestive in the appropriate clinical situation. Lower values must be interpreted with caution because, in certain regions, the prevalence of positive titers in unaffected children is high. Ellis, et al, found 23.1% of normal kindergarten children in a rural western North Carolina county to have positive titers at 1:32 or greater. In selected situations, ELISA tests may be performed on aqueous or vitreous samples. The pres-

ence of eosinophils in these fluids also strongly supports the diagnosis of toxocariasis. Since ocular toxocariasis and VLM are rarely present simultaneously, investigating the presence of peripheral blood eosinophilia in not warranted.

Treatment Treatment of ocular toxocariasis can be challenging. Quiet, peripheral lesions may not require treatment. Topical, periocular, and systemic corticosteroids can be effective when there is active inflammation. The role of antihelminthic agents such as thiabendazole is unclear; if utilized, steroids should be given concurrently to minimize the inflammation caused by the death of the organisms. Surgery is performed to treat vitreous membranes, retinal detachment, cyclitic membranes, cataracts, and glaucoma.

Vogt-Koyanagi-Harada Syndrome (VKH)

Vogt-Koyanagi-Harada syndrome (VKH) is a multisystem disorder of unknown etiology that can cause severe bilateral panuveitis. Young children are not typically affected; teenagers and adults are most often affected. The term *Harada's disease* is reserved for cases in which only the eyes are involved. The common systemic findings in VKH syndrome are given in Box 9-8. The highest prevalence is among Asians, Hispanics, American Indians, and blacks. In Japan, at least 8% of cases of endogenous uveitis are due to VKH.

The disease progresses through three stages. The first, or prodromal, stage, which may last only a few days, is characterized by neurologic findings such as neck stiffness, headache, hearing loss, and vertigo. At this time, many patients will have CSF pleocytosis consisting of predominantly lymphocytes and monocytes, but such findings are transient.

The next stage, the uveitic or ophthalmic stage, comes shortly after the prodrome, with a typically bilateral, granulomatous inflammation that starts posteriorly and then affects the anterior structures. Initially, only one eye may be affected, but the other becomes involved shortly thereafter. First, retinal and choroidal edema, then multifocal choroidal inflammation develops. Overlying retinal pigment epithelium (RPE) changes are present, and RPE dysfunction leads to serous retinal detach-

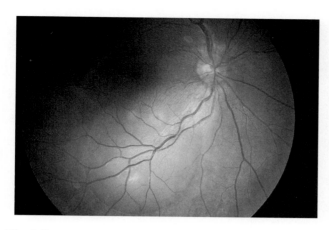

Fig. 9-7 Serous retinal detachment in a patient with Vogt-Koyanagi-Harada syndrome. See color plate.

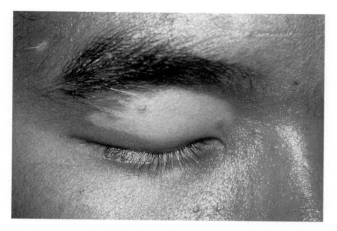

Fig. 9-8 VKH syndrome. Note vitiligo and eyelash poliosis. See color plate.

ments (Fig. 9-7). Subsequently, granulomatous anterior segment inflammation begins, with cell and flare, mutton-fat keratic precipitates, iris nodules, posterior synechiae, and edema of the iris. Angle-closure glaucoma may complicate this uveitis.

Dermatologic changes predominate the convalescent stage, which follows the uveitic stage by weeks to months. Poliosis, especially of the eyelashes, eyebrows, and scalp hair occurs, as does vitiligo (Fig. 9-8). Patients develop depigmentation of the choroid as well; this is responsible for the characteristic orange-red appearance of the fundus (sunset-glow fundus). Dalen-Fuchs nodules, which appear as small, well-circumscribed, yellow-white lesions, also develop in this stage. Sugiura's sign, perilimbal vitiligo, occurs predominantly in Japanese patients and is felt to be a highly specific sign of VKH.

Some authors refer to a fourth, or recurrent, stage that is characterized by episodes of anterior uveitis. The important long-term complications of VKH are glaucoma,

cataract, subretinal neovascular membrane formation, and optic atrophy.

The incidence of the various findings varies in VKH, depending on the race of the patient. For example, poliosis is common in Japanese patients but rare in Hispanic and white patients. As noted earlier, the etiology of VKH is unknown, but autoimmune or hypersensitivity processes are postulated. Patients with the following HLA haplotypes have been found to have an increased risk for developing VKH: HLA-DR4; HLA-B53; HLADQWa; and, HLADw53.

The diagnosis of VKH is predominantly made on clinical grounds, with supporting information from fluorescein angiography, ultrasonography, and spinal fluid analysis. The fluorescein angiographic findings are distinctive, with multiple pinpoint or placoid areas of hyperfluorescence at the RPE level early; later phases demonstrate subretinal accumulation of dye and serous retinal detachments, which may be multiple (Fig. 9-9). Echographic signs of VKH include: diffuse, low-to-medium reflective thickening of the posterior choroid; serous retinal detachments; vitreous opacity; and posterior scleral and episcleral edema. Note that these findings are not pathognomonic, and may also occur in sympathetic ophthalmia. Finally, as noted previously, if the timing of the lumbar puncture is correct, a predominantly lymphocytic pleocytosis will be present. The differential diagnosis of VKH in children includes sarcoidosis, sympathetic ophthalmia, and Lyme disease.

Systemic corticosteroids are the mainstay of treatment for VKH. Most authors recommend high systemic doses followed by a relatively slow taper. Such treatment usually leads to resolution of the serous retinal detachments. Anterior uveitis is treated with topical corticosteroids. Oral cyclosporine may be useful for its steroid-sparing effect.

Sympathetic Ophthalmia

Sympathetic ophthalmia is a bilateral granulomatous uveitis that occurs following accidental penetrating trauma or surgery to the eye. Children constitute a significant proportion of affected patients. The injured, or "exciting" eye, develops a characteristic granulomatous panuveitis, and induces an identical reaction in the fellow eye. Up to two thirds of cases follow accidental trauma. The reported incidence has varied from 0.19% to 0.7% of cases of penetrating trauma and from 0.007% to 0.015% of ophthalmic surgeries. Seventy percent of cases occur within 3 months of the injury or surgery, and 90% of cases occur within 1 year.

The early symptoms are not severe, with mild photophobia, pain, and visual loss in both eyes, although the exciting eye may harbor damage from the trauma or surgical changes. Impairment of accommodation may also

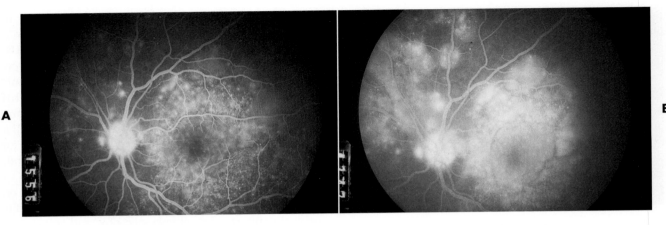

Fig. 9-9 Fluorescein angiography in a case of VKH syndrome. **A,** Early phase angiogram demonstrating multiple pinpoint areas of hyperfluorescence at the level of the RPE. **B,** A later phase displaying subretinal pooling indicating serious retinal detachment.

be an early sign. The condition progresses with worsening symptoms and granulomatous changes throughout the eyes. The anterior segment characteristically shows aqueous cell and flare, mutton-fat keratic precipitates, posterior synechiae, and so on. The posterior eye may develop multiple Dalen-Fuchs nodules, vitreitis, vascular sheathing, choroidal thickening, and disc edema. Note that Dalen-Fuchs nodules are present in only about one third of all cases of sympathetic ophthalmia and are not required to make the diagnosis. Untreated cases go on to develop iris neovascularization, cataracts, secondary glaucoma, retinal detachment, and phthisis. Rare patients have systemic findings similar to those seen in VKH, such as meningismus.

The etiology of sympathetic ophthalmia is not known. T cells predominate in the cellular infiltrate, but the inciting process is unclear. Histopathologically, there is uveal infiltration and expansion by lymphocytes, with nonnecrotizing granulomas. The choriocapillaris is typically not affected. This distinguishes it from VKH, which does involve the choriocapillaris.

Treatment consists primarily of systemic corticosteroids, and initially, high doses are given. Prolonged courses are often required. Cyclosporine may be useful as a second-line agent. Traditional teaching held that enucleation of the exciting eye after the onset of inflammation in the sympathizing eye would not improve the course. Despite the presence of some evidence to the contrary, very few would advocate the removal of an exciting eye with useful vision in an attempt to treat the sympathizing eye.

Ocular Manifestations of AIDS

The primary ocular and periocular complications of HIV infection and AIDS are Kaposi's sarcoma, microsporidial keratoconjunctivitis, molluscum contagiosum, her-

> ### MAJOR POINTS
>
> Pauciarticular juvenile rheumatoid arthritis is the most common type of JRA.
>
> Seventy-eight to 91% of patients with JRA-associated uveitis have the pauciarticular form of arthritis.
>
> In JRA-associated uveitis, cataracts occur in up to 42% of patients and glaucoma occurs in 14% to 22% of patients.
>
> Patients whose juvenile rheumatoid arthritis presents with uveitis have a worse visual prognosis than those who develop uveitis after arthritis.
>
> Anterior uveitis as a result of sarcoidosis must be distinguished from that associated with juvenile rheumatoid arthritis.
>
> The uveitis associated with the HLA-B27 haplotype tends to be an anterior uveitis that is acute and recurrent.
>
> The major causes of visual loss in intermediate uveitis are cataract and cystoid macular edema.
>
> Treatment of toxoplasmosis retinochoroiditis is suggested for lesions within the temporal arcades, lesions adjacent to the optic nerve, cases with severe vitreitis or visual loss, and persistent lesions.
>
> Toxocariasis tends to present with endophthalmitis in young patients and granulomas in older patients.
>
> Intravenous fluorescein angiography is usually diagnostic in VKH, demonstrating multiple small serous retinal detachments.

pes zoster ophthalmicus, HIV retinopathy, cytomegalovirus (CMV) retinitis, toxoplasma retinochoroiditis, and infectious multifocal choroiditis resulting from *Pneumocystis carinii, Cryptococcus neoformans,* and *Mycobacterium avium-intracellulare.* Children with AIDS are at risk for all of these complications, but the single most important one is probably CMV retinitis. It should be understood, however, that most of the available information concerning CMV retinitis in AIDS is derived from the study of adults.

CMV retinitis occurs in up to 40% of patients with AIDS, but there is evidence to suggest that this figure is significantly less in children, both in AIDS and in other immune deficiency states. The retinitis is diagnosed by its characteristic clinical appearance of retinal necrosis with intraretinal hemorrhages, often present along the temporal arcades. The lesions are well demarcated and progress by advancing along an active edge of the retinitis. Adjacent perivascular sheathing may be present. Treatment of CMV retinitis involves antiviral agents; preferred regimens continue to evolve. The primary agents include systemic ganciclovir, foscarnet, and cidofovir, and sustained-release ganciclovir implants.

SUGGESTED READINGS

Aaberg TM: The enigma of planitis, *Am J Ophthalmol* 103:828-830, 1987.

Baarsma GS, LaHey E, Glasius E, et al: The predictive value of serum angiotensin converting enzyme and lysozyme levels in the diagnosis of ocular sarcoidosis, *Am J Ophthalmol* 104:211-217, 1987.

Beniz J, Forster DJ, Lean JS, et al: Variations in clinical features of the Vogt-Koyanagi-Harada syndrome, *Retina* 11:275-280, 1991.

Chylack Jr LT, Bienfang DC, Bellows R, et al: Ocular manifestations of juvenile rheumatoid arthritis, *Am J Ophthalmol* 79:1026-1033, 1975.

Cohen KL, Peiffer Jr RL, Powell DA: Sarcoidosis and ocular disease in a young child: a case report and review of literature, *Arch Ophthalmol* 99:422-424, 1981.

Ellis Jr GS, Pakalnis VA, Worley G, et al: Toxocara canis infestation: clinical and epidemiological associations with seropositivity in kindergarten children, *Ophthalmology* 93:1032-1037, 1986.

Flynn Jr HW, Davis JL, Culbertson WW: Pars plana lensectomy and vitrectomy for complicated cataracts in juvenile rheumatoid arthritis, *Ophthalmology* 95:1114-1119, 1988.

Fox GM, Flynn Jr HW, Davis JL, et al: Causes of reduced visual acuity on long-term follow-up after cataract extraction in patients with uveitis and juvenile rheumatoid arthritis, *Am J Ophthalmol* 114:708-714, 1992.

Giles CL: Pediatric intermediate uveitis, *J Pediatr Ophthalmol Strabismus* 26:136-139, 1989.

Hagler WS, Pollard ZF, Jarrett WH, et al: Results of surgery for ocular Toxocara canis, *Ophthalmology* 88:1081-1086, 1981.

Hemady RK, Baer JC, Foster CS: Immunosuppressive drugs in the management of progressive, corticosteroid-resistant uveitis associated with juvenile rheumatoid arthritis, *Int Ophthalmol Clin* 32:241-252, 1992.

Hetherington S: Sarcoidosis in young children, *Am J Dis Child* 136:13-15, 1982.

Hofley P, Roarty J, McGinnity G, et al: Asymptomatic uveitis in children with chronic inflammatory bowel diseases, *J Pediatr Gastroenterol Nutr* 17:397-400, 1993.

Holland GN, O'Connor GR, Belfort Jr R, et al: Toxoplasmosis. In Pepose JS, Holland GN, Wilhelmus KR, editors: *Ocular infection and immunity,* St Louis, 1996, Mosby.

Hoover DL, Khan JA, Giangiacomo J: Pediatric ocular sarcoidosis, *Surv Ophthalmol* 30:215-228, 1986.

Kanski JJ, Shun-Shin GA: Systemic uveitis syndromes in childhood: an analysis of 340 cases, *Ophthalmology* 91:1247-1252, 1984.

Kanski JJ: Juvenile arthritis and uveitis, *Surv Ophthalmol* 34:253-267, 1990.

Lakhanpal V, Schocket SS, Nirankari VS: Clindamycin in the treatment of toxoplasmic retinochoroiditis, *Am J Ophthalmol* 95:605-613, 1983.

Shields JA: Ocular toxocariasis: a review, *Surv Ophthalmol* 28:361-381, 1984.

Wan WL, Cano MR, Pince KJ, et al: Echographic characteristics of ocular toxocariasis, *Ophthalmology* 98:28-32, 1991.

Weinreb RN, Tessler H: Laboratory diagnosis of ophthalmic sarcoidosis, *Surv Ophthalmol* 28:653-664, 1984.

Wolf MD, Lichter PR, Ragsdale CG: Prognostic factors in the uveitis of juvenile rheumatoid arthritis, *Ophthalmology* 94:1242-1248, 1987.

CHAPTER 10

Pediatric Retinal Disease

RETINOPATHY OF PREMATURITY

Retinopathy of prematurity (ROP), previously referred to as retrolental fibroplasia, is a retinovascular disease that affects premature babies. The earliest description of this entity came from Terry in 1942 who observed a fibroblastic proliferation posterior to the lens in premature babies. Since then, a better understanding of the natural history of ROP has emerged, as have treatments aimed at eliminating the neovascularization characteristic of advanced cases. ROP usually is not confused with other conditions but occasionally can resemble familial exudative vitreoretinopathy (FEVR). FEVR is an autosomal dominant condition characterized by incomplete peripheral retinal vascularization. Advanced ROP must also be differentiated from other entities associated with leukocoria, including Coats' disease, retinoblastoma, PHPV, and Norrie's disease.

Risk Factors

Developing retinal vessels reach the nasal ora serrata by 8 months of gestation, and reach the temporal ora shortly after the birth of full-term babies. Since ROP occurs only in the setting of immature retinal vasculature, essentially only premature babies are at risk. Furthermore, the more premature the baby, the greater the risk

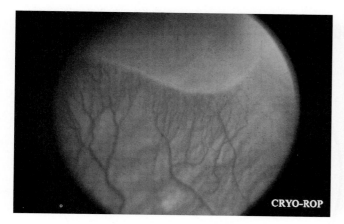

Fig. 10-1   Stage 1 retinopathy of prematurity showing demarcation line. See color plate. (Courtesy of Cryotherapy for Retinopathy of Prematurity Cooperative Group.)

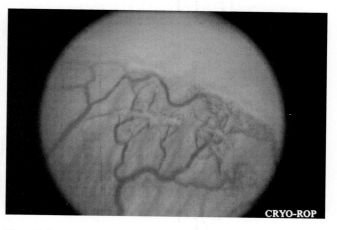

Fig. 10-2   Stage 2 retinopathy of prematurity. An elevated ridgelike structure is present. See color plate. (Courtesy of Cryotherapy for Retinopathy of Prematurity Cooperative Group.)

of developing ROP. Similarly, the lower the birthweight, the greater the risk of developing ROP. The other main risk factor is exposure to supplemental oxygen.

Pathogenesis

Although a complete understanding of the pathogenesis of ROP is not yet at hand, prematurity and exposure to supplemental oxygen are clearly the most important risk factors. High oxygen tensions are believed to cause vasoconstriction and even obliteration of the immature retinal vasculature. Presumably, angiogenic substances are then released, inducing neovascularization. The role of a variety of factors is currently under investigation. Among these, those most likely to be implicated with ROP pathogenesis are the family of the vascular endothelial growth factors (VEGFs), endothelins, and angiopoietins. An additional possible risk factor for the development of ROP is deficiency of antioxidants such as vitamin E. Neonates are susceptible to vitamin E deficiency. Studies of supplemental vitamin E have shown variable results. Exposure to the bright lighting present in neonatal units has also been proposed as a potential risk factor. However, a recent prospective, randomized, multicenter study found that early reduction of light exposure did not reduce incidence of ROP.

Clinical Features and Grading Scheme

The extent and severity in cases of ROP must be defined to determine the risk of poor visual outcome and to decide whether or not treatment is required. The International Classification of Retinopathy of Prematurity (ICROP), published in 1984, continues to be widely used. In this system, outlined in the following, the stage refers to specific characteristics and indicates the sever-

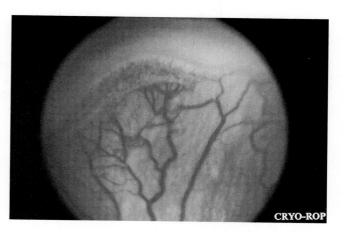

Fig. 10-3   State 3 retinopathy of prematurity demonstrating extraretinal fibrovascular proliferation. See color plate. (Courtesy of Cryotherapy for Retinopathy of Prematurity Cooperative Group.)

ity of the disease, and the zone denotes the region of the retina affected.

Normal premature retina: a region of unvascularized retina that extends posteriorly toward vascularized retina, without a distinct transition.

Stage 1: A distinct demarcation line composed of mesenchymal cells that demarcates vascularized retina from the nonvascularized periphery. The line is white and flat, and the vessels approaching it are abnormally branched (Fig. 10-1).

Stage 2: The demarcation line is now elevated, forming a white or pink ridgelike structure. Vessels may extend to the apex of the ridge, and small tufts of neovascular tissue may occur posterior to the ridge (Fig. 10-2).

Stage 3: Frank neovascularization emanating from the ridge and extending into the vitreous is present (Fig. 10-3).

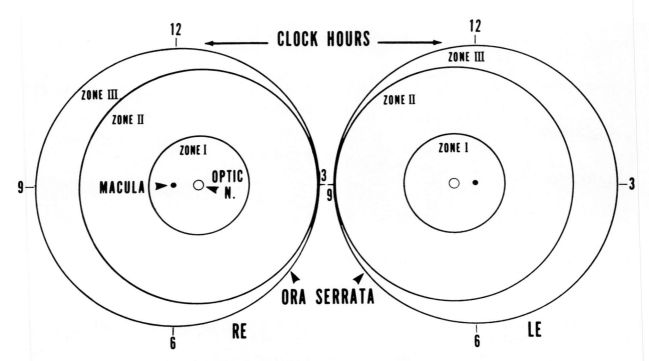

Fig. 10-4   Diagram of the retina of right eye (RE) and left eye (LE) showing zone borders and the clock hours employed to describe location and extent of retinopathy of prematurity. (From The Committee for the Classification of Retinopathy of Prematurity: *Arch Ophthalmol* 102:1130-1134, 1984.)

Stage 4: A subtotal retinal detachment is present, usually as a result of traction arising from the ridge extending anteriorly.

Stage 5: A total retinal detachment is present with retinal folds, drawing of the retina anteriorly, and development of a funnel configuration. The funnel may be open or closed.

The location of ROP is divided into three zones, which were defined by the ICROP for use in the CRYO-ROP study (Fig. 10-4 and Box 10-1).

The extent of ROP is denoted by the number of clock hours (i.e., 30-degree sectors) involved, whether contiguous or total. Treatment decisions often depend on how many clock hours are affected, covered in the following discussion. ROP at any stage may regress spontaneously for reasons that are still unknown.

CRYO-ROP Study

The CRYO-ROP study was a multicentered prospective study that provided important information regarding treatment and natural history of ROP. "High-risk" babies, those with a birthweight of less than 1251 g, were screened. The effect of cryotherapy treatment of the peripheral immature retina was compared to observation in the 291 babies who developed what was and continues to be referred to as threshold retinopathy. Threshold retinopathy was defined as the presence of at least 5 con-

---

Box 10-1   The Three Zones of ROP

ZONE 1

Refers to the region of the posterior pole that includes a circular area centered on the disc, extending for a radius of twice the distance between the disc and the fovea in all directions.

ZONE 2

Encompasses most of the remaining retina and is defined as an annular region extending from zone 1 to the ora nasally and that same distance temporally.

ZONE 3

Includes the area of temporal crescent not included in zone 2.

---

tiguous or 8 total clock hours of grade 3+ (with plus disease) retinopathy present in zones 1 or 2 (Fig. 10-5). Plus disease is defined as dilation of the posterior veins or tortuosity of the posterior arterioles (Fig. 10-6). Eyes reaching threshold were randomized to treatment or observation; if both eyes in a given patient reached threshold, only one was treated. The study evaluated the efficacy of treatment in preventing unfavorable anatomic

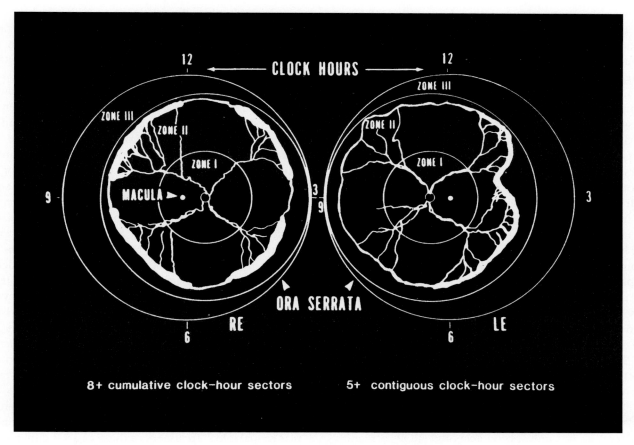

Fig. 10-5   Diagrams of two eyes that show minimum degrees of changes of threshold retinopathy. The right eye demonstrates at least eight total clock hours of stage 3 disease. The left eye shows five contiguous hours of stage 3 disease. The thin line represents stage 1 or 2 disease, and the broad line signifies stage 3 disease. (From Cryotherapy for Retinopathy of Prematurity Cooperative Group:*Arch Ophthalmol* 106:471-479, 1988.)

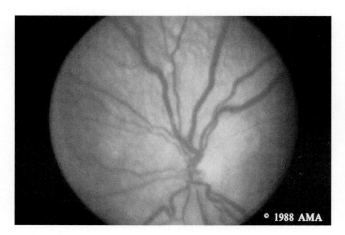

Fig. 10-6   Mild "plus" disease. In the CRYO-ROP study this was the minimum amount of tortuosity and vascular dilation required to categorize the eye as having a "plus" disease. See color plate. (Courtesy of Cryotherapy for Retinopathy of Prematurity Cooperative Group.)

outcomes (posterior retinal detachment or fold or dense retrolental mass) and functional (visual) outcomes.

After 1 year, 47.4% of the untreated eyes developed unfavorable structural outcomes, compared to 25.7% of the treated eyes. Thus cryotherapy for threshold ROP reduced the incidence of poor structural outcomes by about one half. The 5½-year follow-up found approximately the same result. Unfortunately, the outcomes in eyes with zone 1 threshold disease was poor in both groups, with 90% unfavorable outcomes in the control eyes at 1 year and 75% in the treated eyes. The 5½-year visual results showed that 47.1% of the treated eyes had a visual acuity of 20/200 (Snellen or equivalent) or worse compared to 61.7% of control eyes. Although cryotherapy clearly improved the outcome in babies with zone 2 disease, it should be clear that treatment is far from perfect. Retinopathy of prematurity is still a huge problem.

The Cryotherapy for Retinopathy of Prematurity Group reported that the incidence of any degree of retinopathy was 90% when the birthweight was less than 750 g; 78.2% when the birthweight was 750 to 999 g; and 46.9% in newborns weighing 1000 to 1250 g. Threshold retinopathy occurred in 15.5% of patients with a birthweight less than 750 g; 6.8% in those with a birthweight of 750 to 999 g; and 2% if the birthweight was 1000 to 1250 g.

Screening and Examination

There is no universally accepted ROP screening protocol. However, a nursery that accepts premature babies must adhere to a defined policy to ensure that an examination is performed on at-risk babies. The American Academy of Pediatrics and the American College of Obstetrics and Gynecology suggest that examinations be performed, at age 5 to 7 weeks, on babies born at 35 weeks gestational age or born weighing less than 1800 g, if supplemental oxygen was used. Babies delivered at 30 weeks gestational age or weighing less than 1300 g should be examined regardless of oxygen use.

Good pupillary dilation is essential, and can usually be obtained with cyclopentolate 0.2% and phenylephrine 1.0%. Remember that in neonates the concentrations used in adults can lead to systemic toxicity, such as hypertension. Indirect ophthalmoscopy is performed with the aid of a lid speculum, a small scleral depressor, and an assistant. Congestion of the iris vessels may indicate rapidly progressive ROP. The posterior pole should be viewed first, to determine whether or not plus disease is present. The scleral depressor is used to rotate the eye and to gently depress as needed. The findings are noted diagrammatically.

Treatment of ROP

Most ophthalmologists who treat babies with ROP adhere fairly closely to the treatment guidelines in the CRYO-ROP study in the timing of treatment. However, because so many of the treated eyes in the CRYO-ROP study did poorly, there continues to be growing interest in earlier treatment. Transscleral cryotherapy to the peripheral, avascular retina has been the usual therapy for ROP. It may be performed through the conjunctiva, with local or general anesthesia. Indirect ophthalmoscopy is performed to properly localize the cryoprobe and to visualize the freeze. Contiguous, nonoverlapping treatments are given, extending from the ora serrata to the anterior edge of the ridge. Cryotherapy can be quite stressful to these small babies and can cause bradycardia, cyanosis, hypoxemia, and cardiac arrest. Immediate ocular complications include conjunctival hemorrhage and chemosis and preretinal hemorrhage. Note that the neovascular ridge is not directly treated because of the associated high incidence of vitreous hemorrhage. Laser photocoagulation treatment, using an indirect ophthalmoscope delivery device, is now more commonly used than cryotherapy. Laser treatments are probably less stressful for the patients and do not require general anesthesia. Laser photocoagulation appears to be at least as effective as cryotherapy. No randomized prospective study comparing these two treatments has been performed.

About 30% of treated eyes in the CRYO-ROP study developed advanced disease (retinal detachment or macular retinal fold). Treatment of these cases is difficult and may require scleral buckling, vitrectomy, or both. Scleral buckling may be preferred in stage 4 eyes in which the macula is attached; stage 5 cases usually require vitrectomy, either using a closed system or an open-sky technique.

Complications and Findings in ROP

Eyes with spontaneously regressed ROP have a greater incidence of myopia, astigmatism, anisometropia, amblyopia, and strabismus. Eyes with advanced ROP, even if treated, are prone to a variety of additional severe complications, including angle-closure glaucoma, late retinal detachments, high myopia, and visual field loss.

COATS' DISEASE

Coats' disease is a disorder of the retinal vasculature characterized by exudation from defective, telangiectatic vessels. It is nonhereditary, unilateral in about 80% of cases and three times more common in boys than in girls. Two thirds of cases present in the first decade.

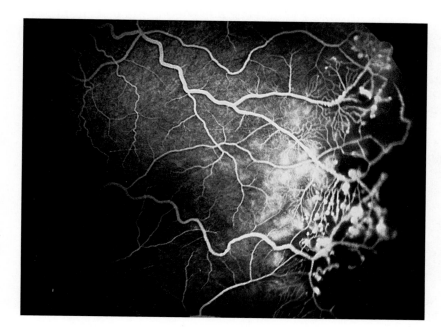

Fig. 10-7   Fluorescein angiogram of a patient with Coats' disease. Note telangiectasia and vascular nonperfusion.

Clinical presentation varies, depending on the severity of the condition. As in retinoblastoma, leukocoria and strabismus are common early signs. Externally, the eyes appear quiet. Typically, early cases show retinal vascular telangiectasias and aneurysms, with subretinal exudate. In the usual case, the abnormal vessels are in the retinal periphery, but the exudate forms some distance from these vessels, in the posterior pole. Intraretinal and vitreal hemorrhages also may be present. The process may fill the eye, with exudative retinal detachment and cholesterol precipitation or be mild and found incidentally. Fluorescein angiography demonstrates the vascular abnormalities nicely, which include leakage and nonperfusion of the surrounding retina (Fig. 10-7). Coats' disease is progressive if untreated. The goal of treatment is to eliminate the vascular exudation. Anterior telangiectatic lesions may be treated with cryoablation and more posterior ones with argon laser photocoagulation using an indirect delivery system. Multiple treatments may be needed, as new lesions may develop. Advanced Coats' disease must be differentiated from retinoblastoma and toxocariasis.

RETINOBLASTOMA

Retinoblastoma is the most common intraocular malignancy of childhood. The most recent estimate of its incidence is 1 per 20,000 live births. Worldwide, the yearly incidence is about 11 per one million children under the age of 5 years. About 5% of childhood blindness is due to retinoblastoma. Untreated, retinoblastoma is almost always lethal. Significant advances have been made in recent years in the treatment of the cancer, and survival rates in patients with retinoblastoma are now greater than 90%. About 1% of deaths from cancer in children younger than 16 years old is attributable to retinoblastoma. Optimal management requires a multispecialty team, consisting of ophthalmologists, oncologists, and radiation oncologists. One of the most important obstacles to successful management of retinoblastoma is that it is too often discovered at an advanced stage.

Clinical Features and Manifestations

On presentation, about 60% of cases of retinoblastoma are unilateral and 40% are bilateral. Children with bilateral involvement have germinal mutations; the average age of presentation is 13 to 15 months. Those with unilateral cases are older at presentation, with an average age of 24 months. Females and males are affected at the same rate. Most cases confined to the eye are painless and do not bother the young patients at all. The most common presenting signs of retinoblastoma are leukocoria (Fig. 10-8) and, in the case of macular lesions, strabismus. The third most common presenting sign is intraocular inflammation, which may cause ciliary injection, pseudohypopyon, secondary glaucoma, and so on. Younger patients tend to develop tumors in the posterior pole, compared to the retinal periphery. Other presenting signs are listed in Box 10-2. It is remarkable how often a parent will notice the white or asymmetric pupillary reflex, either in dim illumination or in photographs, which brings the problem to medical attention.

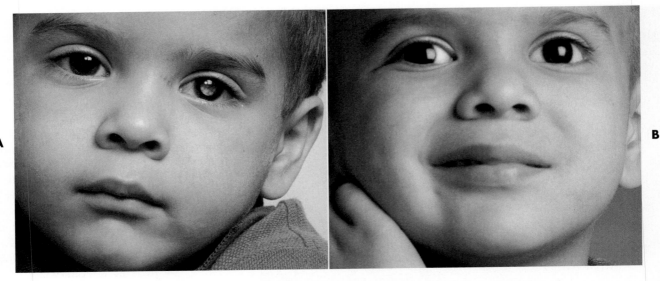

Fig. 10-8   A, Retinoblastoma. Note leukocoria. **B,** Same patient following enucleation with ocular prosthesis. See color plate. (Courtesy of Dr. Barrett Haik.)

Box 10-2   Presenting Signs in Retinoblastoma

Leukocoria (white reflex) (most common)
Strabismus
Inflammation
Positive family history
Glaucoma
Hyphema
Preseptal cellulitis
Nystagmus
Routine examination (rare)

Of course, it is the responsibility of the primary care physician to understand the importance of this sign and immediately refer the child to the ophthalmologist.

Often, retinoblastoma may be diagnosed, with good certainty, solely on its clinical appearance. A classic appearance is the presence of one or multiple white to cream nodular masses, often with associated vascularization. The vitreous may be clear or diffusely hazy resulting from microscopic tumor seeding, or display larger aggregates. The two primary clinical patterns of growth of retinoblastoma are referred to as endophytic and exophytic. Endophytic tumors grow forward into the vitreous, and may fill the vitreous. Associated vitreous seeding is common, with resulting anterior chamber involvement, inflammation, and glaucoma. Exophytic tumors grow subretinally and cause retinal detachment. Extension to the choroid may occur. Rarely, older patients (average age, 6.1 years) will show a third growth pattern, in which a posterior tumor diffusely infiltrates, without developing discrete masses. Small retinoblastoma lesions may be encountered when screening a family member of an affected patient or when examining patients with asymmetric, bilateral disease. Such tumors appear as barely perceptible, nearly transparent, slightly elevated, circular lesions. They have no feeder vessels and resemble early lesions of tuberous sclerosis. As they grow, they become more opaque and more vascularized.

Differential Diagnosis

Most ophthalmologists can easily recite the differential diagnosis of retinoblastoma, listed in Box 10-3; this is the same list of causes of leukocoria. However, on initial inspection, the ophthalmologist usually can narrow down the possibilities significantly. One point that is often brought up concerns the microphthalmic eye. Leukocoria in a small eye suggests congenital cataract or persistent hyperplastic primary vitreous (PHPV, also known as persistence of the fetal vasculature) rather than retinoblastoma. Bilateral involvement, not caused by cataracts, strongly suggests retinoblastoma, whereas PHPV is usually unilateral.

Overall, the entities that present the greatest challenge for the ophthalmologist to differentiate from retinoblastoma are PHPV, toxocariasis, and Coats' disease. Certain aspects of diagnosis deserve mentioning. First, differentiating advanced cases of Coats' disease from retinoblastoma can be challenging. Like retinoblastoma, Coats' disease may fill a quiet eye with a mass of material associated with neovascularization. However, in Coats' disease, the color of the exudate is more yellow than

Box 10-3   Differential Diagnosis of Leukocoria

Retinoblastoma
Persistent hyperplastic primary vitreous (PHPV)
Cataract
Retinopathy of prematurity
Toxocariasis
Coloboma of choroid
Uveitis
Coats' disease
Vitreous hemorrhage
Retinal dysplasia
Tumors other than retinoblastoma
Retinal detachment
Corneal opacity
Myelinated nerve fibers

white, as a result of the presence of cholesterol. Second, ultrasonography and computed tomography (CT) scanning are important tools in the evaluation of suspected cases of retinoblastoma because of their ability to demonstrate calcification. The presence of intraocular calcium in suspected cases strongly supports the diagnosis of retinoblastoma and argues against other disorders such as Coats' disease, toxocariasis, and persistent hyperplastic primary vitreous. Ultrasound and CT scanning can delineate intraocular structures and assist in diagnosing PHPV.

Inheritance

As noted previously, about 60% of cases of retinoblastoma are unilateral. Such cases are usually, but not always, sporadic and nonhereditary. This means that the mutational events that led to the development of the retinoblastoma (see the following discussion) occurred only in a single retinal cell and not in that patient's germ cells. Consequently, the children of such a patient (without a germinal mutation) have no increased risk of developing retinoblastoma because the affected patient does not transmit a mutation to their offspring.

About 40% of new cases are bilateral, and such cases come about in one of two ways. First, more commonly, mutational events occur in the very young embryo and are subsequently carried within all of the patient's cells. Second, in about 10% of the bilateral cases, the heterozygous germinal mutation is transmitted from an affected parent. The result of either of these situations is that all of the child's cells have one normal retinoblastoma (Rb) gene and one abnormal one. The children of such patients will have a high risk of developing retinoblastoma, as outlined in the following.

The previous description must be viewed in the context of the Knudson's visionary two-hit hypothesis, which correctly predicted that two mutational events would be required for the tumor to develop. The Rb gene is a tumor-suppressing gene found on chromosome 13q14. This gene, identified in 1986, was the first gene known to act as a tumor suppressor. The normal gene product is a 105 kD nuclear phosphoprotein, which can bind to DNA and which may regulate the expression of other genes. It contains two alleles; a mutation in one allele causes no known clinical disease, but loss of the suppressing function of both alleles leads to the development of retinoblastoma. Sporadic cases occur because, by chance, two independent mutations occur in the same retinal cell. Since such coincidences are uncommon, the affected patients tend to be older and the tumors tend to form in isolation. In hereditary cases, all of the patient's retinal cells harbor one faulty allele; the second hit (or the second hits) occur because the rate of such spontaneous mutations is about one per one million developing retinal cells. Hence, affected patients are younger, have multiple tumors, and have both eyes involved in 85% of cases. In hereditary cases, the tendency to develop retinoblastoma is transmitted as an autosomal dominant trait with high penetrance. However, both copies of the Rb gene have to be inactivated to cause disease, which is an autosomal recessive process at the cellular level.

Of all new cases of retinoblastoma, only about 6% have a positive family history. However, of all the patients with heritable disease, only 25% have a positive family history. This means that the remainder of heritable cases (young, bilateral, and multifocal) occurred either as de novo germinal mutations, or less commonly, as mutations transmitted from an unaffected carrier parent. Hereditary retinoblastoma is 90% penetrant; hence, 10% of individuals who carry one mutation do not develop retinoblastoma, but their offspring are at high risk for developing retinoblastoma. Furthermore, not all cases of unilateral retinoblastoma are the nonheritable type. Indeed, about 15% of unilateral cases occur in patients who harbor germ-line mutations, but simply did not develop tumors in both eyes, even though each retinal cell contained one faulty allele. Consequently, the clinical finding of a unilateral tumor cannot be used to conclude that the mutation is nonheritable.

In summary, unilateral cases tend to be sporadic and nonheritable and bilateral cases (or unilateral cases with multiple tumors) tend to be heritable. However, family counseling must take into account incomplete penetrance, the presence of a carrier state, and the fact that not all persons with germ-line mutations get bilateral tumors. Data concerning the risk to subsequent family members for the development of retinoblastoma are presented in Table 10-1.

Table 10-1 Empiric recurrence risk in retinoblastoma

Family history	Frequency	Frequency (unilateral vs bilateral)	Phenotype	Mutation (somatic vs germline)	Genetics	Empiric risk for siblings	Empiric risk for offspring
Sporadic	90%	Unilateral 60%	Unilateral	85% Somatic 15% New germline	Nonhereditary 56%	<1%	1%-5%
		Bilateral 40%	Bilateral	New germline	Hereditary 44%	~2%	45%
Familial	10%		Bilateral or unilateral	Transmitted germline		45%	45%

From Murphee AL: *Ophthalmol Clin North Am* 8:156, 1995.

Box 10-4 Reese-Ellsworth Classification

GROUP 1: VERY FAVORABLE

A. Solitary tumor less than 4 disc diameter (DD) in size, at or behind equator.
B. Multiple tumors, none over 4 DD in size, all at or behind equator.

GROUP 2: FAVORABLE

A. Solitary tumor, 4 to 10 DD in size, at or behind equator.
B. Multiple tumors, 4 to 10 DD in size, behind equator.

GROUP 3: DOUBTFUL

A. Any tumor anterior to equator.
B. Solitary tumor, larger than 10 DD, behind equator.

GROUP 4: UNFAVORABLE

A. Multiple tumors, some larger than 10 DD in size.
B. Any lesion extending anteriorly to the ora serrata.

GROUP 5: VERY UNFAVORABLE

A. Massive tumors involving over half the retina.
B. Vitreous seeding.

Staging

The Reese-Ellsworth classification (Box 10-4), developed in the 1950s, was intended to estimate the visual prognosis in affected eyes and not, as some have used the classification, to estimate mortality risks. Since the primary modes of treatment at that time, other than enucleation, were external beam radiation and cryopexy, the prognosis assigned to these groups is worse than is currently the case. However, precise anatomic classification is valuable because it guides treatment decisions and provides uniformity for research and statistical purposes.

Eyes with large or multiple tumors and with extensive vitreous seeding have the poorest prognosis.

Pathology and Natural History

Histopathologically, retinoblastoma cells are small and stain blue with hematoxylin and eosin (H&E). Flexner-Wintersteiner rosettes, characteristic but not required to make the diagnosis, appear as a ring of cells forming as lumen. Fleurettes are formed by cells undergoing photoreceptor differentiation. Necrosis is extremely common and occurs as the tumor outgrows its blood supply. Necrotic areas appear pink with H&E. Finally, as noted previously, calcification is very common. In eyes enucleated for retinoblastoma, the main questions that must be answered are (1) is the cut end of the optic nerve free from tumor; (2) is the choroid involved or spared; and (3) is there any other evidence of extraocular tumor extension? Clearly, if any of the above findings are present, the likelihood of the disease being fatal are greatly increased.

Untreated, retinoblastomas tend to grow relentlessly, and fill the eye with tumor. The eye becomes inflamed and painful, with the appearance resembling endophthalmitis. Further progression leads to extraocular disease, producing a picture that can be confused with preseptal or orbital cellulitis. Direct extension along the optic nerve will involve the brain with tumor. Hematogenous metastases preferentially involve bone and marrow. The pineal gland may be affected by tumor, forming the so-called trilateral retinoblastoma. Such tumors arise in the pineal and may lead to obstructive hydrocephalus. Tumors felt to be spontaneously regressed retinoblastomas are rarely seen.

Evaluating the Patient Suspected of Having Retinoblastoma

As noted earlier, imaging is a key step in the evaluation of patients with retinoblastoma. CT scanning and, sometimes, ultrasonography are performed, primarily to determine whether calcium is present. We also obtain magnetic resonance imaging (MRI) scans of the brain and orbits on all patients, primarily to assess the presence of macroscopic optic nerve extension. Not all practitioners feel the routine MRI scanning is required. The pineal is also imaged. In cases in which extraocular extension is suspected, evaluation of the spinal fluid and bone marrow is performed. However, if the retinoblastoma appears confined to the eye, no further laboratory testing is required. Direct tumor biopsy may be performed in highly unusual cases (if there is visual potential), but this is risky due to the chance of seeding the tumor outside the eye. Most authorities no longer measure aqueous level of lactate dehydrogenase. In many cases, examination under anesthesia may be required to adequately inspect the patient for the purpose of diagnosis and clinical staging.

Treatment

The treatment of retinoblastoma is rapidly changing and significant advances are being made because of the use of effective systemic chemotherapeutic agents, in addition to more conventional methods. It should be kept in mind that the specific agents used continue to evolve, and treatment protocols differ from center to center. Which treatments are implemented depend on the stage of the tumor, whether it is bilateral or unilateral and, to a certain extent, the wishes of the parents. Currently, the available treatment modalities include external beam irradiation, systemic chemotherapy, enucleation, retinal cryopexy, laser photocoagulation and hyperthermia, and plaque irradiation.

Although treatment decisions are made on an individual basis, certain general guidelines can be made. Patients with one unaffected eye and one eye harboring a large tumor, without reasonable prospect for useful vision in that eye, usually undergo enucleation of the affected eye. Other indications for enucleation include associated total retinal detachment, iris or ciliary body involvement, and extensive vitreous seeding. In monocular cases with smaller tumors, the options include treatment with external beam irradiation, plaque radiotherapy, and systemic chemotherapy with or without local measures. By the time most monocular cases are diagnosed, the tumor or tumors are too large to be treated with laser or cryoablation as the primary modality. However, when patients with positive family histories are screened, very small tumors may be discovered, and these tumors may be amenable to photocoagulation or cryoablation. Bilateral cases with advanced disease (Reese-Ellsworth stage V) have traditionally been treated with external beam irradiation to both eyes or enucleation of the more severely affected eye and external

beam irradiation to the remaining eye. Such treatment typically consists of a total of 3500 to 4000 cGy given over the course of 3 to 4 weeks. Unfortunately, this treatment has severe complications, which are listed in Box 10-5. Chemotherapy and radiation are used in cases of orbital extension.

A genuine revolution in retinoblastoma treatment has occurred within the past few years with the use of systemic chemotherapeutics that have the ability to penetrate the globe. Such treatment may be useful in unilateral and bilateral cases and often is performed in concert with other focal modalities. The commonly used agents include carboplatin, etoposide, and vincristine, given according to various protocols. Therapy utilizing these agents, overall, appears to improve treatment results and can avoid the disfiguring consequences of external beam irradiation. However, the usual immediate side effects of chemotherapy do occur, and no long-term information concerning efficacy exists. Alkylating agents may be associated with an increased incidence of secondary malignancies, such as leukemia, and with infertility.

Tumor Regression Patterns

Three ophthalmoscopically visible patterns of tumor regression have been described. In type 1 regression, tumor necrosis occurs, resulting in a white, calcific mass resembling cottage cheese. In type 2 regression, the tumor shrinks and takes on a translucent appearance resembling fish flesh. It is difficult to distinguish such tumors from viable ones, and it is important to carefully document the size and number of each tumor during each examination. Type 3 regression is a combination of types 1 and 2.

Prognosis and Follow-up Care

In large part, the prognosis for life in retinoblastoma is related to posterior extension of the tumor. Patients who undergo enucleation and have tumor cells at the cut end of the optic nerve have approximately an 80% mortality rate. If the tumor is found to involve the lamina cribrosa, even without involvement of the transected optic nerve, the mortality rate is about 40%. With tumors confined to the globe when enucleated, the survival rate is greater than 90%. Preservation of vision depends on the size and location of the tumor. In one study of children with bilateral disease undergoing conservative treatment, 50% demonstrated a visual acuity of 20/40 or better in at least one eye at 8 years of age.

Patients with hereditary tumors lack an allele of a tumor suppressor gene in all their cells and therefore are at an increased lifetime risk for developing a variety of cancers throughout the body. Osteosarcoma is the most common secondary tumor, followed by melanoma, fibrosarcoma, and pineal tumors. Patients who have received radiation are at a significantly higher risk for secondary tumors, especially osteosarcomas, in the field of treatment.

About 15% of patients with monocular involvement harbor a germ-line mutation. These patients may develop involvement of the fellow eye, especially in the first 2 years of life. Since it is usually not known if a patient with a monocular tumor has a germ-line mutation, complete retinal examinations of the unaffected eye, typically under anesthesia, are required. One recommended schedule calls for examinations every 3 to 6 months until age 2 to 3 years, followed by awake examinations thereafter. Offspring of a patient with unilateral or bilateral retinoblastoma and siblings of an affected patient also require regular screening examinations.

Molecular genetic techniques may be used to determine whether or not a patient with a unilateral tumor, or a parent of a patient with retinoblastoma, harbors the Rb gene, but such testing is not yet in wide use. This information would be of obvious value in family planning and assessing the risk for secondary tumors. Most of the mutations are small and cannot be identified with conventional karyotyping. The commonly used techniques are Southern blotting, restriction fragment length polymorphism analysis, and single strand conformational polymorphism.

RETINAL HEMORRHAGES (SHAKEN BABY SYNDROME)

Injury in the shaken baby syndrome occurs when violent acceleration/deceleration causes ocular and intracranial hemorrhages in a child up to 3 years of age. The most common ocular findings are intraretinal and preretinal hemorrhages (Fig. 10-9). Severity of the ocular injury varies greatly, and a victim of shaking may have no hemorrhage or near confluent hemorrhages. Findings that may be seen on ophthalmoscopy are listed in Box 10-6.

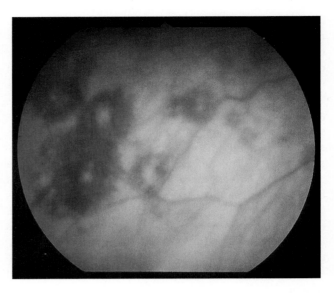

Fig. 10-9   Shaken baby syndrome. Note multiple white-centered intraretinal hemorrhages. See color plate.

Box 10-6   Shaken Baby Syndrome: Ophthalmoscopic Findings

Intraretinal and preretinal hemorrhages
Retinal detachment
Circular perimacular retinal folds
Peripheral retinoschisis
Optic nerve hemorrhage

It is thought that the rapid acceleration and deceleration of the infant or young child's eye leads to tearing of retinal vessels. Young children are predisposed because they have very strong vitreoretinal adhesions, and relatively poor muscular control of the head. Additional ocular manifestations in battered children include subconjunctival hemorrhage, lid ecchymoses, and lens subluxation. A comprehensive and systematic evaluation of a child suspected of being abused is undertaken, typically including a skeletal survey and careful scrutiny of the child's social situation. Violent shaking also causes brain injuries. Such injuries are also thought to result from rapid acceleration and deceleration, with resultant tearing of bridging blood vessels, as well as contusive injury to the parenchyma.

As an isolated finding, the presence of retinal hemorrhage is highly suggestive of shaken baby syndrome but is not diagnostic. Retinal hemorrhages occur following normal childbirth, but they are faint and resolve by 3 to 4 weeks of age. Retinal hemorrhages may occur (rarely) following CPR, as well as in leukemia, bacterial endocarditis, and idiopathic thrombocytopenia.

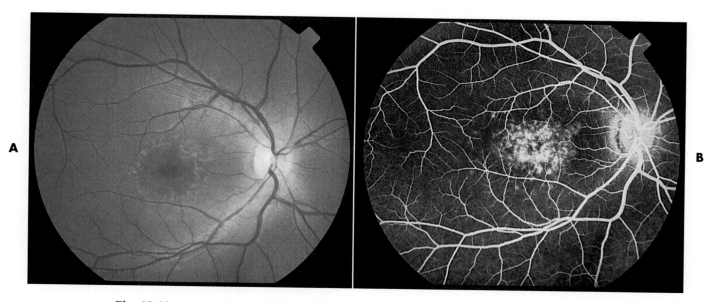

Fig. 10-10   **A,** Fundus pigmentary changes in Stargardt's disease. **B,** Fluorescein angiogram of same patient.

STARGARDT'S DISEASE (FUNDUS FLAVIMACULATUS)

Stargardt's disease is an uncommon, bilateral, progressive maculopathy that appears during the first three decades. It is usually inherited in an autosomal recessive pattern, and a history of consanguinity can sometimes be obtained, although autosomal dominant forms have been described. Early symptoms include bilateral, painless, decreased central vision. Although more frequently symmetric, more severe visual loss in one eye in the early stages of the disease is not uncommon. Often, there is a history that the vision was normal previously. Initially, the fundus may appear entirely normal, and early cases may be mistaken for feigned or nonorganic visual loss. Eventually, however, yellow flecks appear perifoveally, in the periphery, or both. Progressive macular atrophy, with or without pigmentary clumping, is the most common typical end-stage finding (Fig. 10-10). Widespread geographic atrophy may develop, leading to the characteristic "beaten bronze" fundus appearance. However, the clinical appearance does not always mirror the visual function, since some patients with typical findings can retain good vision. Fundus flavimaculatus (FF) is the term usually reserved for cases in which peripheral pisciform flecks predominate.

Most autosomal recessive cases of Stargardt's disease and FF should be considered allelic diseases, that is, different manifestations of distinct mutations of the same gene. In fact, one gene located on chromosome 1, known as ABCR or STGD1, has been recently identified. This gene is expressed in rod outer segments. Compound heterozygote ABCR gene mutations have been

identified both in patients with Stargardt's maculopathy and FF. In other words, different levels of activity yielded by the various mutations of the same gene appear to cause distinct phenotypes. Another locus associated with Stargardt's disease is localized on chromosome 6.

Most often, the vision falls to the level of legal blindness. A relative or absolute central scotoma is present, but the extent of the peripheral visual fields is preserved. A red-green color defect may be present early. The most useful laboratory test in establishing the diagnosis of Stargardt's disease is the fluorescein angiogram. The classic finding, present in 50% to 80% of cases, is the *"dark"* or *"silent" choroid*, whereas the retinal vessels fill normally, but the choroidal fluorescence is absent or attenuated. Presumably, this is due to blocking by the RPE engorged with large amounts of lipofuscin. Electroretinographic testing is less valuable in diagnosing Stargardt's disease, because it is most often normal or mildly abnormal. But, severe ERG amplitude reduction argues against the diagnosis of Stargardt's disease, and suggests a cone or a cone-rod dystrophy. The electro-oculogram is often subnormal. The pathophysiology of Stargardt's disease remains unknown. The primary differential diagnoses include cone dystrophy, pattern dystrophy, dominant optic atrophy, and juvenile ceroid lipofuscinosis. No specific medical treatment exists.

BEST'S DISEASE (VITELLIFORM MACULAR DYSTROPHY)

Best's disease is a rare, usually bilateral, autosomal dominant maculopathy, that displays variable expressivity; therefore, although the average age of onset is 6 years, it may not be detected until much later. The predominant symptom is the painless, gradual loss of acuity, but this may be accompanied by paracentral scotomas and metamorphopsia. The appearance of the macular lesions in Best's disease is described as evolving through four stages. Initially, the normal appearing fundus is called "previtelliform." This is followed, usually in early childhood, by the second or vitelliform stage in which a yellow "egg yolk" lesion develops in the macula. This striking lesion appears yellow, homogeneous, opaque, and elevated, with sharply delineated margins. Later, this evolves into a stage 3 lesion, in which a fluid layer appears, creating a "pseudohypopyon." Stage 4 lesions show atrophic macular pigmentation and may also have scarring and subretinal neovascularization. This stage may be associated with poor vision. There has been no histopathologic study of an eye with an early vitelliform lesion, but it is likely that the yellow material is lipofuscin beneath the RPE. This is consistent with the good vision that can be seen in patients with ophthalmoscopically striking lesions. Eyes with more advanced stages have shown lipofuscin in the sub-RPE space and within RPE cells.

The electro-oculogram is the best test to confirm the diagnosis of Best's disease, giving Arden ratios less than 1.5 in affected patients, even very early in the course. The diagnosis should be questioned if the EOG is normal. The full-field flash ERG remains normal, whereas abnormal focal ERGs responses have been documented. In most cases, patients retain vision as good as 20/30 to 20/50. The etiology of Best's disease is unknown, but genes on chromosome 11 and 8 have been shown to cause a vitelliform-type disease. Pseudo-vitelliform lesions have been observed in families harboring mutations of the peripherin/RDS gene, implicated in various forms of retinitis pigmentosa and pattern dystrophies of the macula. Because of the potentially worse prognosis associated with this latter genotype, this condition needs to be differentiated from true Best's disease. There is no known treatment.

RETINITIS PIGMENTOSA

Symptoms and Clinical Features

Retinitis pigmentosa (RP) comprises a group of retinal disorders characterized by poor night vision, reduced peripheral vision, predominantly rod photoreceptor degeneration, and peripheral bone spicule pigmentary changes. Different hereditary patterns occur, and new causative molecular defects continue to be identified; thus it should not be surprising that the clinical manifestations vary widely. It is hoped that further characterization of specific molecular defects will pave the way for trials of specific treatments. In the United States the incidence of RP is approximately 1 in 3700 people. Most of

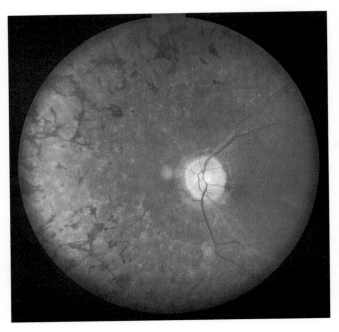

Fig. 10-11   Retinitis pigmentosa. Note bone spicule pigmentation and marked vascular attenuation. See color plate. (Courtesy of Dr. Alessandro Iannaccone.)

these patients, 71% to 84%, have either autosomal recessive disease or are sporadic, "simplex" cases (which may include de novo dominant mutations). Between 10% and 20% of cases are autosomal dominant and 6% to 9% are X-linked. In the United States about 35% of new cases have no family history.

Although the age of onset will vary, depending on the specific type of RP, the most important early features are nyctalopia and visual field constriction. The classic fundus finding is retinal bone spicule-like pigmentation, caused by pigmentary migration along retinal vessels. Other posterior pole findings include variable degrees of retinal vascular narrowing, waxy pallor of the optic disc, RPE atrophy, cystoid macular edema, and, occasionally, optic disc drusen (Fig. 10-11). Vitreous cells and posterior subcapsular cataracts are also common. The degree of central acuity loss is variable, and excellent acuity is often retained even in cases of severe peripheral field loss. Color vision is usually good until late in the course of the disease. Visual acuity may subsequently decrease as a result of degenerative changes or cystoid macular edema. The latter may respond to systematically administered carbonic anhydrase inhibitors. Many patients with X-linked RP are highly myopic. In general the autosomal dominant type is the least severe and the recessive types (both autosomal and X-linked) the most severe.

Types of Retinitis Pigmentosa

The ability to correctly identify the inheritance pattern of heredity for a given patient will provide useful

Box 10-7 Autosomal Recessive Retinitis Pigmentosa Syndromes

Usher's syndrome
Bardet-Biedl syndrome
Laurence-Moon syndrome
Refsum's disease

prognostic information. *Autosomal dominant RP* accounts for 10% to 20% of cases of RP. The most common forms of autosomal dominant RP in North America tend to be less severe and have a later onset than the autosomal recessive and X-linked types, although more severe subtypes of autosomal dominant RP exist. Mutations in rhodopsin, peripherin/RDS, and other proteins have been identified.

Autosomal recessive RP is probably the most common type, but often it is difficult to establish this pattern of heredity, and many patients who are labeled as "simplex" surely have autosomal recessive RP. Patients with autosomal recessive RP differ from those with autosomal dominant disease in that up to 40% of the AR patients have associated systemic disease, including 18% with deafness or hearing loss. Specific RP syndromes are covered in the following. Box 10-7 lists the autosomal recessive RP syndromes.

X-linked recessive RP is the rarest and the most severe type of typical RP and causes visual loss to the level of legal blindness by age 30. Affected patients tend to be more myopic and have greater degrees of astigmatism than other RP patients. Also, they are more likely to have early macular involvement. Carriers of X-linked recessive RP most often demonstrate patchy retinal pigmentary changes (Fig. 10-12). The degree of involvement from patient to patient varies widely. Most carriers are asymptomatic but have mildly decreased ERG amplitudes.

Usher's syndrome is an autosomal recessive condition characterized by the association of congenital hearing loss of variable severity and retinitis pigmentosa. It is the most common syndrome in which RP and another defect coexist. About one half of persons in the United States who are both deaf and blind have Usher's syndrome. On clinical grounds, the two primary types of Usher's syndrome are designated as type 1 and type 2. Type 1 Usher's syndrome is characterized by progressive visual loss from childhood or adolescence, with worsening visual fields, ERGs, and dark adaptation. By age 40, severe visual loss is expected. Hearing loss is most often profound, and speech barely intelligible. Associated features include absent vestibular reflexes and, occasionally, ataxia. Several distinct chromosomal loci associated with type 1 Usher syndrome have been identified. Mutations in the myosin VIIA gene were recently reported in a sub-

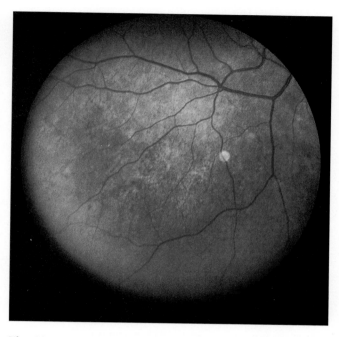

Fig. 10-12 Carrier of X-linked retinitis pigmentosa showing patchy retinal pigmentary changes. See color plate. (Courtesy of Dr. Alessandro Iannaccone.)

set of type 1 patients. The product of this gene is expressed in the inner ear, in the RPE and in the photoreceptors. Type 2 Usher syndrome is somewhat milder and has a later onset. These patients have milder hearing loss and therefore have intelligible speech. Visual problems come on in the later teen years and there is no vestibular dysfunction. Genetic heterogeneity also has been documented for type 2 Usher's syndrome.

In *Bardet-Biedl syndrome*, retinitis pigmentosa is accompanied by congenital obesity and dystrophic extremities (polydactyly, syndactyly or brachydactyly of the hands and feet). Renal disease is an additional feature present in most patients. Dental abnormalities are also frequent, as is hypogenitalism, especially in males (in whom cryptorchidism often coexists). Mental retardation, another reportedly cardinal feature of the syndrome, is often absent. Incomplete presentations are very common. Since extra digits are typically removed surgically in infancy, the parents must be specifically questioned about polydactyly when the diagnosis is being considered. Careful examination may reveal fine linear scars on the ulnar aspect of the hands as the only sign of such surgery. The retinal degeneration is not a typical RP in that hyperpigmentation is not a prominent feature; rather, the clinician finds coarse granularity of the periphery. Atrophic macular lesions and optic nerve atrophy are common, and loss of acuity occurs early in the disease. Severe visual loss occurs by middle age. Electroretinography typically reveals usually early, severe rod and cone dysfunction. Inheritance is autosomal recessive, and at least five distinct chromosomal loci linked to

Bardet-Biedl syndrome have been found. Causal genes have yet to be identified. *Laurence-Moon syndrome* differs from Bardet-Biedl syndrome in that in the former, there is no obesity or polydactyly. Laurence-Moon patients develop spasticity later in the course of the disease. Choroidal atrophy is reported as a fundus feature peculiar to this rarer syndromic variant.

Refsum's disease (phytanic acid storage disease) is a rare, autosomal recessive condition in which the enzyme, phytanic acid oxidase is deficient or absent. Consequently, phytanic acid accumulates in tissues. In addition to retinitis pigmentosa, the main features are peripheral polyneuropathy and ataxia. Most patients become symptomatic before age 20 with nyctalopia, ataxia, or both. Other features that are variably present include anosmia, deafness, and cardiac arrhythmias. Cerebrospinal fluid protein elevation is typical. Determination of phytanic acid blood levels is usually diagnostic. Dietary phytanic acid restriction will prevent the development of most systemic manifestations, but the retinal degeneration is progressive, despite this treatment.

Clinical Evaluation

Electroretinography is the primary test used to diagnose and to monitor RP. End-stage eyes produce an extinguished ERG, when tested with a single flash, without computer averaging. Electroretinography should be performed in accordance with standardized criteria and permits the assessment of the rod and cone systems separately. RP patients show a progressive reduction in the amplitudes of the rod-driven responses, in contrast to patients with cone dystrophies, who show primarily cone dysfunction. ERG testing will also help differentiate RP from other photoreceptor disorders such as congenital stationary night blindness (CSNB). Young children may be tested under chloral hydrate or propofol sedation or, if needed, general anesthesia.

Kinetic visual field testing is an important test to help diagnose and follow patients with RP. Perimetric findings include bilateral midperipheral (ring) scotomas, which eventually break out into the periphery, paracentral scotomas, and peripheral contraction, with preservation of the central fields. Progressive loss of the peripheral field occurs over the course of years to decades. Patients with greater cone than rod dysfunction will show greater central field loss. The ultimate reason for legal blindness is most often visual field loss. Fluorescein angiography is performed in selected cases and reveals RPE transmission defects and CME.

Management

Little is available specifically to treat most types of RP. Modest decreases in rate the deterioration of cone ERGs

---

Box 10-8   Primary Diagnostic Features of Leber's Congenital Amaurosis

Severe congenital visual deficit
A nonrecordable or highly attenuated electroretinogram since birth
Absence of another systemic abnormality

---

were found with vitamin A treatment in one study. The role of the ophthalmologist is to accurately characterize the type of retinal degeneration to provide sound advice regarding prognosis and risk to other family members. The carrier state in X-linked cases may be identified by ophthalmoscopy, fluorescein angiography, or electroretinography. Identifying the type of retinal degeneration also permits referral to the proper specialists. For example, recognition of a case of Bardet-Biedl syndrome should prompt a visit to the nephrologist, since renal failure is a significant cause of morbidity in affected patients. The ophthalmologist must rule out the possibility of a treatable syndrome such as abetalipoproteinemia, Refsum's disease, or, in some cases, gyrate atrophy. Another role of the ophthalmologist is the treatment of secondary problems such as CME, which may be responsive to acetazolamide, and cataracts. Patients should be provided with the most effective optical aids and be referred to a low vision specialist, if required. Many patients and their families may benefit greatly from association with a support group. Referral of these patients to specialized centers for retinal degenerations is also appropriate.

LEBER'S CONGENITAL AMAUROSIS

Leber's congenital amaurosis (LCA) is the most severe form of congenital retinal dystrophy or degeneration. The three main diagnostic features are listed in Box 10-8.

The typical affected patient presents in the first few months of life with extremely poor vision or blindness and nystagmus. Ultimately, the final visual acuity varies from 20/200 to no light perception. However, most patients have vision in the count fingers to no light perception range. The parents may report the presence of the *oculo-digital sign*, whereas the child presses his or her globes with the hands or fingers. This common habit is felt to cause orbital fat atrophy with subsequent enophthalmos in many of the patients with LCA. It also might contribute to the development of keratoconus in some patients. The pupils react sluggishly or not at all. However, a paradoxical pupil response is not found in LCA. The anterior eye structures are usually normal with the exception of the occasional patient who has, or subsequently develops, cataracts. A great deal has been written about the posterior pole findings. Approximately half the patients have a normal-appearing fundus during the first year of life. Others show retinal pigmentary changes, including peripheral pigmentary mottling, macular pigmentation, macular "coloboma," and retinal vascular attenuation. As affected patients age, retinal pigmentary changes develop. Also, optic atrophy is found in some patients. Refractions may vary from myopia to hyperopia, but there is a definite tendency toward moderate to high degrees of hyperopia.

Other neurologic abnormalities are present in approximately 20% of patients and include developmental delay and mental retardation, cerebral palsy, and deafness. Other systemic findings are rare.

Inheritance is autosomal recessive. LCA likely consists of a variety of different defects that await further characterization. Recently, mutations in two distinct genes have been associated with LCA. One of the genes encodes for the phototransduction cascade enzyme guanylate cyclase, which is expressed in photoreceptors. Another causal gene, known as RPE65, is expressed in the RPE.

The constellation of fundus findings, refractive error, family history, and the behavior of the patient can strongly suggest the correct diagnosis. Electroretinography reveals a completely extinguished or severely attenuated ERG. Although pigmentary retinal changes progress with time, in many instances vision does not deteriorate further, except for the subgroup of patients with macular colobomas. Lambert and colleagues reviewed 75 cases in which the diagnosis of LCA had been previously made. On reexamination, they revised the diagnosis in 40% of the cases. The most common new diagnoses were congenital stationary night blindness, Joubert's syndrome, retinitis pigmentosa, and achromatopsia. Knowledge of the patients' course, review of the family history, and repeating the ERGs with more sensitive equipment provided the information necessary to make the correct diagnoses.

CHOROIDEREMIA

Choroideremia is an X-linked recessive disorder characterized by degeneration of the retina and choroid. Patients typically present in childhood or the teens, with poor night vision. Examination at that time reveals pigmentary mottling or regions of chorioretinal atrophy at the equator. Over time, these regions coalesce and enlarge to involve the anterior and posterior eye. Remaining RPE demonstrates a characteristic scalloped appearance. Early in the course, choroideremia may be confused with RP. Fluorescein angiography will aid in diagnosis by demonstrating clearly defined regions of profound atrophy of the choroid and retina. Early cases

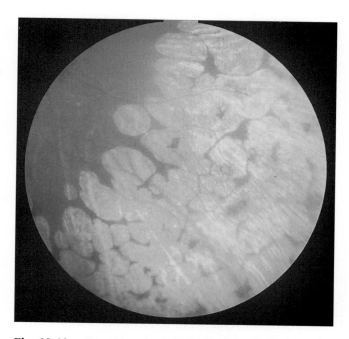

Fig. 10-13   Gyrate atrophy. Note the large regions of chorioretinal atrophy. See color plate. (Courtesy of Dr. Alessandro Iannaccone.)

show decreased ERG amplitudes, and in late cases, ERGs become extinguished. Similar to RP, visual field loss is progressive, with peripheral loss and relatively spared central vision until late in the course. Female carriers have pathognomonic streaks of peripheral RPE mottling but normal visual function. The acuity falls to the 20/200 range by the fourth decade. Several mutations in the CHM gene, which maps to chromosome Xq21, have been identified. The disease mechanism is related to an abnormal trafficking and accumulation in the RPE of byproducts of the metabolism of the diseased protein. There is no known treatment.

GYRATE ATROPHY

Gyrate atrophy is an autosomal recessively inherited condition caused by mutations in the ornithine aminotransferase (OAT) gene, which maps to chromosome 10. It is quite rare in the United States, but in Finland, the estimated frequency is 1/50,000. The characteristic fundus abnormality is characterized by well-defined areas of chorioretinal atrophy, starting in the mid-periphery and coalescing and extending anteriorly and posteriorly (Fig. 10-13). The lesions are first visible in the first or second decade. Patients present with nyctalopia and subsequently demonstrate visual field loss, corresponding to the atrophic regions. High myopia and astigmatism are common. The fovea and central vision is usually spared until the fifth or sixth decade. Both the ERG and EOG amplitudes are reduced.

Elevated levels of plasma ornithine, resulting from decreased ornithine aminotransferase activity, are found and confirm the diagnosis. However, the precise pathophysiology of gyrate atrophy is unknown. In fact, there are cases reported in the literature of gyrate atrophy-like retinal degenerations not associated with the characteristic hyperornithinemia. Treatment attempts have been made by restricting the dietary intake of arginine, with or without pyridoxine supplementation. Not is only this regimen quite difficult to maintain, but it also is not equally effective in all subjects. Unfortunately, many patients are nonresponders to these dietary measures.

CONE DISORDERS

Cone disorders are a heterogeneous group of conditions in which the cone system is preferentially involved and include progressive disease entities referred to as cone dystrophies and nonprogressive conditions such as achromatopsia (rod monochromatism) and blue cone monochromatism. Achromatopsia and blue cone monochromatism are congenital, whereas the other cone dystrophies develop later in life.

Progressive Cone Dystrophies

The *cone dystrophies* are progressive degenerations of the cones that occasionally can become symptomatic in teens. They may occur sporadically or display an autosomal dominant or X-linked recessive inheritance pattern. Early symptoms are mildly decreased central acuity and color perception, and a slowly progressive course ensues. Since fundus findings may remain virtually absent for many years after the onset of symptoms, the real challenge for the clinician is to consider the diagnosis and to obtain an ERG. Even in early cases, the ERG will usually reveal very attenuated or absent cone responses. Some forms also affect rod function (cone-rod dystrophies), although to a far lesser extent. Subsequently, over a variable time, and depending on the severity of the case, macular degenerative changes will appear; the final expected visual acuity is in the 20/200 to 20/400 range. Bull's eye maculopathy or patches of macular atrophy with pigmented margins are characteristic of these conditions in the later stages of the diseases. Affected patients have normal visual function during infancy; therefore nystagmus is not a common feature of the cone dystrophies. Like RP, cone dystrophies are genetically heterogeneous. A variety of loci have been identified, and some causal genes have been recently cloned. One of these, called CRX, is actually a gene regulator of photoreceptor cell development, and not a gene exerting a function in the adult retina.

Achromatopsia and Blue Cone Monochromatism

In achromatopsia there is a profound congenital reduction in the number of cones, with normal rod function. Affected patients have marked light aversion, congenital nystagmus, paradoxical pupil responses, virtually absent color vision, and poor visual acuity. ERG testing shows normal rod-driven responses, but absent (complete forms) or severely attenuated (incomplete forms) cone responses. In the complete form, the visual acuity is about 20/200, and in the incomplete form, the acuity ranges from about 20/50 to 20/200. Most patients are hyperopic. The fundi may appear normal, but most often a characteristic foveal aplasia can be appreciated. Late in the course of the complete form bull's eye macular changes may occasionally be seen. As the patients age, both the light aversion and the amplitude of the nystagmus tend to lessen. Inheritance is autosomal recessive.

Patients with the rare entity, blue cone monochromatism, may present with congenitally poor vision and nystagmus. However, some patients are less severely affected. The rod ERG response is normal, although the cone response is significantly reduced. This condition is transmitted in an X-linked manner, and affected males are usually myopic. Titled discs are frequently observed in blue cone monochromats. Both blue cone monochromatism and achromatopsia may be incorrectly diagnosed as idiopathic "congenital nystagmus" if an ERG is not performed.

CONGENITAL STATIONARY NIGHT BLINDNESS

Congenital stationary night blindness (CSNB) refers to a group of retinal disorders in which visual function in good illumination is normal or only slightly impaired, but the night vision is poor. Two major groups of CSNB exist, one with normal or nearly-normal appearing fundi and one with abnormal fundi. The second of these two groups includes the entities, Oguchi's disease and fundus albipunctatus and will not be discussed further here.

Three patterns of inheritance exist for CSNB with normal appearing fundi: X-linked (most common), autosomal dominant, and autosomal recessive. The main clinical feature of CSNB is abnormal scotopic vision, which is demonstrated by dark adaptometry. Typically, the thresholds are 2 to 3 log units above normal. The X-linked form is characterized by moderate to very high myopia and nystagmus. The autosomal recessive form also can be associated with a myopia but not with nystagmus. Autosomal dominant CSNB (the Nougaret or Riggs type) differs in that there is no excess tendency

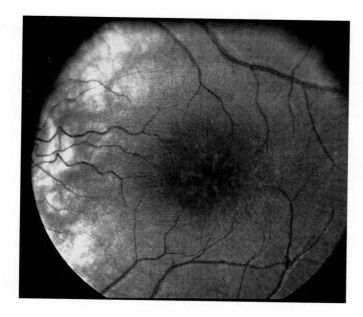

Fig. 10-14   X-linked juvenile retinoschisis. Red-free photograph of macula.

toward myopia. Rod responses are unrecordable, and cone responses are normal or nearly normal.

Determination of the type of CSNB is most often achieved by electroretinography. In X-linked and recessive forms, a characteristic electronegative shape of the maximal ERG response is seen: when tested with a bright white flash, the a-wave appears normal or nearly normal but the b-wave is nearly absent. This distinctive waveform is peculiar to the so-called *Schubert-Bornschein* form of CSNB, and is not observed in the dominant (*Nougaret-Riggs*) form, in which ERGs are subnormal in amplitude under all testing conditions but normal in waveform. Schubert-Bornschein CSNB includes two subtypes, the complete and the incomplete form. These are also easily distinguished by ERG testing. X-linked forms are best confirmed by examining female carriers, who show reduced oscillatory potentials of the ERG.

Congenital stationary night blindness typically presents by school age, when the parents or child realize that the night vision is impaired. The visual acuity in good illumination is usually normal but may be as poor as 20/200. Nystagmus may be present, especially in males with X-linked forms. Patients previously thought to have congenital "motor" nystagmus may actually have CSNB and electrophysiologic testing should be considered. In other patients with CSNB, an erroneous diagnosis of spasmus nutans may be made. Another important feature, often present in CSNB, is a *paradoxical pupillary light response*. Although this is best demonstrated using infrared videography, so that one may observe constriction of the pupil in darkness, a dim light from the side will usually permit observation of this sign. The importance in distinguishing CSNB, a static condition, from

retinitis pigmentosa, a progressive condition, should be evident.

VITREORETINAL DYSTROPHIES

This group of diseases includes many clinically and genetically heterogeneous familial conditions that share degenerative processes involving the vitreous and the retina. Because of their high potential to result in rhegmatogenous retinal detachments, vitreoretinal dystrophies must be distinguished from other more benign conditions or retinal degenerations not typically associated with retinal detachments, such as RP or choroideremia. The most important and common vitreoretinal disorders are described below.

X-Linked Juvenile Retinoschisis

X-linked juvenile retinoschisis (XLJR) is a rare, bilateral condition affecting only boys in which there is a splitting of the nerve fiber layer. This results in both foveal and peripheral retinal findings. In the fovea, early signs are a slight elevation of the retina with microcystic changes and stellate maculopathy, retinal folds that radiate out from the fovea (Fig. 10-14). The best way to visualize these changes is with slit-lamp biomicroscopy, using a contact lens and red-free light. Although infantile cases have been documented, patients usually present in early childhood with mildly impaired vision in the 20/50 range and, at times, with strabismus. Since the foveal schisis may be subtle, affected children may be misdiagnosed with amblyopia. Although previously the peripheral changes of bilateral inferotemporal schisis were the emphasized feature in X-linked juvenile retinoschisis, peripheral changes are found only in half of the cases, whereas virtually all of the cases have foveal schisis. The split peripheral nerve fiber layer results in a very fine, membranous, domed elevation, which may contain both blood vessels and large oval holes. Vitreous veils represent fragmented areas of nerve fiber layer adherent to the posterior hyaloid. Another frequently observed phenomenon is the presence of a peripheral patchy metallic reflex at the vitreoretinal interface. Vitreous hemorrhage may result from tearing of vessels bridging across inner retinal layer tears, but the foveal disease is usually responsible for the visual loss in this condition. Retinal detachments frequently complicate this disease, caused by full-thickness retinal tears, vitreoretinal traction, or a combination of both.

Electroretinography early in the disease shows normal or moderately reduced a-waves and markedly decreased b-wave amplitudes producing electronegative ERGs as in Schubert-Bornschein CSNB. Oscillatory potentials are also virtually absent in every case, confirming the selective impairment of the inner retina. Reduced ERG amplitudes are observed for both rod-driven and cone-driven responses, as XLJR is believed to be caused by a defect in K^+ ion transport mechanisms in Müller cells. Perimetric testing reveals absolute scotomas corresponding to the areas of peripheral schisis. Such testing is not usually required to confirm the diagnosis since the foveal findings are quite specific. XLJR progresses slowly, resulting in macular atrophic changes by the fifth to sixth decade. At this stage of the disease, RP-like pigmentary changes of he retinal periphery also ensue, making the distinction between the two conditions very difficult. Treatment is reserved for frank retinal detachment and cases of vitreous hemorrhage. The differential diagnosis of XLJR is given in Box 10-9. The responsible gene has been mapped to the Xp22 region and has been recently cloned. Investigations are in progress to characterize the retinal localization and the function of the gene product.

Stickler Syndrome

Stickler syndrome (hereditary progressive arthro-ophthalmopathy) is a dominantly inherited, heterogeneous condition caused by a defect in collagen formation. Its incidence is about 1/20,000. Stickler syndrome is genetically heterogeneous. One of the causal genes, known as COL2A1, maps to chromosome 12q and encodes for type II procollagen, accounting for the multisystemic manifestations of the disease. Patients with COL2A1 mutations tend to have a high incidence of retrolenticular vitreal abnormalities.

The primary ocular findings include vitreoretinal degeneration, with peripheral lattice retinal degeneration

Box 10-9   X-Linked Juvenile Retinoschisis—Differential Diagnosis
Goldmann-Favre vitreoretinopathy Retinitis pigmentosa Senile retinoschisis Retinopathy of prematurity Eales disease

and perivascular pigmentation, congenital high myopia, cataracts, and glaucoma. Liquifaction of the vitreous leads to its becoming optically empty, and vitreous condensates form bands. The retinal changes include chorioretinal degeneration, with the formation of retinal breaks. The lifetime risk for retinal detachment is about 50%. By definition, Stickler syndrome includes systemic anomalies. Some patients have a flattened face and depressed bridge of the nose. Others have the Pierre-Robin anomaly or appear marfanoid. Progressive hearing loss is the most common systemic defect. A progressive arthropathy is also common, but may not become apparent until adulthood. Bone epiphyseal dysplasia and articular cartilage degeneration are typically observed on routine roentgenograms. Identification of associated systemic features is key to proper diagnosis. Stickler syndrome must be distinguished from two less common autosomal dominant conditions, Wagner disease and erosive vitreoretinopathy. Until recently believed to be a simple variant of Stickler syndrome devoid of systemic manifestations, Wagner disease maps to chromosome 5q, a locus distinct from that of Stickler syndrome. Erosive vitreoretinopathy also maps to chromosome 5, but at a different locus. Besides the absence of systemic abnormalities, both Wagner disease and erosive vitreoretinopathy cause a more severe form of retinopathy, with prominent RPE and retinal atrophy and frankly subnormal ERG responses. The distinction is also important because rhegmatogenous retinal detachments are far less common in true Wagner disease compared to Stickler disease and erosive vitreoretinopathy. Retinal detachments in all three of the above conditions are notoriously difficult to manage. Frequent periodic retinal examinations are suggested for all diseases, with laser photocoagulation treatment applied to retinal breaks as they appear.

Familial Exudative Vitreoretinopathy

Familial exudative vitreoretinopathy (FEVR) is a rare, typically bilateral, autosomal dominantly inherited condition first described in 1969. The clinical appearance is similar to retinopathy of prematurity; however, there is no history of premature birth or use of oxygen in the neonatal period. The primary clinical features are incomplete peripheral retinal vascularization, particularly temporally, with telangiectasia and vascular engorgement. The severity of FEVR varies widely. Many patients are asymptomatic, whereas others are bilaterally blind. Mild forms of FEVR (stage 1) reveal a peripheral avascular zone, best demonstrated with fluorescein angiography. The adjacent vasculature is telangiectatic, abnormally arborized, and contains arteriovenous shunts. Intraretinal crystal-like deposits in the avascular areas are frequently observed. The peripheral avascular zone may remain stable for life. More advanced stages of FEVR show neovascularization and vascular exudation in the subretinal and intraretinal space (stage 2). The temporal periphery is, again, most affected. Peripheral traction retinal detachments occur and lead to dragging of the macula and optic disc. Temporally, a fibrovascular mass may be present. In the most advanced forms of FEVR (stage 3), the peripheral fibrovascular mass causes frank traction retinal detachments, associated with retinal folds and secondary rhegmatogenous detachments. In fact, retinal detachment is the most significant cause of visual loss in FEVR. The reported incidence of retinal detachment varies from 4% to 30%. Vitreous hemorrhage is also a possible complication, as well as extension of neovascular processes to the anterior segment, with rubeosis and neovascular glaucoma.

The primary entity from which FEVR must be distinguished is retinopathy of prematurity. Other diagnoses that, at times, must be considered include Eales disease, sickle retinopathy, and Toxocara canis.

The primary abnormality is thought to be one of retinal vasculature maturation, but the precise genetic defect has not yet been identified. A locus for the disease has been mapped to chromosome 11q. Penetrance is extremely high, but, as mentioned in the previous discussion, the expression of disease is highly variable. Thus minimally affected parents can have children with severe disease. FEVR is thought not to progress significantly after 10 years of age.

SUGGESTED READINGS

Aldred MA, Dry KL, Sharp DM, et al: Linkage analysis in X-linked congenital stationary night blindness, *Genomics* 14:99-104, 1992.

Berson EL, Simonoff EA: Dominant retinitis pigmentosa with reduced penetrance: further studies of the electroretinogram, *Arch Ophthalmol* 97:1286-1291, 1979.

Campo RV, Aaberg TM: Ocular and systemic manifestations of the Bardet-Biedl syndrome, *Am J Ophthalmol* 94:750-756, 1982.

Carr RE, Siegel IM: *Electrodiagnostic testing of the visual system: a clinical guide,* Philadelphia, 1990, F.A. Davis.

Dryja TP, Li T: Molecular genetics of retinitis pigmentosa, *Hum Mol Genet* 4:1739-1743, 1995.

Fishman GA, Alexander KR, Anderson RJ: Autosomal dominant retinitis pigmentosa, *Arch Ophthalmol* 103:366-374, 1985.

Fishman GA, Farber M, Patel BS, et al: Visual acuity loss in patients with Stargardt's macular dystrophy, *Ophthalmol* 94(7):809-814, 1987.

Fishman GA, Kumar A, Joseph ME, et al: Usher's syndrome: ophthalmic and neuro-otologic findings suggesting genetic heterogeneity, *Arch Ophthalmol* 101:1367-1374, 1983.

Fishman GA, Sokol S: *Electrophysiologic testing in disorders of the retina, optic nerve, and visual pathway: AAO Ophthalmology Monograph #2,* San Francisco, 1990, American Academy of Ophthalmology.

Fishman GA, Weinberg AB, McMahon TT: X-linked recessive retinitis pigmentosa: clinical characteristics of carriers, *Arch Ophthalmol* 104:1329-1335, 1986.

George NDL, Payne SJ, Bill RM, et al: Improved genetic mapping of X-linked retinoschisis, *J Med Genet* 33(11):919-922, 1996.

George NDL, Yates JRW, Moore AT: X-linked retinoschisis, *Br J Ophthalmol* 79(7):697-702, 1995.

Heckenlively JR, Arden GB: *Principles and practice of clinical electrophysiology of vision,* St Louis, 1991, Mosby.

Heher KL, Traboulsi EI, Maumenee IH: The natural history of Leber's congenital amaurosis, *Ophthalmol* 99(2):241-245, 1992.

Kaplan J, Bonneau D, Frézal J, et al: Clinical and genetic heterogeneity in retinitis pigmentosa, *Hum Genet* 85:635-642, 1990.

Leppert M, Baird L, Anderson KL, et al: Bardet-Biedl syndrome is linked to DNA markers on chromosome 11q and is genetically heterogeneous, *Natur Genet* 7:108-112, 1994.

Murphree AL: Molecular genetics of retinoblastoma, *Ophthalmol Clin North Am* 8(1):155-166, 1995.

Phillips PH, Repka MX: Current concepts in the treatment of retinopathy of prematurity, *Semin Ophthalmol* 12(2):72-80, 1997.

Reynolds JD: Retinopathy of prematurity, *Pediatric Ophthalmol* 9(2):149-159, 1996.

Reynolds JD, Hardy RJ, Kennedy KA: Lack of efficacy of light reduction in preventing retinopathy of prematurity, *N Engl J Med* 338:1572-1576, 1998.

Scott IU, O'Brien JM, Murray TG: Retinoblastoma: a review emphasizing genetics and management strategies, *Semin Ophthalmol* 12(2):59-71, 1997.

Sieving PA: Diagnostic issues with inherited retinal and macular dystrophies, *Semin Ophthalmol* 10(4):279-294, 1995.

Stone EM, Nichols BE, Streb LM: Genetic linkage of vitelliform macular degeneration (Best's disease) to chromosome 11q13, *Nat Genet* 1:246-250, 1992.

Pediatric Systemic Disease with Ocular Involvement

PHAKOMATOSES

Neurofibromatosis I

Neurofibromatosis I (NF-I), the prototypical neurocutaneous disorder, is an autosomal dominantly inherited, clinically variable, progressive, multiorgan disorder with frequent ophthalmic manifestations. Although multiple cutaneous neurofibromas are characteristic and give the syndrome its name, numerous other defects, such as malignancies and skeletal deformities, are responsible for significant morbidity in this disease. NF-I is the most common of the phakomatoses, with an incidence of 1:3500 to 1:4000. The defective gene is found on the long arm of chromosome 17 (17q11.2) and is very large, contributing to its high mutation rate. One of the gene's functions is as a guanosine dephosphatase–activating protein (GAP), which helps to regulate and to control cell growth. Thus mutations in the NF-I gene may lead to the development of neoplasms and hamartomas. Penetrance in NF-I is almost 100%, with remarkable phenotypic variability, even within families. The spontaneous mutation rate is high, with about half of the new cases having no family history.

Ophthalmologists are often asked to examine the irides for the presence of Lisch nodules, which are melanocytic hamartomas. They appear as yellow or brown, slightly raised, well-circumscribed lesions on the iris surface. They usually are bilateral and multiple, and are quite specific for NF-I (Fig. 11-1). Lisch nodules are usually absent at birth, but about 50% of affected patients develop them by age 5, and greater than 75% of affected children 15 years of age have them. Other anterior segment changes include enlarged corneal nerves, seen in up to 25% of patients, and conjunctival neurofibromas. Glaucoma is an important complication of NF-I and occurs in about half of patients with orbital or eyelid neurofibromas. It may manifest as juvenile glaucoma, with buphthalmos, or it may develop later. Infiltration of the angle by neurofibromatous material is probably the most common mechanism of glaucoma. Patients with orbital or eyelid neurofibromas are at high risk for developing ipsilateral glaucoma and should be followed regularly for life. Retinal findings include astrocytic hamartomas and combined hamartomas of the retina and RPE.

The plexiform neurofibroma is the most common orbital lesion in NF-I. This tumor is composed of Schwann

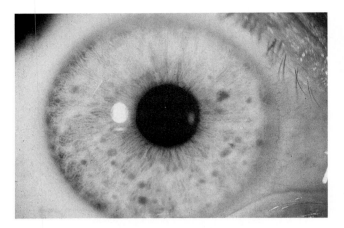

Fig. 11-1 Lisch nodules in neurofibromatosis I. See color plate.

cells, with surrounding axons and fibroblasts. The feel of such lesions, when the eyelid is involved, has been likened to a "bag of worms." Orbital and eyelid plexiform neurofibromas infiltrate the normal orbital tissues and, consequently, are extremely difficult to excise without damaging normal structures. Subcutaneous neurofibromas may be seen throughout the body, including the eyelids. About 15% of patients with NF-I develop optic pathway gliomas, most in the first decade of life. In NF-I, gliomas affecting the chiasm are more common than those limited to the optic nerve. Usually, they are low-grade, pilocytic astrocytomas, and many children are asymptomatic with respect to the glioma when it is discovered. Optic pathway gliomas are best characterized by magnetic resonance imaging (MRI) (see Chapter 4). Congenital dysplasia or absence of the greater wing of the sphenoid is also seen and may be associated with pulsatile exophthalmos.

Various other systemic changes are found in NF-I, and may aid in diagnosis. Café-au-lâit spots are hyperpigmented skin macules, which may be congenital but often increase in size. Many normal persons have one such lesion, but NF-I patients tend to have multiple spots (Box 11-1). Axillary and inguinal freckling are present in 90% to 95% of patients with NF-I and are highly specific signs. Neurofibromas may occur anywhere in the central or peripheral nervous system, and intracranial tumors such as meningiomas and ependymomas occur at increased rates. Mild mental retardation is found in 45% of patients. Other osseous lesions, such as pseudoarthroses and tibial bowing, are sometimes found.

Neurofibromatosis II

Neurofibromatosis II (NF-II), despite its historical connection and similar name, is a completely different disease than NF-I and should not be confused with NF-I. NF-II, previously referred to as central neurofibromatosis

or bilateral acoustic neurofibromatosis, has bilateral vestibular schwannomas as its hallmark. It has been suggested that the term *acoustic neuroma* be abandoned since the tumors do not arise from the acoustic nerve and the tumors are not neuromas. The gene for neurofibromatosis II is on chromosome 22q11, and the gene product, called merlin or schwannomin, is thought to be a tumor suppressor. The diagnostic criteria for NF-II are given in Box 11-2.

Neurofibromatosis II is much less common than NF-I, with an incidence of about 1:50,000. It is a highly penetrant, autosomal dominant condition, with a high spontaneous mutation rate. Most often, patients present with bilateral hearing loss; other early signs are tinnitus, imbalance, and facial paresthesia. As the schwannomas grow, hydrocephalus, brainstem compression, and death may occur. The schwannomas are best identified with MRI (Fig. 11-2). Other tumors frequently present in NF-II include intracranial and optic nerve sheath meningiomas and ependymomas, as well as spinal meningiomas, ependymomas, and schwannomas. Ocular manifestations include early posterior cortical cataracts, epiretinal membranes, and combined hamartomas of the retina and the RPE.

Sturge-Weber Syndrome

The possibility of Sturge-Weber syndrome (encephalotrigeminal angiomatosis), a sporadic condition, is indicated at birth by the presence of a facial hemangioma (nevus flammeus) (Fig. 11-3). Further examination may

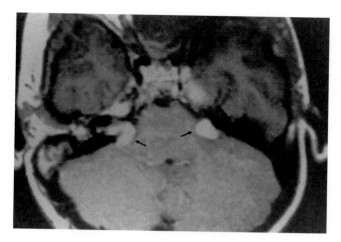

Fig. 11-2 Bilateral vestibular schwannomas in neurofibromatosis II. (From Grossman RI, Yousem DM: *Neuroradiology: the requisites,* St Louis, 1994, Mosby.)

The diagnostic criteria for neurofibromatosis II (NF-II) are met by an individual who has:
1. Bilateral eighth nerve masses seen with appropriate imaging techniques (e.g., CT or MRI)
   or
2. A first-degree relative with NF-II and either
   a. Unilateral eighth nerve mass or
   b. Two of the following:
      neurofibroma
      meningioma
      schwannoma
      juvenile posterior subcapsular lenticular opacity

Note: An individual must have one of these criteria to diagnose NF-II.

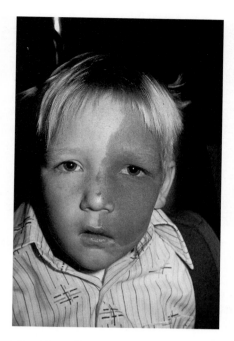

Fig. 11-3   Nevus flammeus in Sturge-Weber syndrome.

reveal the presence of ophthalmic and central nervous system (CNS) abnormalities. The facial angioma occurs in the regions supplied by the first and second divisions of the trigeminal nerve and is usually unilateral. It is composed of dilated, telangiectatic capillaries in the dermis and may be associated with facial hemihypertrophy.

Ipsilateral leptomeningeal angiomatosis, associated with gyral calcification and cortical atrophy, leads to contralateral seizures, which are present in up to 80% of patients. Eventually, hemiparesis may result. Developmental delay is common, with mental deficiency present in about 50% of affected parentis. Various ophthalmic abnormalities may be found. Diffuse choroidal hemangiomas (mixed capillary/cavernous) are present in up to 40% of patients. The hemangiomas in Sturge-Weber syndrome are flat and, initially, only slightly elevated. The fundus appears a deeper red than that of the fellow eye,

which may be the only sign of the hemangioma. This has been called the *"tomato catsup fundus."* Progressive hyperopia, retinal and choroidal degeneration, and serous retinal detachment may result. Glaucoma is the ocular complication of greatest concern in Sturge-Weber syndrome. Overall, it occurs in 30% of affected patients, most often in those with upper eyelid involvement. In about 60% of cases, it presents with buphthalmos. Increased episcleral venous pressure, a congenital chamber anomaly, and acquired obstruction of the trabecular meshwork all may contribute to the glaucoma. Intraocular surgery in affected patients carries increased risks of choroidal effusion, expulsive hemorrhage, and hyphema.

Tuberous Sclerosis

The classic description of tuberous sclerosis (tuberous sclerosis complex, TSC) is a triad consisting of adenoma sebaceum, seizure disorder, and mental retardation. However, the features of tuberous sclerosis are much more complex and variable than suggested by the triad. Only about 30% of patients now considered to have tuberous sclerosis display each of the three features. Furthermore, many additional abnormalities occur as part of the complex.

Tuberous sclerosis shares some general features with neurofibromatosis. Both are highly penetrant, autosomal dominant disorders with great variability within a family. Both NF and TSC have a high spontaneous mutation rate of about 50%. And, of course, both have cutaneous and neurologic manifestations. The reported incidence of

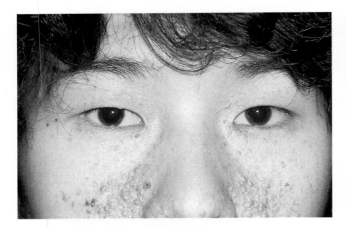

Fig. 11-4   Facial angiofibromas in tuberous sclerosis.

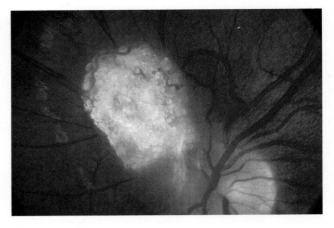

Fig. 11-5   Retinal astrocytic hamartoma in tuberous sclerosis. See color plate.

TSC has ranged from 1:20,000 to 1:300,000, with males and females affected at equal rates. About 75% have no family history, and there is no racial predilection. The most common presenting feature is infantile spasms (salaam spasms), and, ultimately, about 90% of patients eventually demonstrate abnormal EEGs. Mental retardation is present in about 60% of patients. Adenoma sebaceum refers to the skin lesions that appear in a butterfly distribution on the cheeks and face. Since these lesions are actually *angiofibromas*, both parts of the term *adenoma sebaceum* are misnomers (Fig. 11-4). Hypopigmented skin macules *(ash leaf spots)* are seen in 15% to 50% of older patients and are best demonstrated with a Woods' lamp. The melanocytes in ash leaf spots have decreased tyrosinase activity. *Shagreen patches* are caused by fibromatous infiltration of the skin and are seen in about 20% of patients. Other systemic manifestations include subungual fibromata, foci of sclerosis in the calvarium and spine, rhabdomyomata and cardiac arrhythmias, renal angiomyolipomas, and pulmonary and subpleural cysts.

Retinal hamartomas are seen in up to 50% of patients with TSC. Early, they are flat, smooth, transparent, superficial gray-yellow lesions that form in the posterior pole. These lesions are easily missed during examination, and a region where the retinal reflex is altered may be a signal to look more carefully. More mature hamartomas may calcify and appear as white or yellow, elevated lesions, with a mulberry appearance (Fig. 11-5). The CNS manifestations include cortical tubers, white matter heterotopias, and subependymal giant cell nodules. Cortical tubers are areas of disordered lamination and gliosis. Their frequency in tuberous sclerosis is unknown. White matter heterotopias are areas of disorganized, enlarged neurons in the white matter, which represent zones of arrested migration. Subependymal giant-cell nodules, from which giant cell astrocytoma arise, are seen most often in the region of the basal lateral ven-

tricles and contain glial processes, blood vessels, and calcium.

Visual loss from tuberous sclerosis is rare; when it occurs, usually it is from obstructive hydrocephalus and resultant papilledema. The retinal lesions rarely impair vision. Defects on chromosome 9 and 11 have been demonstrated in TSC.

Von Hippel-Lindau Disease

Von Hippel-Lindau disease *(retinal and cerebellar hemangiomatosis)* is an autosomal dominantly inherited disease, with irregular penetrance, and an incidence of about 1:40,000. The incidence in males and females is equal, and only about one quarter of cases are familial. The gene is located on chromosome 3p25.5 and is a tumor-suppressor gene. Various variations of the gene, which may lead to different patterns of tumor formation, have been identified. This disease is also characterized by marked clinical variability. The primary features are cerebellar, spinal, medullary, or cerebral *hemangioblastomas*; retinal hemangioblastomas; renal cysts and adenocarcinoma; pancreatic cysts and islet cell tumors; pheochromocytomas; and epididymal cystadenomas. Von Hippel-Lindau disease rarely has cutaneous manifestations, and often diagnosis is not made until adulthood. Retinal angiomas (retinal hemangioblastomas) are found in most patients, causing symptoms of visual loss, floaters, and metamorphopsia and may be the first signal of the disease. They are capillary tumors, usually in the midperiphery and are up to three disc diameters across. They have a dilated, tortuous feeding artery and a draining vein and associated intraretinal leakage and exudation is common (Fig. 11-6). Fluorescein angiography shows early hyperfluorescence and leakage. Retinal angiomas typically become symptomatic in the third decade. Untreated, retinal detachment, neovascularization, glaucoma, and phthisis may occur. Argon laser photoco-

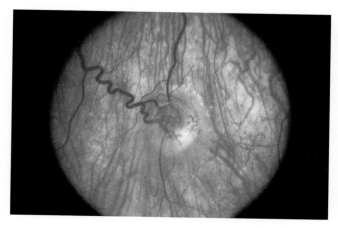

Fig. 11-6   Retinal angioma in von Hippel-Lindau disease. See color plate.

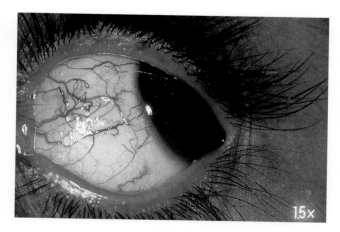

Fig. 11-7   Conjunctival telangiectasias in ataxia-telangiectasia.

agulation is the preferred treatment for posterior lesions, applying direct treatment to small lesions and treating the feeder vessel of larger ones. Cryotherapy or diathermy is used for more anterior lesions. Cerebellar hemangioblastomas, usually cystic lesions, are the most common CNS finding in von Hippel-Lindau disease. Most often they are found in the posterior and lateral cerebellum, causing gait disturbance, vertigo, vomiting, and headache as the initial symptoms. Less commonly, the medulla, spinal cord, or cerebrum are affected. Visceral involvement includes renal cell carcinoma in up to 25% of patients, pheochromocytoma in 3% to 10% of patients, and, less commonly, renal and pancreatic cysts. Because of the multiorgan and progressive nature of this disease, ongoing surveillance, with physical examinations and specialized testing, is required. Biannual or annual ophthalmic examinations are suggested.

Ataxia-Telangiectasia

Ataxia-telangiectasia *(Louis-Bar syndrome)* is a rare, autosomal recessive disease caused by a mutation on chromosome 11q22-23. The normal gene product aids in cellular recovery following DNA damage. The first clinical sign is usually ataxia, which becomes apparent about the time the child begins to walk. As the child ages, the ataxia progresses to include choreoathetosis, dysarthria, and myoclonus. Ultimately, affected children are confined to a wheelchair. Bilateral conjunctival telangiectasias develop by age 7. Examination reveals dilated, corkscrew vessels of the interpalpebral bulbar conjunctiva (Fig. 11-7). Cutaneous telangiectasia is also seen. Ocular motility disturbance, such as ocular motor apraxia, saccadic dysfunction, nystagmus, and strabismus may appear later. Cerebellar degeneration is the primary neurologic finding, and cerebellar atrophy can be demonstrated with MRI. Affected patients also are prone to

recurrent sinopulmonary and skin infections, because there is thymic hypoplasia with decreased levels of IgA, IgE, and IgG. Increased rates of leukemia, lymphoma, and other neoplasms are found.

Racemose Hemangiomatosis

Racemose hemangiomatosis *(Wyburn-Mason syndrome)* is a syndrome consisting of arteriovenous anastomoses (arteriovenous malformations, AVMs) in the retina and brain, particularly the midbrain; the thalami and cerebrum are less often involved. The etiology is unknown, and females are affected as often as males. Usually, only one eye is affected and, at times, ipsilateral facial angiomas are seen. The retinal vessels, particularly the temporal ones, are dilated, distorted, and tortuous (Fig. 11-8). The vessels are thought to be congenitally malformed, and the changes nonprogressive. The malformed vessels may extend posteriorly into the orbit and may even connect to the intracranial AVM.

The condition usually becomes evident by age 30, either with ocular or CNS signs. The vision of the affected eye may be normal or significantly decreased. Causes of visual loss include retinal and vitreous hemorrhage and vascular exudation. Ipsilateral midbrain AVMs can cause a variety of problems, including subarachnoid hemorrhage, hemiparesis, oculomotor nerve dysfunction, and hydrocephalus. Unfortunately, such AVMs are very difficult to treat.

METABOLIC DISORDERS

This section primarily deals with diseases caused by defects of lysosomal catabolic enzymes. Such defects are responsible for a variety of systemic diseases with ocular involvement. The primary types are the mucopolysac-

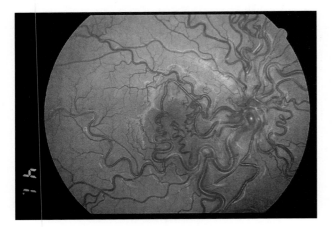

Fig. 11-8   Tortuous and dilated retinal vessels in Wyburn-Mason syndrome.

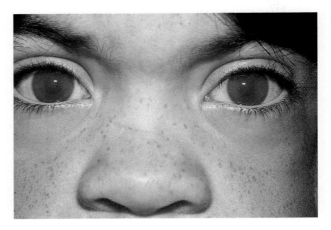

Fig. 11-9   MPS I H (Hurler syndrome) showing bilateral corneal clouding. See color plate. (Courtesy of Dr. Delmar Caldwell, Tulane University School of Medicine.)

charidoses, the sphingolipidoses, the gangliosidoses, the mucolipidoses, the galactosialidoses, mannosidosis, and fucosidosis. Tissue accumulation of various compounds results in a progressive disease course. Only the more common entities, and those of most interest to ophthalmologists, are covered in the following. Wilson's disease and cystinosis are also covered in this section.

Mucopolysaccharidosis I H

Mucopolysaccharidosis I H (MPS I H) *(Hurler's syndrome)* is caused by a deficiency in the enzyme L-iduronidase, leading to accumulation of dermatan sulfate and heparan sulfate. This is the most common of the MPS syndromes. The inheritance pattern is autosomal recessive. Affected patients have a severe and early disease, with corneal clouding by age 6 months to 3 years, as well as retinal degeneration and optic atrophy (Fig. 11-9). Slit-lamp examination reveals fine, punctate opacities in the stroma. The patients are short in stature, demonstrate progressive psychomotor retardation, are severely mentally retarded, and have progressive facial dysmorphism, with coarsening of the features, heavy brows, synophrys, and coarsening of the lashes. Death usually occurs by the second decade; thus penetrating keratoplasty is usually not performed.

Mucopolysaccharidosis I S

Mucopolysaccharidosis I S *(Scheie's syndrome)* is similar to MPS I H but is milder and rarer. Systemic findings include facial coarsening, hand deformities, hearing loss, and cardiac abnormalities. The intelligence is normal, and many patients have a normal life span. The ocular manifestations are similar to those in Hurler's syndrome and include corneal clouding, optic nerve swelling and atrophy, and pigmentary retinopathy. Penetrating kera-

toplasty can be performed with success, but, ultimately, blindness from retinal degeneration ensues.

Mucopolysaccharidosis II

Mucopolysaccharidosis II *(Hunter's syndrome)* differs from the other MPS syndromes in that it is inherited in an X-linked recessive manner. Deficiency of the enzyme L-iduronase sulfate sulfatase causes tissue accumulation of dermatan sulfate and heparan sulfate. The more severe form, type A, resembles Hurler's syndrome, and affected patients succumb early. Patients with the milder form, type B, have coarse faces and heart abnormalities. The corneas are clear in Hunter's syndrome, a finding that will differentiate these patients from those with MPS I H. Retinal degeneration occurs, to a variable degree. Swelling of the optic nerves, resulting from increased ICP, as well as other causes, is a feature of MPS II.

Other MPS syndromes of interest to ophthalmologists are MPS VI (Maroteaux-Lamy syndrome) and MPS IV (Morquio's syndrome). Patients with *MPS VI (Maroteaux-Lamy syndrome)* have normal or near-normal intellect and may have a relatively long life span. Glaucoma and corneal clouding, as well as optic atrophy, may occur. *MPS IV (Morquio's syndrome)* does not cause retinal degeneration, but corneal clouding does occur. These patients have dwarfism and vertebral defects and are of normal intelligence.

GM2 Type I Gangliosidosis

GM2 type I gangliosidosis *(Tay-Sachs disease)* is one of a class of disorders caused by deficiency of hexosaminidase A or B, or beta-galactosidase, leading to deposition of gangliosides. Tay-Sachs disease presents in the first year of life with loss of acquired developmental milestones, blindness, seizures, and an increased startle response. Death usually comes by 4 years of age. The defect is an absence of hexosaminidase A, which leads to accumulation of gangliosides in the retina and brain. The characteristic *cherry red spot* develops because of ganglioside deposition in the retinal ganglion cells (Fig. 11-10). A ring of opacified retina, surrounding a normal fovea, develops because the ganglion cells are densest in the perifoveal macula and absent in the foveal center. Cherry red spots are not specific for Tay-Sachs disease and may be seen in other storage diseases, as well as in retinal artery occlusions, following trauma and with macular hemorrhages. In Tay-Sachs disease, as the retinal degeneration proceeds, the cherry red spot fades and optic atrophy develops. The gene frequency is highest among Ashkenazi Jews.

Fabry's Disease

Fabry's disease is a multisystem disorder in which, as a result of deficient alpha-galactosidase A, trihexosylceramide is deposited throughout the body. It is inherited as an X-linked recessive trait. The deposits are relatively abundant in vascular endothelium and smooth muscle and, to a lesser extent, in connective tissue. Conjunctival vessels (especially the inferior bulbar portion) and retinal vessels are tortuous and telangiectatic. Such changes are present in about 70% of affected patients and 25% of carriers. Whorl dystrophy of the cornea *(corneal verticillata)* appears as fine, linear opacities near the level of the Bowman's membrane and is seen in most patients and carriers (Fig. 11-11). The corneal changes are similar in appearance to those caused by amiodarone, chloroquine, and phenothiazines and do not degrade the vision. Cataracts are less frequent, but have an extremely characteristic spoke-like configuration. They occur in the posterior cortex and are best visualized with retroillumination.

Affected males develop recurrent episodes of pain in the extremities, beginning in childhood. Also seen in the bathing trunk area are small skin lesions, called angiokeratoma diffusum, which are composed of telangiectasias. Diagnosis can be made with enzyme assays of white blood cells or fibroblasts or by conjunctival biopsy.

Wilson's Disease

Wilson's disease (hepatolenticular degeneration) is a rare, autosomal recessive disorder of copper metabolism. Copper accumulates in the liver, causing cirrhosis; in the basal ganglia, causing tremor, choreoathetosis and psychiatric disease; and in the kidneys, causing aminoaciduria. Untreated, Wilson's disease is fatal. In the eyes, deposition is in the peripheral Descemet's membrane, creating a peripheral brown ring—the *Kayser-Fleischer ring.* In fewer cases, pigment deposition in the anterior

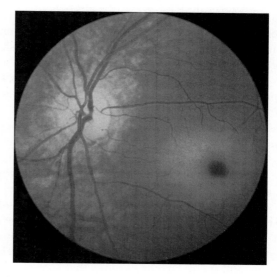

Fig. 11-10 Cherry red spot of Tay-Sachs disease. See color plate. (From Rosen ES, Cumming WJK, Eustace P, et al: *Neuro-Ophthalmology,* St Louis, 1997, Mosby.)

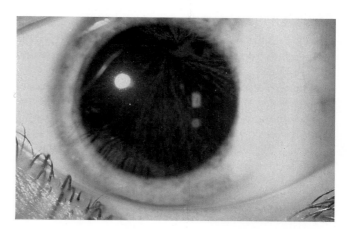

Fig. 11-11 Corneal verticillata in Fabry's disease. See color plate.

subcapsular lens occurs, referred to as a sunflower cataract.

The ophthalmologist is often asked to examine a child or teenager with liver disease to determine if a Kayser-Fleischer (KF) ring is present. KF rings occur relatively late in the disease; thus determining the serum copper and ceruloplasmin levels are better diagnostic tests. Also, other types of liver disease may cause a KF ring. However, patients with neurologic involvement from Wilson's disease generally have KF rings, and the rings can be seen to regress with treatment. Early Kayser-Fleischer rings are best seen with gonioscopy.

Cystinosis

In cystinosis, lysosomal accumulation cystine, the dimeric form of cysteine, occurs in many organs, but the significant morbidity results from renal and ocular involvement. Infantile, juvenile, and adult forms occur, all of which are autosomal recessive disorders, and all showing corneal crystals. However, the systemic manifestations vary widely in severity; the adult form causes no symptoms and may be found incidentally, and the infantile form causes early, life-threatening renal failure.

Infantile cystinosis presents by the end of the first year of life, with episodes of fever and dehydration resulting from renal tubular dysfunction. Eventually, metabolic bone disease develops. The corneal crystals are not present at birth but uniformly become visible by 1 year of age, sometimes before the onset of severe renal disease. Fine needle-like or rectangular iridescent crystals are first seen in the anterior, peripheral cornea and eventually progress to involve the entire stroma (Fig. 11-12). These deposits, and the recurrent erosions that sometimes occur, lead to severe photophobia. Peripheral pigmentary retinopathy may also occur. Other systemic findings seen in the infantile form include growth retardation and skin hypopigmentation. In the less severe adolescent form of cystinosis, the retina may be spared, and the renal disease is variable. Growth and skin are normal. Patients with the adult form have no significant renal disease and no retinopathy.

Affected infants require oral cysteamine, which delays renal damage, or undergo renal transplantation, but neither treats the corneal disease. However, frequent application of topical *cysteamine* drops has been shown to cause corneal clearing. Diagnosis of cystinosis can be made with conjunctival tissue, either by demonstrating increased cystine or with electron microscopy.

CHROMOSOMAL ANOMALIES

Trisomy 13

Patients with trisomy 13 *(Patau's syndrome)* very often have bilateral, severe congenital ocular defects. Affected patients have widespread anomalies, most notably, cleft lip and palate, polydactyly, and hypotonia. Brain anomalies are present in 70% to 80%. Many die in the perinatal period, and 95% die by age 3 years. The common ocular findings are listed in Box 11-3.

Trisomy 21

Trisomy 21 *(Down syndrome)* occurs in about 1 in 700 live births and is the most common trisomy syndrome. The incidence increases with increased maternal age. The systemic findings include brachydactyly, flattened facial features, depressed nasal bridge, a large protruding tongue, transverse palmar crease, and mental retardation. Many ocular features may require attention, including cataracts, myopia, strabismus (present in

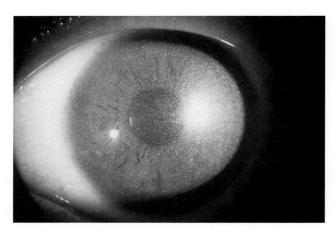

Fig. 11-12   Corneal crystals in cystinosis. See color plate.

Box 11-3   Common Ocular Findings in Patients with Trisomy 13
Colobomatous microphthalmia Cataracts PHPV Cyclopia Glaucoma Retinal dysplasia Intraocular cartilage Corneal opacities

14% to 23%), blepharitis, keratoconus, and ectropion. *Brushfield spots* of the iris occur in 85% of those with Down syndrome and consist of an area of normal or slightly hypercellular iris surrounded by an area of iris hypoplasia.

CONNECTIVE TISSUE DISORDERS

Marfan Syndrome

Marfan syndrome is an autosomal dominantly inherited condition, primarily involving the eyes, aorta, and skeleton. The incidence is 1:10,000 to 1:20,000, with males and females affected at the same rate. A number of responsible mutations of the fibrillin gene, on chromosome 15q21.1, have been found. Affected patients are tall, with arachnodactyly (elongated digits), kyphoscoliosis, joint laxity, and pectus excavatum. Aortic aneurysm, dilation of the aortic root, and mitral valve prolapse may be present. At least 60% of affected patients have ocular findings, the most common of which are listed in Box 11-4.

Lens subluxation usually occurs in the superior and temporal direction, but any direction is possible. The

Box 11-4   Common Ocular Findings in Patients with Marfan Syndrome

Ectopia lentis
Cataracts
High myopia
Retinal detachment
Strabismus

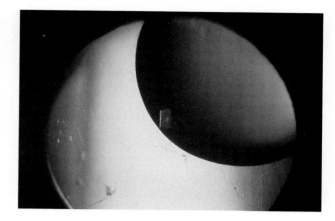

Fig. 11-13   Dislocated lens in Marfan syndrome, showing stretched zonules. See color plate.

degree of dislocation varies widely among patients, and pupillary dilation may be required to visualize mildly dislocated lenses (Fig. 11-13). Note that evaluation and treatment of patients with Marfan syndrome is hindered because the pupils tend to dilate poorly with pharmacologic agents. In most patients, ectopia lentis does not progress. Aberrations caused by the edge of the lens within the pupillary aperture may prompt lens removal, but more often, cataract is the reason for lens extraction. However, cataract surgery, whether it is done with a pars plana approach and vitrectomy instruments or with an intracapsular technique, carries a very high risk of postoperative retinal detachment and should be avoided, if possible. Ophthalmic care consists of providing the best spectacle correction possible and treating amblyopia and strabismus as needed.

Pseudoxanthoma Elasticum

Pseudoxanthoma elasticum (PXE) is a rare, usually autosomal recessive disorder affecting the elastic component of connective tissue. The organs most often affected are the skin, heart, blood vessels, gastrointestinal tract, and eyes. Xanthomatous skin lesions coalesce to form the peau d'orange lesions found in skin folds of the neck, axilla, and inguinal regions. Skin biopsy of these plaques reveals fragmentation of the elastic fibers and scattered calcification. Similar changes in the heart and blood vessels lead to peripheral vascular disease, coronary atherosclerosis, and gastrointestinal hemorrhage. *Angioid streaks,* discontinuities in Bruch's membrane, which appear as vessel-like irregular lines radiating from the disc, are found in 85% of patients with PXE but are usually not seen until the fourth decade. (Remember the other systemic conditions associated with angioid streaks: Paget's disease of bone, sickle-cell anemia, Ehlers-Danlos syndrome, and acromegaly.) However, children with PXE often show the *peau d'orange fundus* appearance as an early fundus manifestation.

Juvenile Xanthogranuloma

Juvenile xanthogranuloma is a condition of infants and young children in which proliferations of *non-*

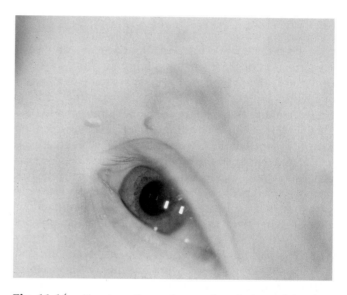

Fig. 11-14   Two juvenile xanthogranuloma lesions of the skin. See color plate.

Langerhans' histiocytes develop on the skin and, less commonly, in the eye. Rarely, only the eye is affected. The iris is the ocular structure most commonly affected. The skin lesions are small, yellow to orange, slightly raised nodules. In about 30% of patients, they are present at birth. These may be biopsied to provide a presumptive diagnosis of intraocular lesions and will show the characteristic Touton giant cells, as well as lymphocytes, plasma cells, and histiocytes. Iris lesions appear as yellow to white, localized masses. They may bleed spontaneously because of their high vascularity. In such cases, the differential diagnosis includes hyphemas as a result of trauma, other tumors, rubeosis, and iris arteriovenous malformations. Skin and iris lesions ultimately regress spontaneously, but, because of the risk of hyphema, topical corticosteroids are usually prescribed to treat iris lesions.

Box 11-5   Ocular Features of Albinism

Foveal hypoplasia
Foveal hypopigmentation
Iris transillumination defects
Nystagmus
Decreased visual acuity
Strabismus
Delayed visual maturation
Photophobia
Increased proportion of chiasmal crossing fibers

ALBINISM

In albinism, there is a reduction or absence of normal pigmentation of the eye, skin, and other structures as a result of decreased melanin. The prevalence of all types of albinism is 1:10,000 to 1:20,000. Albinism may broadly be divided into two main types: ocular albinism and oculocutaneous albinism. Within these broad classes, a number of subtypes exist. However, since there is great clinical heterogeneity in the albinism syndromes, molecular genetic techniques are required to determine with certainty which type is present. Ocular features and severity vary, but most patients with ocular or oculocutaneous albinism have foveal hypoplasia, nystagmus, and reduced vision. The ocular features of albinism are listed in Box 11-5. The enzyme *tyrosinase* is responsible for the first step of melanin synthesis, hydroxylating tyrosine to form DOPA. In the past, much emphasis was placed on determining whether a given case of albinism was tyrosinase positive or negative, as determined by the hair bulb assay. Tyrosinase negative cases were thought to have absent or non-functioning tyrosinase, and tyrosinase-positive cases had at least some enzyme function. It has become clear that this approach was oversimplified and that there is more to melanin biosynthesis than simply tyrosinase activity and that there is more to albinism than melanin biosynthesis.

Melanosomes are intracellular structures normally filled with melanin. In oculocutaneous albinism, melanosomes are normal in number but incompletely filled with melanin. In contrast, patients with ocular albinism have fewer than usual, but normally pigmented, melanosomes. The hair bulb tyrosinase assay determines tyrosinase activity by incubating hair bulbs in L-tyrosine or L-DOPA and observing any darkening of the bulbs. Currently, this test is rarely performed.

Most albinos have, as mentioned earlier, anomalous chiasmal decussation of retinal projections, whereby too many fibers cross. The reason for this defective routing and its exact relationship to hypopigmentation is unclear. Misrouting can be demonstrated in patients by performing monocular visual-evoked potentials and measuring the simultaneous responses from both occipital cortices. In affected patients, the contralateral response is significantly greater than the ipsilateral response. Since the techniques utilized in different laboratories vary, the sensitivity and specificity of VEP testing is unknown, limiting the value of such evaluations.

Oculocutaneous Albinism

Approximately 10 types of oculocutaneous albinism have been characterized. Oculocutaneous albinism 1 A *(OCA 1A)* corresponds to what has previously been called tyrosinase negative albinism. This is an autosomal recessive disorder. Affected patients have no pigment in their melanosomes and no tyrosinase activity, either because of absent protein or production of a faulty enzyme. They have white hair, pale pink skin, blue irides that transilluminate strongly, nystagmus, macular hypoplasia, and absence of fundus pigmentation. The vision is usually reduced to the 20/400 level, and affected patients may have severe photophobia. Carriers may show variable degrees of milder hypopigmentation but have normal visual function. Many mutations in the tyrosinase gene (TYR), which maps to chromosome 11q14-21, have been identified.

Patients with oculocutaneous albinism 1B *(OCA 1B)* resemble OCA 1A patients at birth but, in the first few years of life, develop some pigmentation as a result of residual (2% to 10% of normal) tyrosinase enzyme function. The hair takes on a yellow color; thus these patients are sometimes referred to as "yellow" albinos. Some patients who were previously (incorrectly) diagnosed with autosomal recessive ocular albinism actually have this form of OCA. Other, less common, forms of OCA 1 exist.

Oculocutaneous albinism 2 *(OCA 2)* is an autosomal recessive type of albinism in which there is tyrosinase activity. The defect is in the P gene, on chromosome 15q11.2-12. OCA 2 corresponds to what has been referred to as tyrosinase-positive OCA. The function of the product of the P gene has yet to be determined, but mutations lead to albinism, despite tyrosinase activity. Affected patients have very little pigmentation at birth but gradually develop skin and fundus pigmentation. There is foveal hypoplasia and moderately decreased vision, in the 20/70 to 20/200 range.

Brown OCA patients also have tyrosinase function and clinically look like OCA 2 patients, but they harbor a different mutation on chromosome nine. *Red OCA* or *Rufous OCA* patients have only been described in Africa and New Guinea. The entity is not well-characterized, but the patients' skin is red-brown, and the hair is red.

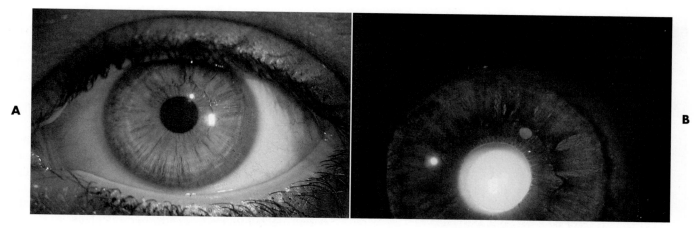

Fig. 11-15   Hermansky-Pudlak syndrome. **A,** The iris is pigmented, but **B,** transilluminates strongly. See color plate. (Courtesy of K.W. Wright, M.D.)

Autosomal dominant OCA is very rare and, in fact, may not be a true entity. *Hermansky-Pudlak syndrome (HPS)* is an uncommon form of OCA, which is associated with a bleeding diathesis, pulmonary fibrosis, and colitis. It is rare in the general population; however, it is common in the Puerto Rican population. The degree of hypopigmentation of the hair, irides, and skin varies widely in HPS (Fig. 11-15). The visual acuity ranges from 20/60 to 20/400. The platelet storage granules in affected patients are deficient or absent, resulting in poor aggregation. Therefore these patients have mild hemorrhagic episodes such as easy bruising, epistaxis, gingival bleeding, and excessive post-partum bleeding. Rarely, severe bleeding occurs. Tyrosinase activity is present, but the mechanism of hypopigmentation is unclear. Inheritance is autosomal recessive.

The *Chédiak-Higashi syndrome* is a rare form of autosomal recessive OCA in which there is an increased susceptibility to bacterial infections. Patients' peripheral blood granulocytes have abnormal giant lysosomal granules. The degree of pigmentation varies.

Ocular Albinism

Albinotic hypopigmentation limited to the eye is referred to as ocular albinism *(OA)*. X-linked and autosomal recessive forms exist. The X-linked recessive form of OA is also called *Nettleship-Falls albinism* or *OA1*. This form of albinism is rare, with a prevalence of approximately 1:50,000 to 1:150,000 males. Affected males have normal skin pigmentation, but variably decreased ocular pigment, with iris transillumination and foveal hypoplasia. Visual impairment is mild to moderate. About 80% of carrier females show patchy RPE pigmentation and, in some, iris transillumination defects. Patients with ocular albinism have melanocytes, but the melanosomes are abnormally large, suggesting that ocular albinism is proba-

bly a form of OCA. Children with nystagmus must be evaluated with the possibility of ocular albinism in mind because the hypopigmentation may be subtle. Fundus examination of the mother of a child with nystagmus may help establish the diagnosis of ocular albinism. The gene has been mapped to Xp22.

OA2 (Åland island eye disease) is an X-linked recessive condition that has similar features to OA1, with the additional findings of axial myopia, astigmatism, poor dark adaptation, and defective color vision. However, there is no axonal miswiring. The gene locus has been mapped to Xp11.3, near the gene for CSNB. *Autosomal recessive ocular albinism, OA3* affects males and females equally, with normal appearing skin and hair but variably decreased ocular pigmentation. The genetic defect or defects have not yet been elucidated.

Clinical evaluation and management Suspected cases of albinism, in most instances, can be confirmed on physical examination by considering the findings reviewed previously. However, determining the exact subtype may be a greater challenge, since genetic tests are not widely available. Obtaining a family history and examining the mother to determine whether or not she is a carrier, may provide important clues. Skin biopsy may demonstrate macromelanosomes in patients with OA. It is important to distinguish true albinism from *albinoidism,* another condition in which the skin and eyes contain little pigmentation. Patients with albinoidism have normal foveae, normal acuity, and no nystagmus.

Albinos should be given the appropriate refractive correction and treated for amblyopia as needed. Low vision aids, such as a hand-held telescope, may be useful, and photophobia may be lessened with tinted lenses. Strabismus surgery is performed if needed. Finally, the use of sunscreen and hats, to lessen the risk of skin cancer, should be encouraged.

◣◣ **MAJOR POINTS** ◢◢

The incidence of neurofibromatosis I is 1:3500 to 1:4000.

About 30% of patients with NF-I demonstrate Lisch nodules by 5 years of age and greater than 90% of affected patients over age 5 have them.

Approximately 15% of patients with NF-I develop gliomas of the optic pathway.

The hallmark of neurofibromatosis II is bilateral vestibular schwannomas.

Diffuse choroidal hemangiomas are found in up to 40% of patients with Sturge-Weber syndrome, and glaucoma is present in 30% of affected patients.

Only 30% of patients with tuberous sclerosis have the complete triad of adenoma sebaceum, seizure disorder, and mental retardation.

Patients with von Hippel-Lindau disease may become symptomatic because of ocular disease (retinal hemangioblastoma) or neurologic disease (cerebellar hemangioblastoma).

In Hurler's syndrome (MPS 1H), tissue accumulation of dermatan sulfate and heparan sulfate occurs.

Hurler's and Scheie's syndromes are autosomal recessive conditions but Hunter's syndrome is an X-linked recessive condition.

Corneal verticillata is present in approximately 70% of patients with Fabry's disease and 25% of carriers of Fabry's disease.

Cysteamine has been shown to be effective in clearing the corneas of patients with cystinosis.

The diagnosis of juvenile xanthogranuloma can usually be made with skin biopsy.

Patients with true albinism demonstrate foveal hypoplasia, nystagmus, and decreased visual acuity.

FETAL ALCOHOL SYNDROME

A constellation of typical dysmorphic features with intellectual impairment resulting from excessive maternal alcohol ingestion composes fetal alcohol syndrome (FAS). Although deleterious effects on the fetus had been previously recognized, it was not until 1973 that Jones et al consolidated the findings and coined the name still used. Risk of the teratogenic effects of ethyl alcohol in humans is evident with maternal ingestion of the daily equivalent of six drinks; however, no daily safe dose has been established. As many as one half or more of the children of alcoholic mothers display some characteristic stigmata, but mild cases often go unrecognized.

The ocular features have been well described. Most common among them is telecanthus, narrowing of the palpebral fissures, epicanthus, and ptosis. The ptosis is remarkable because it is frequently asymmetric or unilateral. Strabismus, poor visual acuity, and high refractive errors occur frequently. Associated anterior segment digeneses, Peters' anomaly in particular, have also been described. An important and frequent finding is optic nerve hypoplasia, reported in 48% of patients. Often, there is accompanying retinal vascular tortuosity with anomalous branching.

Other consistent facial features are a thin vermilion border of the upper lip and a flat philtrum. The external features may be present to a variable degree but taken together produce the distinctive picture of FAS. The systemic effects of maternal alcohol abuse include low birth weight, decreased body length, microcephaly, and a variety of heart, lung, and skeletal defects. Mental retardation is present in most patients with FAS and may be severe.

SUGGESTED READINGS

Abadi R, Pascal E: The recognition and management of albinism, *Ophthal Physiol Opt* 9:3-15, 1989.

Castronuovo S, Simon JW, Kandel GL, et al: Variable expression of albinism within a single kindred, *Am J Ophthalmol* 111: 419-426, 1991.

Charles SJ, Green JS, Grant JW, et al: Clinical features of affected males with X-linked ocular albinism, *Br J Ophthalmol* 77: 222-227, 1993.

Collins MLZ, Traboulsi EI, Maumenee IH: Optic nerve head swelling and optic atrophy in the systemic mucopolysaccharidoses, *Ophthalmol* 97(11):1445-1449, 1990.

Gahl WA, Brantly M, Kaiser-Kupfer MI: Genetic defects and clinical characteristics of patients with a form of oculocutaneous albinism (Hermansky-Pudlak syndrome), *N Engl J Med* 338 (18):1258-1264, 1998.

Hardwig P, Robertson DM: von Hippel-Lindau disease: a familial, often lethal, multi-system phakomatosis, *Ophthalmol* 91(3): 263-270, 1984.

Iwach AG, Hoskins Jr HD, Hetherington Jr J, et al: Analysis of surgical and medical management of glaucoma in Sturge-Weber syndrome, *Ophthalmol* 97(7):904-909, 1990.

Kaiser-Kupfer MI, Gazzo MA, Datiles MB, et al: A randomized placebo-controlled trial of cysteamine eye drops in nephropathic cystinosis, *Arch Ophthalmol* 108:689-693, 1990.

King RA, Hearing VJ, Creel DJ, et al: Albinism. In Scriver CR, Beaudet AL, Sly WS, Valle D, editors: *The metabolic and molecular basis of inherited disease*, New York, 1995 McGraw Hill.

Listernick R, Charrow J: Neurofibromatosis type 1 in childhood, *J Pediatr* 116(6):845-853, 1990.

Mulvihill JJ, Parry DM, Sherman JL, et al: Neurofibromatosis 1 (Recklinghausen disease) and Neurofibromatosis 2 (bilateral acoustic neurofibromatosis), *Ann Intern Med* 113(1):39-52, 1990.

Obringer AC, Meadows AT, Zackai EH: The diagnosis of neurofibromatosis-1 in the child under the age of 6 years, *Am J Diseases Children* 143:717-719, 1989.

Rettele GA, Brodsky MC, Merin LM, et al: Blindness, deafness, quadriparesis, and a retinal malformation: the ravages of neurofibromatosis 2, *Surv Ophthalmol* 41(2):135-141, 1996.

Russell-Eggitt I, Kriss A, Taylor DSI: Albinism in childhood: a flash VEP and ERG study, *Br J Ophthalmol* 74:136-140, 1990.

Sher NA, Letson RD, Desnick RJ: The ocular manifestations in Fabry's disease, *Arch Ophthalmol* 97:671-676, 1979.

Welling DB: Clinical manifestations of mutations in the neurofibromatosis type 2 gene in vestibular schwannomas (acoustic neuromas), *Laryngoscope* 108:178-189, 1998.

In this chapter, important congenital and acquired optic nerve disorders are discussed. Some disc abnormalities, such as optic nerve hypoplasia and morning glory disc anomaly, may indicate the presence of a systemic syndrome. Therefore it is important for the ophthalmologist to be able to correctly identify the various congenital structural abnormalities. Optic neuritis and pseudotumor cerebri, the more common acquired pediatric optic neuropathies, are also covered. Congenital nystagmus is a frequent and important problem in children, which may be an isolated motor dysfunction or may be related to afferent visual system dysfunction. The features and causes of congenital nystagmus are discussed in this chapter. Also covered is another notable variety of childhood nystagmus, spasmus nutans. Cranial nerve palsies are covered in Chapter 19 of this volume, and discussions of other types of nystagmus may be found elsewhere in this series.

OPTIC NERVE DISORDERS

Optic Nerve Hypoplasia

Hypoplastic optic nerves appear as congenitally small optic discs. The magnitude of hypoplasia varies widely, as does the associated level of visual impairment. Additionally, the associated features and configuration of affected nerves may also vary greatly. The ophthalmologist should be able to recognize the different manifestations of optic nerve hypoplasia because it is the most common congenital optic nerve abnormality.

The classic description of the hypoplastic optic nerve is that of a small nerve surrounded by a ring of pigmentation (*double ring sign*), often associated with tortuous retinal vessels. Affected discs may be normal, gray, or pale in color but must be distinguished from optic atrophy, an acquired condition. Histologic study has shown that hypoplastic discs have fewer axons than normal discs, but the glial supporting tissue is normal. The double ring is formed by abnormal retina and retinal pigment epithelium. Severely affected nerves are not difficult to diagnose with the true disc substance appearing as a minute structure at the scleral opening (Fig. 12-1). Mild cases are more difficult to diagnose, and, indeed, there are no universally accepted diagnostic guidelines to distinguish normal optic nerves from mildly hypoplastic ones.

The visual function of eyes with optic nerve hypoplasia may range from essentially normal to no light perception. To a certain extent, the amount of vision can be predicted by the structure of the nerve. However, the

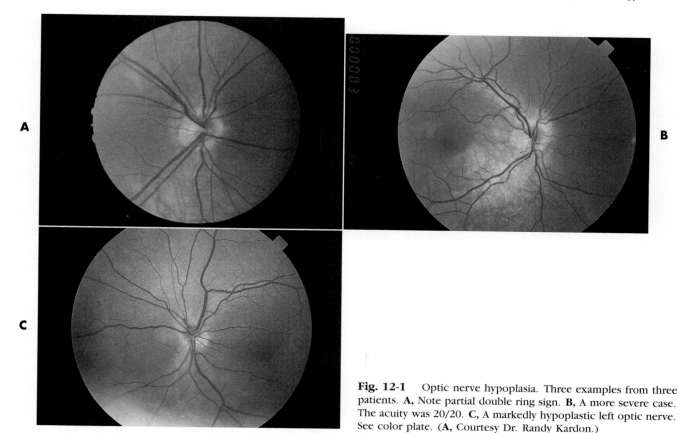

Fig. 12-1 Optic nerve hypoplasia. Three examples from three patients. **A,** Note partial double ring sign. **B,** A more severe case. The acuity was 20/20. **C,** A markedly hypoplastic left optic nerve. See color plate. (**A,** Courtesy Dr. Randy Kardon.)

most important factor, the presence or absence of an intact papillomacular bundle, cannot be predicted by optic nerve appearance. Hence, some eyes with fairly small discs retain good central vision. The clinician should resist the urge to predict the ultimate vision when optic nerve hypoplasia is diagnosed in infancy.

Optic nerve hypoplasia may occur unilaterally or bilaterally. At the present time, most cases are thought to be sporadic, with no known genetic defect or identifiable gestational insult responsible. However, maternal ingestion of alcohol or other drugs may be responsible for some cases. Children of insulin-dependent diabetic mothers may have a specific variety of optic nerve hypoplasia where the superior aspect of the disc is absent, resulting in a predominantly inferior field defect.

Monocular or asymmetric cases present with decreased vision or strabismus. Since amblyopia may complicate such cases, it is important to attempt amblyopia treatment to determine whether or not any of the visual loss is recoverable. High refractive errors, particularly astigmatism, are common in optic nerve hypoplasia and may require correction. Bilateral cases of optic nerve hypoplasia usually present with decreased vision and nystagmus.

The frequent association of optic nerve hypoplasia with other central nervous system (CNS) structural ab-

normalities places the added responsibility of proper diagnosis on the shoulders of the ophthalmologist. The most well known of these abnormalities is called *septo-optic dysplasia (de Morsier's syndrome).* In addition to optic nerve hypoplasia, affected patients have an absent septum pellucidum and agenesis or thinning of the corpus callosum. A variety of other malformations have been identified in association with optic nerve hypoplasia. These include abnormalities of cortical migration, such as schizencephaly and cortical heterotopia, and posterior pituitary ectopia. In the later condition, which is present in approximately 15% of patients with optic nerve hypoplasia, magnetic resonance imaging (MRI) reveals that the normal hyperintense signal of the posterior pituitary gland is not found in the sella turcica but is present superior to the normal pituitary gland. Since many of the patients with midline structural defects will develop hypopituitarism, MRI scanning, particularly of patients with bilateral disease, has been advocated. Another reason to obtain MRIs on such patients is to identify cortical migration defects, which are predictive of developmental deficits.

In septo-optic dysplasia, growth hormone deficiency is the most commonly found endocrine abnormality. Other associated findings include hypothyroidism, diabetes insipidus, and hypopituitarism. Affected babies

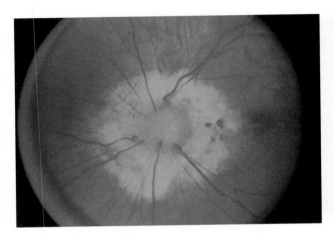

Fig. 12-2 Morning glory disc anomaly. See color plate. (From Rosen ES, Cumming WJK, Eustace P, et al: *Neuro-Opthalmology,* St Louis, 1997, Mosby.)

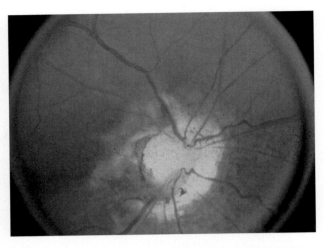

Fig. 12-3 Optic disc coloboma. See color plate. (From Rosen ES, Cumming WJK, Eustace P, et al: *Neuro-Ophthalmology,* St Louis, 1997, Mosby.)

may also have corticotropin deficiency, which can lead to hypoglycemia and dysfunctional thermoregulation. These factors, in combination with diabetes insipidus, can lead to shock and sudden death following relatively minor illness or stress.

Morning Glory Disc Anomaly

The morning glory disc anomaly is a specific type of maldevelopment of the optic nerve and posterior pole that must be differentiated from optic nerve coloboma. It appears as a funnel-shaped excavation of the posterior pole within which an abnormal optic nerve is present. The disc appears enlarged and either may be recessed within the funnel or may contain an overlying tuft of white-gray glial tissue. Elevated retinal folds radiating from the disc are also typical. The blood vessels emanating from this disc are always abnormally straight and the number of vessels increased. Surrounding the excavation, a wide band of chorioretinal hyperpigmentation is often present (Fig. 12-2).

Visual acuity is usually poor, 20/200 or worse, but occasionally patients with better vision are encountered. Almost all cases are unilateral, and females are more commonly affected than males. Amblyopia may accompany eyes with the morning glory disc anomaly; thus a trial of patching is usually warranted. Serous retinal detachments, usually surrounding the disc, are common, but the source of the fluid is debated.

The morning glory disc anomaly is often accompanied with a basal encephalocele. Basal encephaloceles are characterized by a congenital herniation of a midline meningocele through a defect in the sphenoid bone. This herniated tissue may be mistaken for nasal polyps or other masses in the nose or nasopharynx. Hence, neuroimaging of all patients with the morning glory disc anomaly is indicated. The presence of a basal encephalocele may be suggested by other midfacial anomalies, such as hypertelorism, cleft lip, cleft palate, and notching of the upper lip.

Optic Disc Coloboma

Optic disc colobomas comprise another congenital excavated disc anomaly. Such colobomas, like colobomas of the iris and the choroid and retina, are thought to result from faulty closure of the embryonic fissure.

Affected nerves vary widely in appearance, but typically there is a well-defined, white, glistening excavation involving the inferior disc. Larger colobomas may involve the entire nerve, as well as large regions of the posterior pole, resulting in profound visual loss. However, predicting final visual acuity based on optic nerve appearance is difficult. Optic nerve colobomas are often associated with chorioretinal colobomas, iris colobomas, and lens colobomas. Therefore a thorough ocular examination to identify other defects is essential and may serve to confirm the diagnosis. Optic nerve colobomas are often confused with morning glory discs, but a variety of features are useful in distinguishing these entities. Colobomatous discs often occur bilaterally and with known syndromes such as the CHARGE association. The morning glory disc anomaly is rarely bilateral and is unassociated with known coloboma syndromes. Optic disc colobomas have no central glial tuft, no retinal folds, and little, if any, peripapillary pigment disturbance, all of which are present in morning glory discs. Finally, beyond the area of the coloboma, the retinal vasculature in colobomatous eyes is normal, whereas it is abnormal in discs with morning glory anomaly.

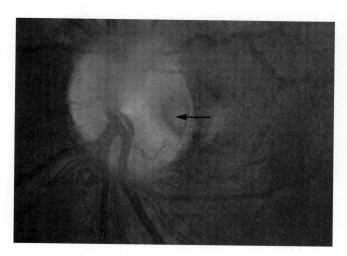

Fig. 12-4   Optic pit. Note the deep hole in the temporal nerve. See color plate. (From Rosen ES, Cumming WJK, Eustace P, et al: *Neuro-Ophthalmology*, St Louis, 1997, Mosby.)

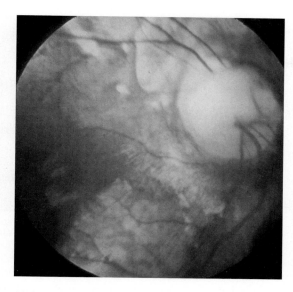

Fig. 12-5   Fundus in Aicardi syndrome, showing large peripapillary lacunae and an anomalous disc.

Optic Pit

Optic pits are congenital disc anomalies characterized by a deep excavation, usually in the temporal aspect of the nerve. They appear as a round or oval, gray to yellow depression (Fig. 12-4). In more than half of affected eyes, a cilioretinal artery emerges from the pit. Optic pits are bilateral in 15% of cases. Serous macular detachments occur in 25% to 75% of eyes with optic pits, but symptoms from such elevations usually do not occur until the third or fourth decade. The source of the fluid is controversial. Since permanent progressive visual loss may develop from the macular detachment and because spontaneous resolution appears to occur less commonly than previously thought, vitrectomy with intraocular gas tamponade has been advocated.

Aicardi Syndrome

Aicardi syndrome is a rare, possibly X-linked syndrome, with primary manifestations in the eye and brain. The major ocular findings include optic nerve hypoplasia and distinctive multiple chorioretinal lacunae. These lacunae appear as round or ovoid regions, usually around the disc, of well-demarcated defects of the RPE and choroid (Fig. 12-5). Overlying retina is present, but abnormal. Associated ocular abnormalities include microphthalmos iris colobomas, and retinal detachment.

The common CNS anomalies in Aicardi syndrome are agenesis of the corpus callosum and cortical migration anomalies, findings that are demonstrated with MRI. Affected patients develop infantile spasms and severe mental retardation. Bony abnormalities also commonly occur,

particularly involving the vertebral column and the ribs. Because no males with Aicardi syndrome have been reported, the condition is thought to be X-linked dominant and lethal in males. However, the specific genetic cause remains undetermined. Patients with the ocular findings suggesting Aicardi syndrome should undergo neuroimaging and be evaluated by a pediatric neurologist.

Hereditary Optic Neuropathies

Dominant optic atrophy   Dominant optic atrophy *(Kjer optic atrophy)* is the most common of the heritable optic atrophies with an incidence of 1:50,000. Typically, visual loss is slowly progressive and insidious, becoming apparent by age 8 years. Often, visual impairment is discovered on routine screening. The acuity ranges from 20/70 to 20/200. Many patients demonstrate a blue-yellow color vision deficit, but others have a generalized color deficiency. The typical optic disc appearance is that of a temporal wedge-shaped region of disc pallor. The remainder of the disc may appear relatively normal, or, in some patients, diffuse atrophy is present (Fig. 12-6). The characteristic visual field defect is the central or cecocentral scotoma. However, the peripheral visual field is usually normal. In most patients with dominant optic atrophy, there are no associated systemic defects. The genetic defect has been mapped to chromosome three. There is no treatment available for this condition.

Recessive optic atrophy   Recessive optic atrophy differs from dominant optic atrophy in that it is significantly less common and typically associated with systemic abnormalities such as mental retardation, spasticity, and hypertonia. When such systemic defects are

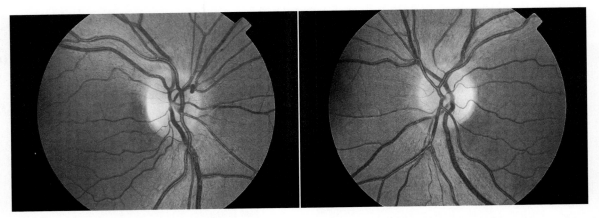

Fig. 12-6   Dominant optic atrophy, with temporal, wedge-shaped disc pallor. See color plate.

present, the condition is referred to as *Behr optic atrophy*. Affected patients have severe bilateral visual loss from an early age, with optic disc pallor and vascular attenuation. Nystagmus is present in approximately half of the patients.

Leber's hereditary optic neuropathy   Leber's hereditary optic neuropathy (LHON) is a bilateral, painless anterior optic neuropathy, which may occur simultaneously in both eyes or sequentially. The second eye is usually affected within 6 months of the first. Most cases develop in males in their twenties, but children and females may also be affected. This condition is inherited exclusively through point mutations in the maternal mitochondrial DNA. Therefore all children of a female carrier are at risk for developing Leber's hereditary optic neuropathy. However, the children of affected men are at no increased risk because sperm contribute no mitochondrial DNA to the zygote.

The classic description of Leber's hereditary optic neuropathy includes mild to moderate optic nerve pseudoedema (no fluorescein leakage present) and characteristic peripapillary telangiectasia. Cecocentral visual field defects are present, and optic atrophy ensues, with permanent visual loss. However, this picture is often absent.

The recent explosion in the understanding of this condition has resulted in improved diagnostic ability and the recognition that LHON is much more clinically heterogeneous than previously thought. The first mitochondrial DNA point mutation to be linked to LHON was a mutation at the 11778 position. Such mutations are responsible for approximately 50% of cases. Mutations at the 3460 position are found in approximately 15% to 30% of affected patients. A smaller proportion of patients are found to have mutations at the 14484 and the 15257 positions. The clinical features may vary, in part, depending on which mutation is present. For instance, about one quarter of patients with the 15257 mutation experience significant visual recovery. Genetic testing has also permitted identification of affected patients who

never had the classic findings in the acute or subacute stages. Rather, they present with painless visual loss and normal appearing nerves that later become atrophic.

Genetic testing is available to all patients by sending blood to a specialized laboratory. All patients with unexplained optic neuropathies, particularly bilateral ones, should be suspected of having LHON and should be offered genetic testing. Overall, children tend to have better visual outcomes than adults, but, unfortunately, no effective treatment has emerged. The pathophysiology may relate to an energy deficit in the cells serving the papillomacular bundle, but the reason for an increased susceptibility of this region remains speculative.

Optic Neuritis

The causes of optic neuritis and its clinical characteristics in children differ significantly from optic neuritis in adults. In adults, episodes of optic neuritis are typically monocular and often occur in association with, or before, the development of multiple sclerosis. Additionally, retrobulbar optic neuritis is common in adults. In contrast, childhood optic neuritis tends to be bilateral and uncommonly is an early manifestation of multiple sclerosis. Most cases of pediatric optic neuritis are thought to be related to preceding systemic viral illnesses such as measles, mumps, and infectious mononucleosis. Noninfectious causes include the optic neuritis associated with *Devic disease* (bilateral optic neuritis with transverse myelitis), sarcoidosis, vasculitis, and multiple sclerosis. Other cases of pediatric optic neuritis are thought to be localized forms of acute disseminated encephalomyelitis.

As noted previously, bilaterality is thought to be common in childhood optic neuritis. However, it is probable that many unilateral cases go unnoticed. The visual loss in childhood optic neuritis may be quite severe, with the acuity often falling to 20/200 or worse. Large central and cecocentral scotomas are typical, and in unilateral or bilaterally asymmetric cases, relative afferent pupillary defects are seen. Evaluation is aimed at determining whether or not an identifiable or treatable cause is present. A general physical examination should be performed, looking for lymphadenopathy or splenomegaly, which might indicate mononucleosis. Ocular examination should, in addition to characterizing the status of the optic nerve, include a careful assessment of the presence or absence of intraocular inflammation, which might indicate sarcoidosis, toxoplasmosis, toxocariasis, or tuberculosis. The presence of an early macular star should be specifically sought because the differential diagnosis of neuroretinitis differs somewhat from optic neuritis. Cranial magnetic resonance imaging is performed on all patients to evaluate for the presence of demyelination or other inflammatory processes. Additionally, in bilateral cases, imaging signs of increased intracranial pressure are also sought because in young children it may be difficult to distinguish papilledema from bilateral optic neuritis. Most authorities suggest performing lumbar puncture to evaluate for the possibility of encephalitis and markers of multiple sclerosis and to measure the cerebrospinal fluid pressure.

Optimal management of presumed post-infectious optic neuritis is uncertain. Many authors suggest using relatively high-dose corticosteroids in the acute phase, and this has been our practice, although scientific data demonstrating its efficacy over observation are lacking. In cases where the optic neuritis is thought to be related to multiple sclerosis (demyelinating plaques present on MRI), it seems reasonable to follow the protocol used in the Optic Neuritis Treatment Trial, keeping in mind that children were not a part of that study. The differential diagnosis of optic disc swelling in the pediatric population is given in Box 12-1.

Pseudotumor Cerebri

In pseudotumor cerebri *(idiopathic intracranial hypertension)*, there is an elevation of intracranial pressure without hydrocephalus, which results in papilledema. Pseudotumor cerebri in adults most often occurs in overweight women in the childbearing years and is associated with headache, visual loss secondary to papilledema, and sixth nerve palsies resulting from the elevated intracranial pressure. The pathophysiology may relate to decreased cerebral spinal fluid absorption or a hindrance of cranial venous outflow; however, the details thus far remain elusive.

Pediatric pseudotumor cerebri (occurring before puberty) equally affects boys and girls and is not strongly associated with obesity. Following puberty, the demographics (and, by inference, the pathophysiology) resemble those of adults. Infants and young children may present with systemic signs such as somnolence and irritability. Esotropia caused by sixth nerve weakness,

---

Box 12-1   Differential Diagnosis of Optic Disc Swelling

PEDIATRIC OPTIC DISC SWELLING

(a) Papillitis
    Post-infectious optic neuritis (usually bilateral)
(b) Toxocara of disc (unilateral)

PAPILLEDEMA

(a) Intracranial mass (bilateral)
(b) Pseudotumor cerebri (bilateral)
(c) Malignant hypertension (e.g., renal failure) (bilateral)
(d) Cranial synostosis (unilateral or bilateral)

OTHERS

(a) Hamartoma of optic disc (e.g., Glial tumors of tuberous sclerosis) (usually asymmetric)
(b) Optic nerve drusen (may be bilateral but usually asymmetric)
(c) Hypermetropia (usually bilateral)

---

with papilledema and variable vision loss are found. MRI should performed to rule out intracranial mass lesions, hydrocephalus, and venous sinus thrombosis. Remember that in children mastoiditis, occurring as a consequence of otitis media, may lead to thrombosis of the adjacent lateral venous sinus, causing increased intracranial pressure and a secondary pseudotumor cerebri. Other risk factors include corticosteroid withdrawal, tetracycline or minocycline therapy (drugs commonly used to treat acne), and vitamin A intoxication (particularly isoretinoin, also used to treat acne). Lumbar puncture should be performed. Formal visual field testing also should be attempted, if the child is old enough. As in adults, treatment is individualized, with the options including acetazolamide, optic nerve sheath fenestration, and lumboperitoneal shunting.

NYSTAGMUS

Congenital Nystagmus

Nystagmus is a rhythmic oscillation of the eyes. Congenital nystagmus is a predominantly horizontal nystagmus, sometimes present at birth but usually present by age 12 weeks. In the past decade, a great deal has been learned about congenital nystagmus, particularly its underlying causes. Thus the evaluation of patients with congenital nystagmus has evolved. Congenital nystagmus is a conjugate, bilateral, predominantly horizontal nystagmus. Its distinctive features permit clinical diagnosis in most cases and are summarized in Box 12-2. Often, a

Box 12-2   Features of Congenital Nystagmus

Bilateral and conjugate
Always uniplanar and usually horizontal
Worsens with attempted fixation
Improves with eye closure or convergence
Null point may be manifested by a head turn
Oscillopsia is not present

conjugate torsional component is present, although magnification or eye movement recordings may be required to make this observation. Congenital nystagmus displays an increased intensity with extreme gaze. In right gaze, the nystagmus beats to the right, and in left gaze, the nystagmus beats to the left. The *null point* is that direction of gaze where the magnitude of the nystagmus is minimal. The presence of a null point is one of the major characteristics of congenital nystagmus. Children naturally find their null points and turn their heads to place the eyes in the direction of the null point. Any head position may result, including combinations of head turn, tilt, and elevation or depression. Another interesting characteristic of congenital nystagmus is that even in up or down gaze the oscillations remain predominantly horizontal. The magnitude of nystagmus tends to increase with attempted fixation but tends to decrease with convergence. Therefore the measured near visual acuity is usually somewhat better than the distance visual acuity. This phenomenon can be exploited by fitting patients with spectacles containing base-out prisms, which induce convergence. *Oscillopsia,* an illusory to-and-fro movement of the environment, is present in many cases of acquired nystagmus but, with exceedingly rare exceptions, is absent in congenital nystagmus. In fact, when patients with congenital nystagmus are forced to view in a gaze direction away from their null point, they report increased blur, rather than oscillopsia, even though the magnitude of the nystagmus clearly may be increased. Some patients with congenital nystagmus display intermittent episodes of involuntary, unconscious, small magnitude head shaking. Previously, such head shaking was thought to be a compensatory mechanism to improve vision, but currently, the movements are thought to be an associated pathologic phenomenon. Strabismus accompanies congenital nystagmus in up to one third of cases, and high degrees of with-the-rule stigmatism are often seen.

Eye movement recordings have demonstrated numerous waveforms and combinations of waveforms in congenital nystagmus. Previously, opinion held that cases of jerk nystagmus were a result of a primary motor dysfunction (hence the designation *congenital "motor" nystag-*

mus) and that cases of congenital nystagmus with pendular waveforms were caused by afferent visual system sensory dysfunction *(sensory nystagmus).* This classification scheme is now known to be incorrect, and various waveforms are seen in congenital nystagmus irrespective of cause.

Currently, the etiology of congenital nystagmus may be broadly divided into those cases caused by a sensory defect and those in which, after careful physical examination and electrophysiologic testing, are found to have no sensory deficit. This latter group, previously referred to as "motor" nystagmus, is now known to account for a small percentage of all cases of congenital nystagmus. The remainder of cases of congenital nystagmus either have obvious sensory defects, as indicated by structural abnormalities visible by physical examination, or sensory defects disclosed by electrophysiologic testing. However, when evaluating a child with congenital nystagmus it is still useful to think in terms of sensory causes versus motor causes; just keep in mind that some sensory etiologies do not cause visible defects.

Examination of an infant or child with congenital nystagmus should therefore focus on identifying ocular signs of afferent dysfunction, such as bilateral optic nerve hypoplasia, bilateral cataracts, iris transillumination defects, and macular hypoplasia, suggesting albinism and other macular problems. Such entities are the common causes of "sensory" nystagmus. If none of these findings is apparent, then further historical points and physical examination findings may provide etiologic clues. Patients with normal ocular examinations very often are found to have a congenital retinal dystrophy. Parents should be asked about the presence of severe photophobia or the *oculo-digital sign.* High levels of myopia and the presence of a paradoxical pupil also suggest a congenital retinal disease. Ultimately, electroretinography is required to diagnose these patients, and, the most common entities found are Leber's congenital amaurosis, achromatopsia, cone dystrophies, and congenital stationary night blindness. It is the recognition that these retinal dystrophies account for a large proportion of patients previously thought to have "motor" nystagmus that has changed the approach to patients with congenital nystagmus.

The primary treatment goals in congenital nystagmus are decreasing the nystagmus amplitude, increasing the foveation time to permit improved visual acuity, and correction of torticollis. Medications are largely ineffective in congenital nystagmus, but prisms are of some value in selected patients. Biofeedback has been reported useful by some authors, and others have advocated the use of contact lenses, which may quiet the nystagmus by providing tactile feedback. Usually, if any treatment beyond spectacles is undertaken, it involves strabismus surgery (see Chapter 19).

Spasmus Nutans

Spasmus nutans consists of a triad of nystagmus, head nodding, and torticollis. Not all patients demonstrate all three features. Although the condition usually comes to attention because of the head nodding, the nystagmus is considered to be the earliest and most constant sign of spasmus nutans. Most often, a bilateral, but asymmetric, pendular, predominantly horizontal nystagmus is seen. It is intermittent, at times appearing with brief bursts of high frequency (7 Hz) oscillations, which have been referred to as having a shimmering quality. At times, oblique or vertical oscillations occur. Characteristically the nystagmus is disconjugate, a feature that increases in extreme gaze. The head nodding is typically a combined movement, consisting of up-and-down movements with side-to-side movements. These also occur intermittently but are larger in amplitude, up to 25°, and slower in frequency, about 3 Hz, than the nystagmus. The head nodding is a compensatory mechanism to decrease the nystagmus. The head tilt is the least constant finding.

Spasmus nutans typically has its onset between age 6 and 12 months, and most cases resolve by age 2 years. Some cases, however, persist for many years longer. The visual acuity is usually good, although mild amblyopia may occur, and associated strabismus is not uncommon. Earlier descriptions of spasmus nutans indicated that it was more prevalent in regions of low socioeconomic conditions. Currently, spasmus nutans is believed to be more prevalent among black patients. The etiology is unknown.

Approximately 1% of patients with what appears to be spasmus nutans actually harbor a suprasellar tumor, usually an *optic pathway glioma* or a thalamic glioma, which is responsible for the clinical syndrome. Technically, such cases are not designated spasmus nutans, but on clinical and oculographic grounds, the nystagmus, head nodding, and torticollis appear identical to patients with the idiopathic condition. Patients with such intracranial tumors often can be identified because of the presence of decreased vision, a relative afferent pupillary defect, or optic disc pallor. Unfortunately, such findings are not always present, and children with typical spasmus nutans–like presentations and normal eye examinations may have such tumors. Therefore routine neuroimaging (MRI) has been advocated, and this has been our practice.

The main clinical entity often confused with spasmus nutans is congenital nystagmus, but many features help distinguish between spasmus nutans and congenital nystagmus. Congenital nystagmus is almost always seen within the first 2 months of age, whereas spasmus nutans usually comes on after 6 months. Head nodding in congenital nystagmus occurs in approximately 10% of cases, and is fairly small in amplitude, whereas it is much more common in spasmus nutans and has a larger amplitude.

MAJOR POINTS

In optic nerve hypoplasia, visual function is difficult to predict solely on the basis of the nerve's appearance.

Cases of monocular optic nerve hypoplasia tend to present with visual loss and strabismus, whereas bilateral cases present with nystagmus.

The primary features of septo-optic dysplasia are optic nerve hypoplasia, absence of the septum pellucidum, and agenesis or thinning of the corpus callosum.

Progressive visual loss may occur in the morning glory disc anomaly as a result of serous retinal detachment.

Dominant optic atrophy is the most common hereditary optic neuropathy, with an incidence of 1:50,000.

Visual loss in recessive optic atrophy is more severe than in dominant optic atrophy.

Leber's hereditary optic neuropathy is a bilateral disease, but the eyes may be affected months apart.

In children, optic neuritis is bilateral much more often than in adults.

In contrast to adults, childhood optic neuritis is not a strong predictor of the development of subsequent multiple sclerosis.

In pediatric pseudotumor cerebri boys are affected at the same rate as girls.

As a rule, patients with congenital nystagmus do not experience oscillopsia.

Many cases of congenital nystagmus thought to be the "motor" type are actually caused by retinal dystrophies.

Children with spasmus nutans may harbor an optic pathway tumor.

The oscillations of congenital nystagmus often contain jerk, as well as pendular waveforms, often have fairly large amplitudes, are conjugate (the eyes are in phase), and are constant. In spasmus nutans, the oscillations are strictly pendular with a variable phase relationship and a definite intermittency. Rarely, patients thought to have spasmus nutans are later found to have a condition such as a congenital retinal dystrophy or even a neurodegenerative disease. Therefore it is prudent to cautiously diagnose spasmus nutans. Some authors contend that the diagnosis of spasmus nutans should only be made in retrospect, after spontaneous resolution.

SUGGESTED READINGS

Babikian P, Corbett J, Bell W: Idiopathic intracranial hypertension in children: the Iowa experience, *J Child Neurol* 9(2): 144-149, 1994.

Brodsky MC, Conte FA, Taylor D, et al: Sudden death in septo-optic dysplasia, *Arch Ophthalmol* 115:66-70, 1997.

Brown Jr J, Fingert JH, Taylor CM, et al: Clinical and genetic analysis of a family affected with dominant optic atrophy (OPA1), *Arch Ophthalmol* 115:95-115, 1997.

Cibis GW, Fitzgerald KM: Electroretinography in congenital idiopathic nystagmus, *Peditr Neurol* 9:369-371, 1993.

Gottlob I, Zubcov A, Catalano RA, et al: Signs distinguishing spasmus nutans (with and without central nervous system lesions) from infantile nystagmus, *Ophthalmology* 97(9):1166-1175, 1990.

Johns DR, Heher KL, Miller NR, et al: Leber's hereditary optic neuropathy: clinical manifestations of the 14484 mutation, *Arch Ophthalmol* 111:495-498, 1993.

Johns DR, Smith KH, Savino PJ, et al: Leber's hereditary optic neuropathy: clinical manifestations of the 15257 mutation, *Ophthalmology* 100(7):981-986, 1993.

Johnston RL, Burdon MA, Spalton DJ, et al: Dominant optic atrophy, Kjer type: linkage analysis and clinical features in a large British pedigree, *Arch Ophthalmol* 115:100-103, 1997.

Lessell S: Pediatric pseudotumor cerebri (idiopathic intracranial hypertension), *Surv Ophthalmol* 37(3):155-166, 1992.

Lincoff H, Lopez R, Kreissig I, et al: Retinoschisis associated with optic nerve pits, *Arch Ophthalmol* 106:61-67, 1988.

Newman NJ: Leber's hereditary optic neuropathy: new genetic considerations, *Arch Neurol* 50:540-548, 1993.

Newman SA: Spasmus nutans: or is it? *Surv Ophthalmol* 34(6):453-456, 1990.

Weiss AH, Biersdorf WR: Visual sensory disorders in congenital nystagmus, *Ophthalmology* 96(4):517-523, 1989.

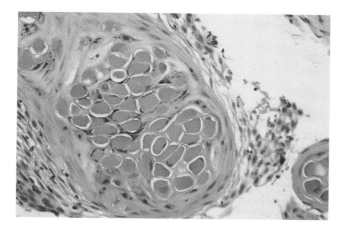

Plate 2-13

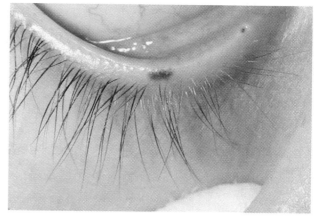

Plate 2-15

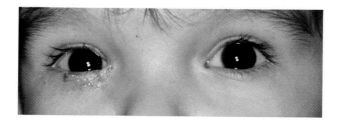

Plate 3-1

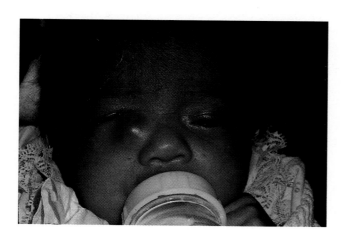

Plate 3-2

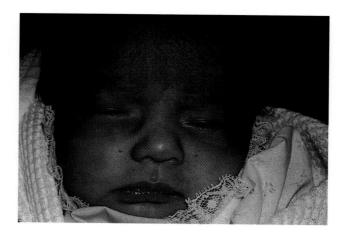

Plate 3-3

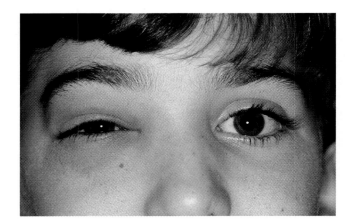

Plate 4-1

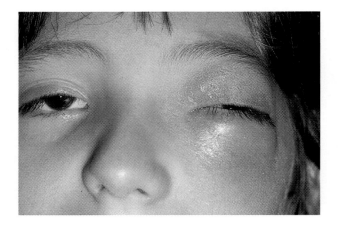

Plate 4-2

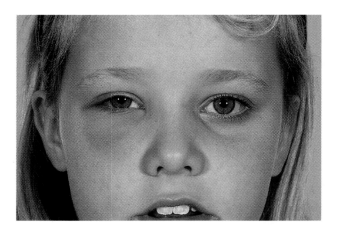

Plate 4-3

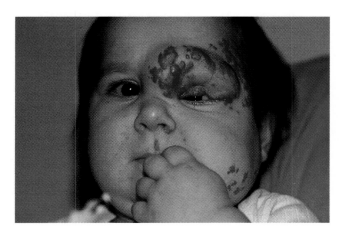

Plate 4-4, A

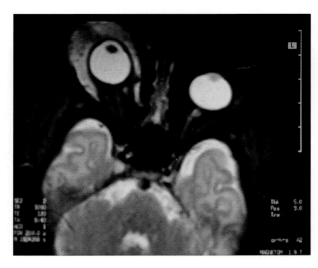

Plate 4-4, B

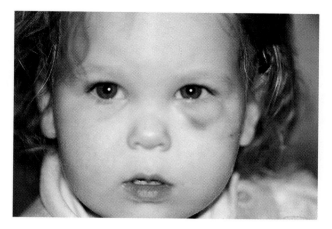

Plate 4-5

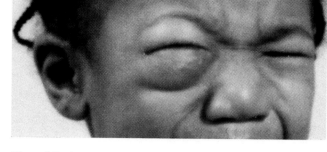

Plate 4-7, A

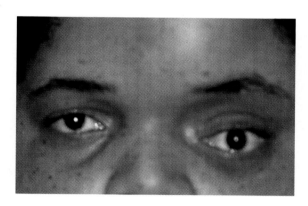

Plate 4-11, A

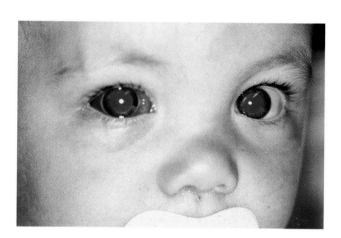

Plate 5-4

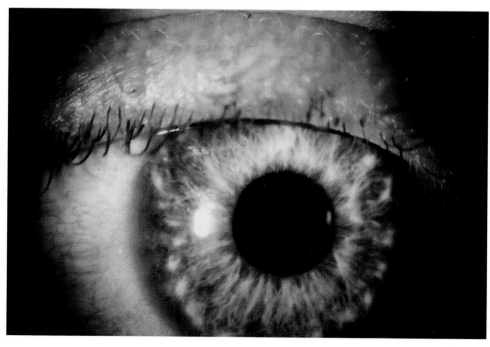

Plate 6-10

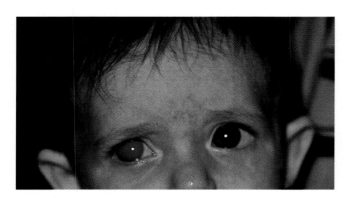

Plate 7-1

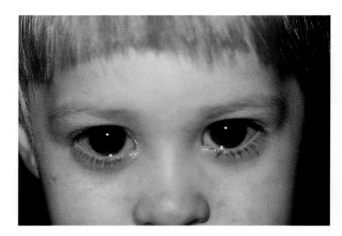

Plate 7-2

Plate 7-3

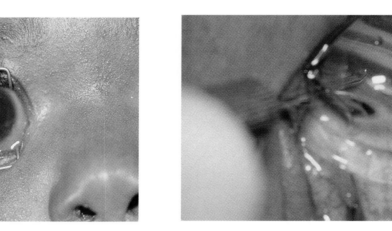

Plate 7-4

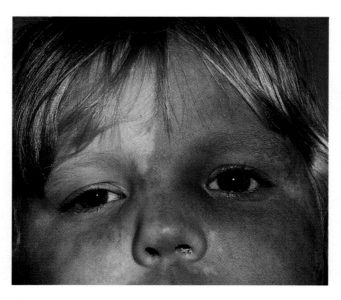

Plate 7-8

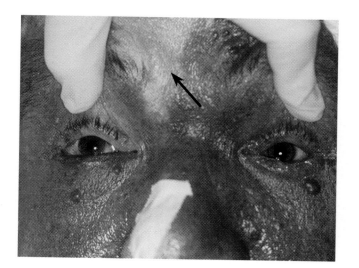

Plate 7-9, A

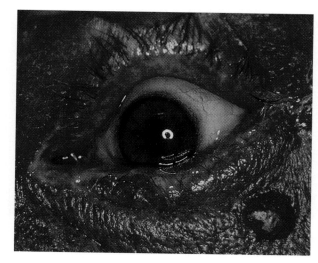

Plate 7-9, B

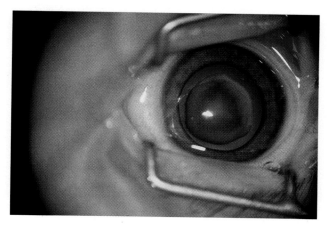

Plate 8-4

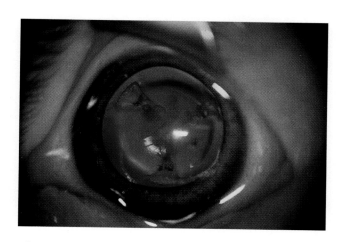

Plate 8-5

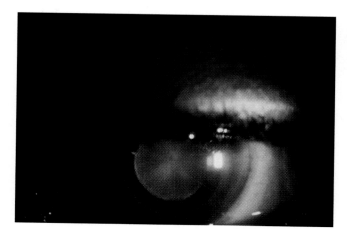

Plate 8-7, A

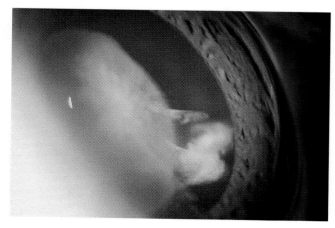

Plate 8-7, B

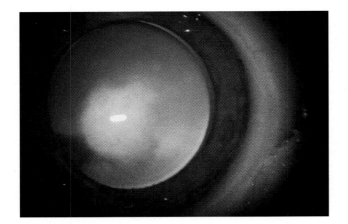

Plate 8-9, B

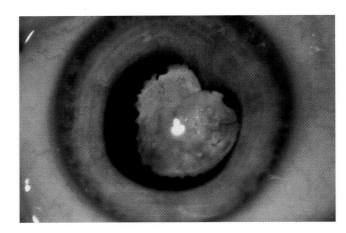

Plate 8-9, C

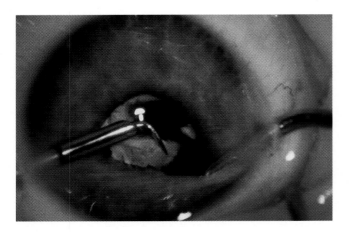

Plate 8-9, D

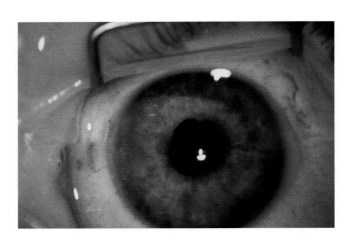

Plate 8-9, E

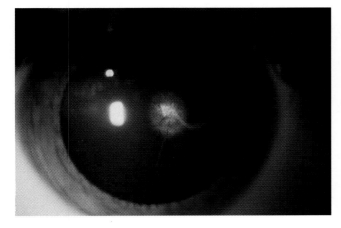

Plate 8-10, A

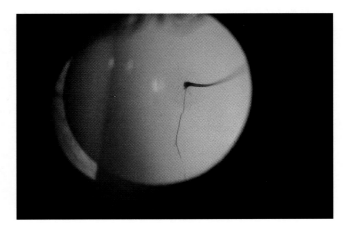

Plate 8-10, B

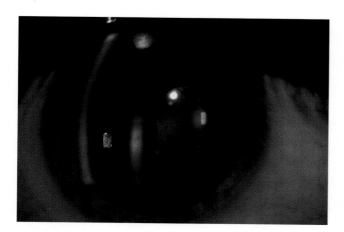

Plate 8-11, A

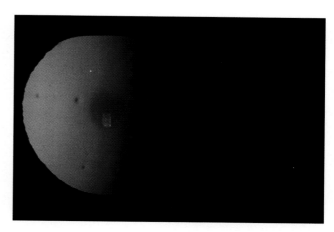

Plate 8-11, B

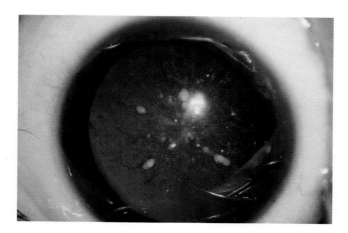

Plate 8-12

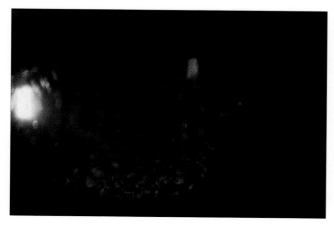

Plate 8-13, A

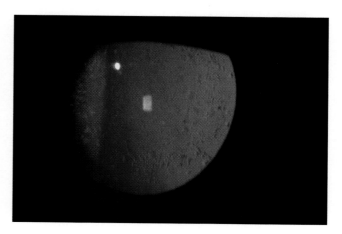

Plate 8-13, B

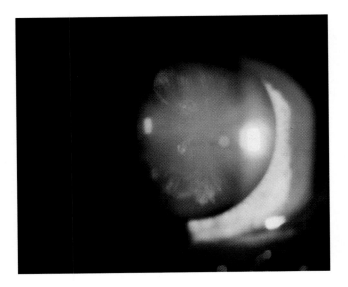

Plate 8-15, A

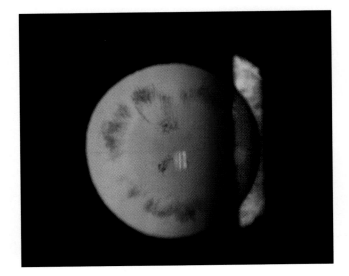

Plate 8-15, B

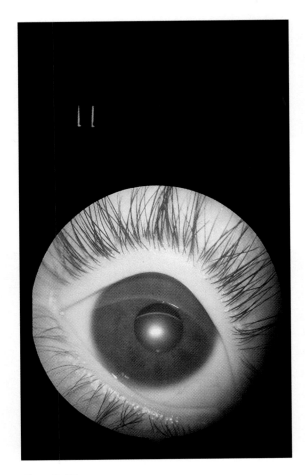

Plate 8-17

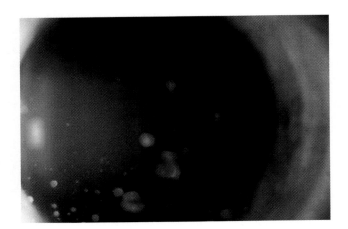

Plate 9-2, A

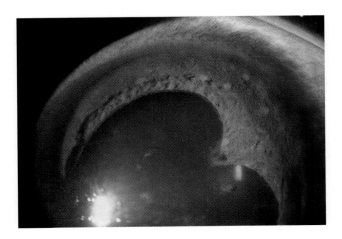

Plate 9-2, B

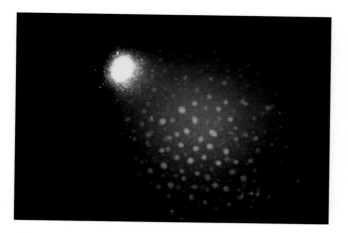

Plate 9-5, A

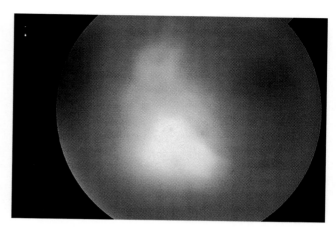

Plate 9-5, B

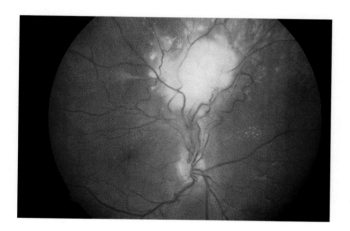

Plate 9-6, A

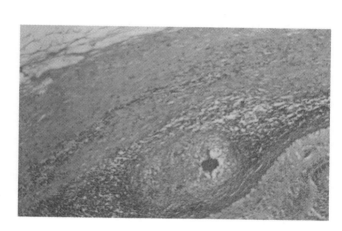

Plate 9-6, B

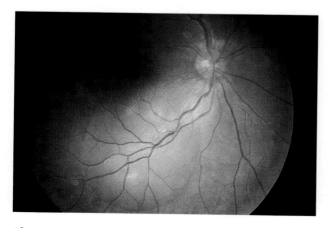

Plate 9-7

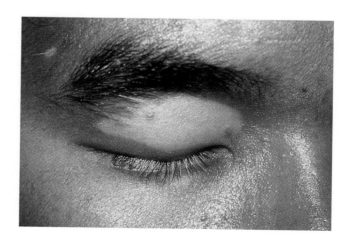

Plate 9-8

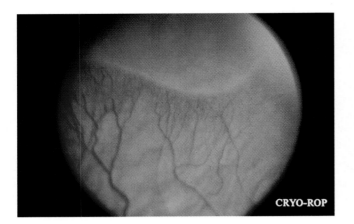

Plate 10-1

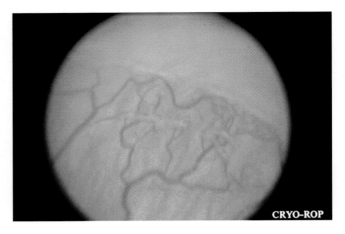

Plate 10-2

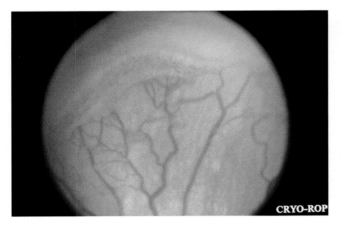

Plate 10-3

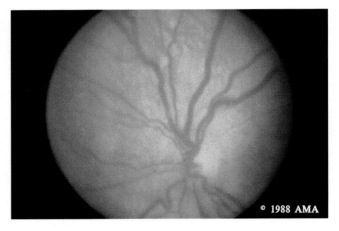

Plate 10-6

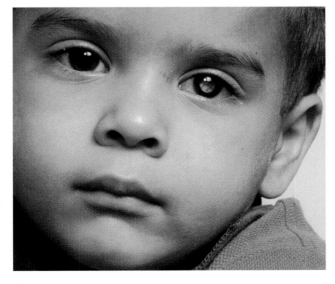

Plate 10-8, A

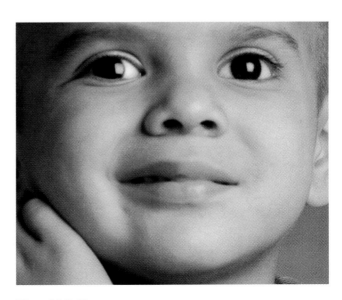

Plate 10-8, B

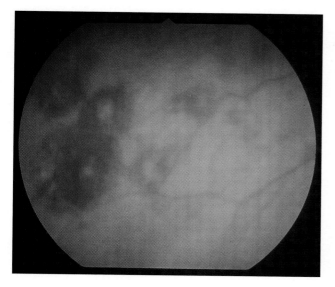

Plate 10-9

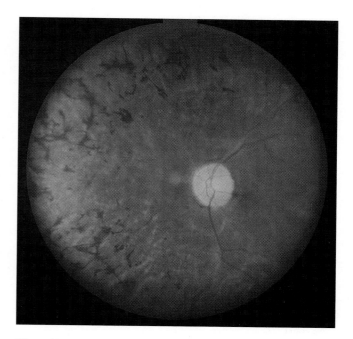

Plate 10-11

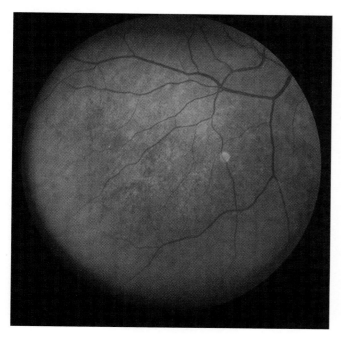

Plate 10-12

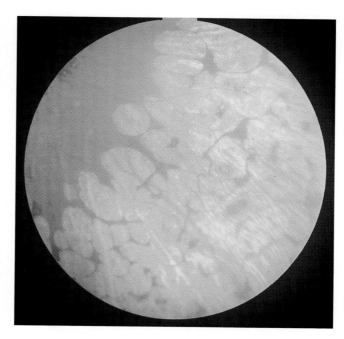

Plate 10-13

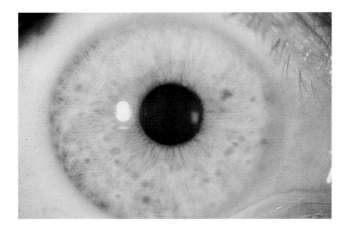

Plate 11-1

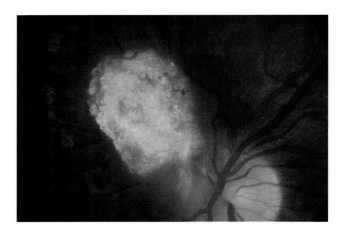

Plate 11-5

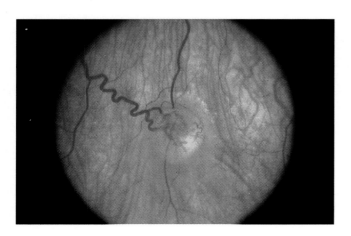

Plate 11-6

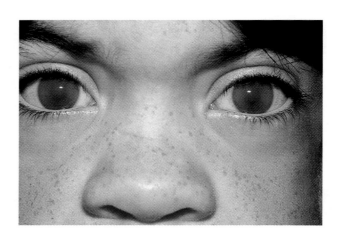

Plate 11-9

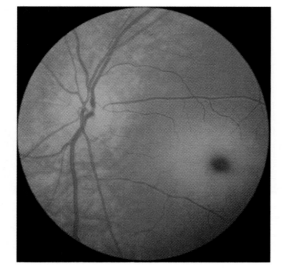

Plate 11-10

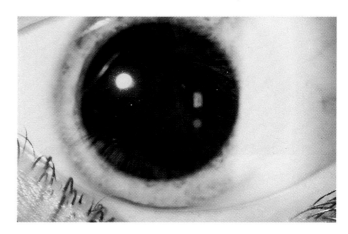

Plate 11-11

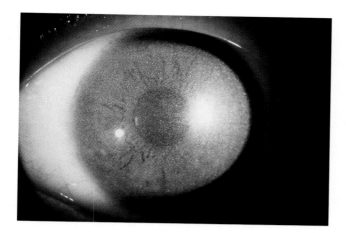

Plate 11-12

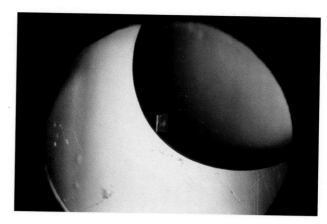

Plate 11-13

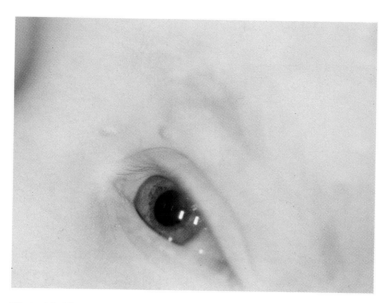

Plate 11-14

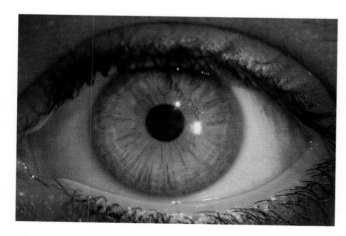

Plate 11-15, A

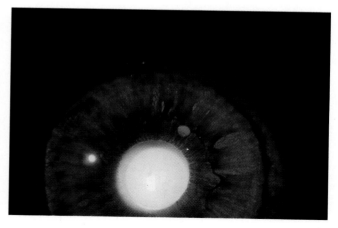

Plate 11-15, B

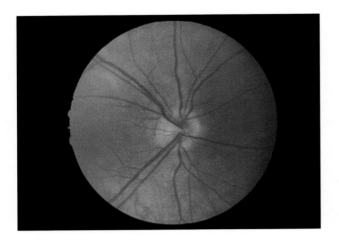

Plate 12-1, A

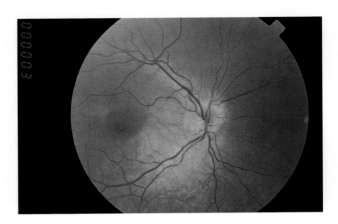

Plate 12-1, B

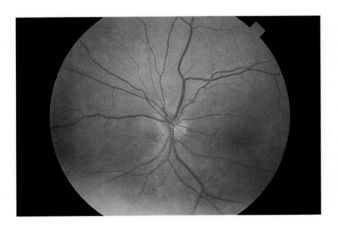

Plate 12-1, C

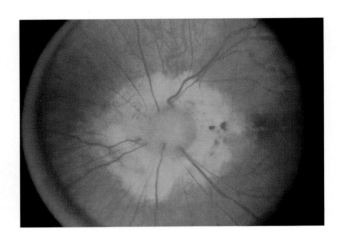

Plate 12-2

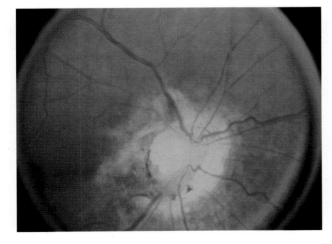

Plate 12-3

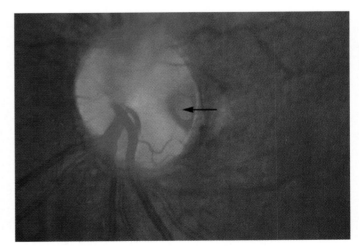

Plate 12-4

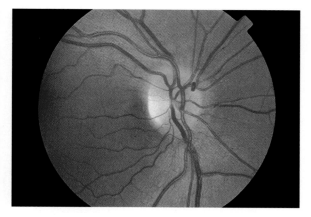

Plate 12-6, A

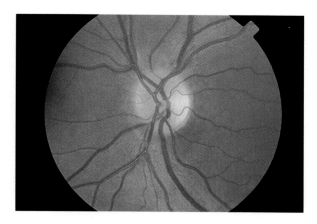

Plate 12-6, B

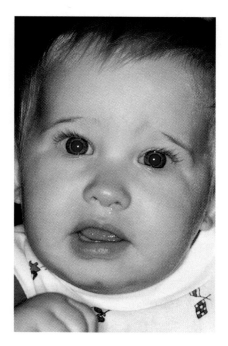

Plate 14-19, A

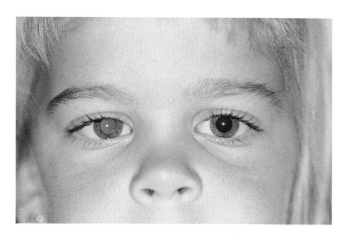

Plate 14-19, B

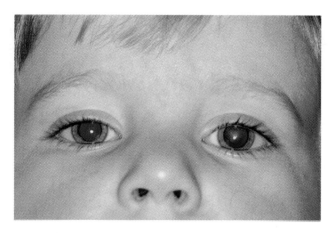

Plate 14-19, C

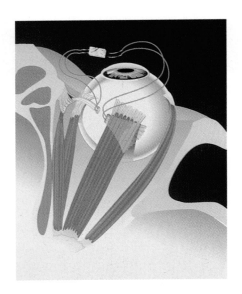

Plate 18-6, A

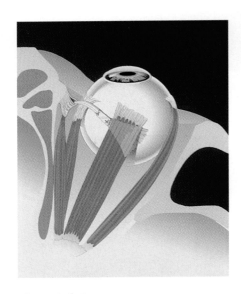

Plate 18-6, B

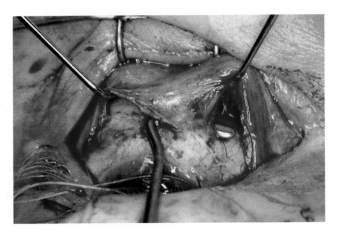

Plate 20-2, Left

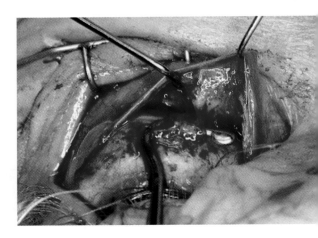

Plate 20-2, Right

There are six extraocular muscles that are responsible for rotating the eye, including two horizontal rectus muscles, two vertical rectus muscles, and two oblique muscles (Table 13-1). The extraocular muscles turn the eye by contracting or shortening, which pulls the muscle insertion towards the muscle's functional origin. Table 13-1 summarizes the functions and anatomy of the extraocular muscles. This chapter covers the anatomy and physiology of the extraocular muscles and basic physiology of eye movements.

EXTRAOCULAR MUSCLE ANATOMY

Relations of Globe, Extraocular Muscles, and Orbit

The eyeball is suspended in the center of the anterior orbit by the six extraocular muscles, the suspensory ligaments of the lids, and the surrounding orbital fat (Fig. 13-1). A tug-of-war exists between the four rectus muscles, which pull the eye posteriorly towards the apex of the orbit, and the two oblique muscles and orbital fat,

which provide counterforces that keep the eye forward. Increased rectus muscle tension pulls the eye posteriorly resulting in relative enophthalmos, whereas decreased rectus muscle tone produces proptosis. Large rectus muscle resections can result in relative enophthalmos and lid fissure narrowing as the tightened rectus muscles pull the eye back into the orbit, while recessions reduce muscle tension and tend to cause mild proptosis producing lid fissure widening. Changes in the size of the lid fissures after strabismus surgery is for the most part very subtle, unless two or more rectus muscles of one eye have had the same procedure (i.e., either a recession or resection). In Duane's retraction syndrome, the clinician can see both globe retraction associated with co-contraction of the medial and lateral rectus muscles and proptosis associated with sixth nerve paralysis (see Duane's syndrome).

When the eye is looking straight ahead with the visual axis parallel to the sagittal plane, the eye is in *primary position*. An important relationship exists between the *orbital axis* and the *visual axis* of the eye when the eye is in primary position (Fig. 13-2). The orbits diverge from the central sagittal plane of the head by approximately 23°; thus the visual axis in primary position is 23° nasal to the orbital axis. Rectus muscles parallel the orbits so the rectus *muscle axis* is in line with the orbital axis. The term *position of rest* relates to the position of the eyes when all the extraocular muscles are relaxed or paralyzed. Normally, the position of rest is in a divergent or exotropic position, with the visual axis in line with the orbital axis. A patient under general anesthesia usually has the eyes deviated in a divergent position.

Ocular Rotations

Monocular rotations are termed *ductions.* Ductions are evaluated clinically under monocular viewing conditions so patients are examined with one eye occluded

Table 13-1   Functions and anatomy of the extraocular muscles

Muscle	Approx. muscle length (mm)	Origin	Anatomic insertion (mm)	Tendon length (mm)	Arc of contact (mm)	Muscle action (from primary position)
Medial rectus	40	Annulus of Zinn	5.5	4	6	Adduction
Lateral rectus	40	Annulus of Zinn	7.0	8	10	Abduction
Superior rectus	40	Annulus of Zinn	8.0	6	6.5	Elevation, Intorsion, Adduction
Inferior rectus	40	Annulus of Zinn	6.5	7	7	Depression, Extorsion, Adduction
Superior oblique	32	Above annulus of Zinn. Functional origin is the trochlea	From temporal pole of superior rectus to within 6.5 mm of optic nerve	26	12	Intorsion, Depression, Abduction
Inferior oblique	37	Lacrimal fossa	Macular area	1	15	Extorsion, Elevation, Abduction

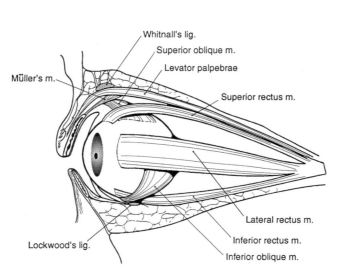

Fig. 13-1   Side view of extraocular muscles. Note that the rectus muscles pull the eye posteriorly while the oblique muscles pull the eye anteriorly.

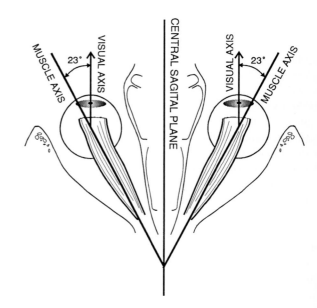

Fig. 13-2   Diagram shows visual axis versus orbital axis. No[] that the visual axes parallel the central sagittal plane while th[] orbital axis of each eye diverges 23° from the visual axis.

(Fig. 13-3). An upward movement of an eye is referred to as *supraduction, elevation,* or *sursumduction*; a downward movement is termed *infraduction, depression,* or *deorsumduction*; a nasalward movement is termed *adduction;* and a temporal movement is termed *abduction*. *Torsional* rotations (twisting movements) are known as *cycloductions,* with *incycloduction (intorsion)* referring to a nasal rotation of the 12 o'clock position of the cornea, and *excycloduction (extorsion)* referring to a temporal rotation of the 12 o'clock position.

Ocular movements are a result of contraction and relaxation of multiple muscle groups, which act to rotate the eye around a fixed center of rotation. There are thre[] axes that pass through the center of rotation of the ey[] and these are termed the *axes of Fick* (Fig. 13-4). Th[] axes of Fick include the Z-axis (vertical orientation) fo[] horizontal rotation, the X-axis (horizontal orientation[] for vertical rotation, and the Y-axis (oriented with th[] visual axis) for torsional rotation. *Listing's plane* is a ve[] tical plane that includes the X-, Z-, and oblique-axes th[] passes through the center of the eye (Fig. 13-5). *Listing[] law* states that virtually all positions of gaze can b[] achieved by rotations around axes that lie on Listing[] plane. *Donder's law* is related to Listing's law and state[]

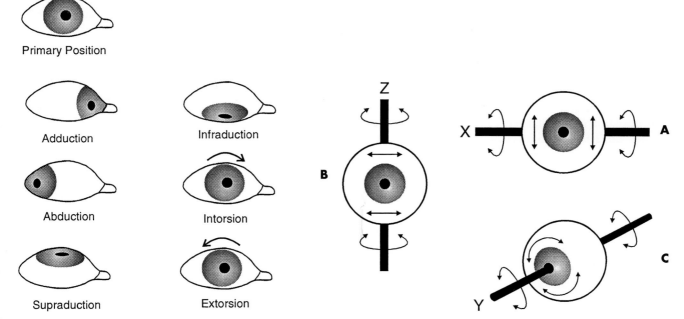

Primary Position

Adduction

Abduction

Supraduction

Infraduction

Intorsion

Extorsion

g. 13-3   Diagram shows ductions, which are monocular eye ovements.

Fig. 13-4   Three axes of Fick. **A,** Z-axis for horizontal rotation. **B,** X-axis for vertical rotation. **C,** Y-axis for torsional rotation.

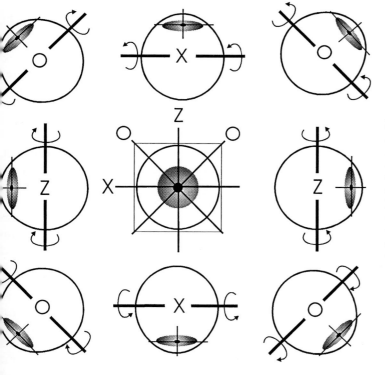

Fig. 13-5   Listing's plane is shown in the center diagram, which includes the Z- and X-axes of Fick. Diagram shows that the eye can reach all positions of gaze by rotations around axes that are on Listing's plane. In the center diagram, the O-axes represent oblique axes that are on Listing's plane and are oriented between the Z- and X-axes of Fick. Note that the oblique axes of rotation seen on the four corners of the diagram allow the eye to rotate obliquely, up and in, up and out, down and in, and down and out. Also, observe the pseudotorsion of the cornea when the eye rotates around the oblique axis.

that there is a specific orientation of the retina and cornea for every position of gaze. This corneal orientation is specific for each position of gaze regardless of the path the eye took to achieve that position of gaze. Fig. 13-5 demonstrates Listing's and Donder's laws showing the specific corneal orientations for ocular rotations around various axes on Listing's plane. Note that when rotations are directly around the X-axis (pure vertical movement), or directly around the Z-axis (pure horizontal movement) there is no associated torsional rotation of the cornea. In contrast, oblique ocular rotations cause a torsional shift in the corneal orientation relative to the planar coordinates of Listing's plane. This torsional shift relative to Listing's plane is not due to true rotation around the Y-axis and is therefore referred to as "pseudotorsion." Active or true torsional rotations around the Y-axis (cycloduction) are created by contraction of vertical and oblique muscles. True torsional movements normally occur to keep the eyes aligned during head tilting or occur pathologically when a vertical or an oblique muscle overacts or underacts.

Muscle Action Versus Field of Action

A *muscle's action* refers to the effect of muscle contraction on the rotation of the eye when the eye starts in primary position. Horizontal rectus muscles have only one muscle action, either adduction for the medial rectus, or abduction for the lateral rectus. This is because the muscle axis is in line with the visual axis of the eye when the eye is in primary position (Fig. 13-6). However, vertical and oblique muscles have vertical, horizontal, and torsional actions. These multiple functions of extraocular muscles are called primary, secondary, and tertiary actions, and occur because the muscle axis and the visual axis are not in line with the eye in primary position (Fig. 13-7). Remember the classic descriptions of primary, secondary, and tertiary actions relate to the eye when it is in primary position.

The *field of action,* on the other hand, is the position of gaze where an individual muscle is the primary mover of eye. For example, when a person looks up and nasal the inferior oblique muscle is the primary mover of the eye, whereas movement up and temporal is primarily a function of the superior rectus muscle. Fig. 13-8 shows the field of action of each muscle of the six extraocular muscles. A muscle's function is best evaluated by having the patient look into the field of action of the muscle. Thus, to evaluate over- or under-action of the inferior oblique, the examiner should have the patient look "up and nasal." Granted, virtually all eye movements are the result of combined contraction and relaxation of multiple muscles, but the six positions of gaze in Fig. 13-8 are where one muscle provides the dominant force. Note that the field of action and the muscle action are the same for the horizontal rectus muscles.

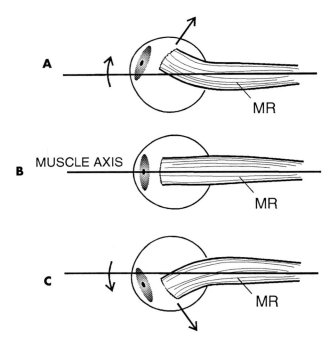

Fig. 13-6   Diagram shows that in primary position (**B**) the horizontal rectus muscles have one function, but when the eye rotates up (**A**), or down (**C**), there are secondary vertical functions. Note in the center, **B**, the medial rectus is a pure adductor since the muscle axis and the visual axis are aligned. When the globe rotates superiorly (**A**) the medial rectus also secondarily functions as elevator and when the eye is rotated down it has a secondary function of depression. These secondary actions also relate to the lateral rectus muscle.

Rectus Muscles

The four rectus muscles originate at the orbital apex the annulus of Zinn, and course straight (thus the term *rectus*) forward to insert anterior to the equator onto the globe. The rectus muscle insertions form a progressive spiral (spiral of Tillaux) around the corneal limbus with the medial rectus being the closest to the limbus (5 mm), inferior rectus next (6.5 mm), the lateral rectus next (7.0 mm), and superior rectus is the furthest from the limbus (8.0 mm) (Fig. 13-9). The muscle-scleral insertion line actually has a horseshoe shape with the rounded apex pointing towards the cornea. The scleral thickness behind the rectus insertions is 0.3 mm the thinnest in the eye. The widths of the rectus insertions are approximately 10 mm and the distance between insertions intermuscular spacing is only 6 to 8 mm. The closeness of the muscle insertions makes it relatively easy hook the wrong muscle during strabismus surgery. Each rectus muscle is 40 mm long, essentially the same length as the orbit. The rectus muscles are innervated from the intraconal side of the muscle belly at the junction of the anterior two thirds and posterior one third of the muscle.

Horizontal rectus muscles   The horizontal rectus muscles consist of the medial and lateral rectus muscles (Fig. 13-10).

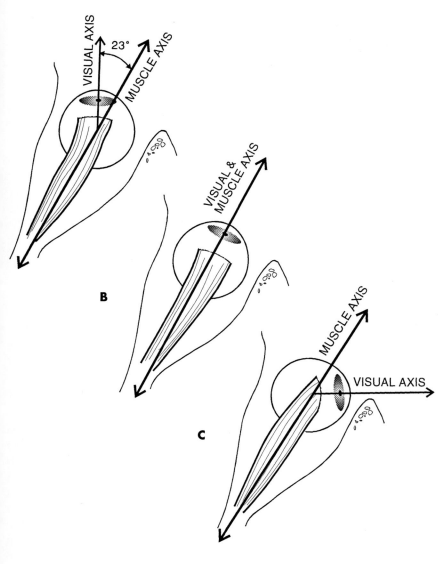

Fig. 13-7 Functions of the vertical rectus muscles change as the eye moves to various positions of gaze. **A,** The eye is in primary position with the visual axis 23° nasal to the muscle axis. Classic muscle actions apply; superior rectus is an elevator, intortor, and adductor, while the inferior rectus is a depressor, extortor, and adductor. **B,** The eye is abducted 23° temporal from primary position and the visual axis is now in line with the muscle axis, and here the superior rectus is a pure elevator and the inferior rectus a pure depressor. **C,** With the eye abducted more than 23° from the primary position the visual axis is now temporal to the muscle axis and the superior rectus is an elevator, extortor, and abductor, while the inferior rectus is a depressor, intortor, and abductor.

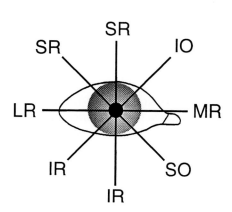

Fig. 13-8 Diagram shows the field of action of the extraocular muscles. The arrows point to the quadrant where the specified muscle is the major mover of the eye. (*S.R.* superior rectus, *I.O.* inferior oblique, *M.R.* medial rectus, *S.O.* superior oblique, *I.R.* inferior rectus, *L.R.* lateral rectus)

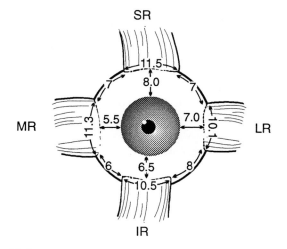

Fig. 13-9 Distance of the rectus muscle insertions from the limbus. Note that the medial rectus inserts closest to the limbus and the distances increase, going counter-clockwise from the medial rectus towards the superior rectus, which inserts furthest from the limbus.

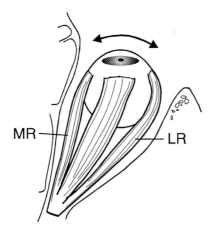

Fig. 13-10   Simple function of the medial and lateral rectus muscles with the eye in primary position.

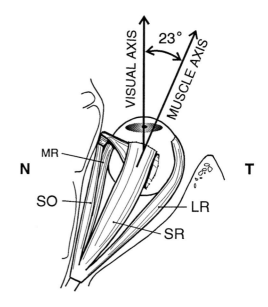

FROM ABOVE

Fig. 13-11   Eye and orbit from a top view looking down on the superior rectus muscle. Note that the superior rectus muscle overlies the superior oblique.

Medial rectus   The medial rectus is innervated by the lower division of the oculomotor nerve (third cranial nerve). It has the shortest tendon length of the rectus muscles (4 mm). The medial rectus is a pure adductor when the eye is in primary position. Because of the divergent angle of the orbit versus the visual axis, the medial rectus muscle has the shortest arc of contact to sclera (6 mm) (see Fig. 13-10). It is the only rectus muscle that does not have fascial connections to an adjacent oblique muscle. During strabismus surgery, if a medial rectus muscle is inadvertently disinserted and released from the globe, it can retract completely off the eyeball, making retrieval extremely difficult.

Lateral rectus muscle   The lateral rectus muscle is innervated by the sixth cranial nerve. It has the longest arc of contact (10 mm) (see Fig. 13-10) and the longest tendon (8 mm). In primary position, the lateral rectus is a pure abductor. The inferior border of the lateral rectus muscle courses just superior to the inferior oblique insertion, and there are connective tissue bands that connect the lateral rectus to the inferior oblique muscle. This is an important anatomic relationship since a lost or slipped lateral rectus muscle will come to rest at the insertion of the inferior oblique muscle (see inferior oblique muscle in the following discussion). The surgeon can often find a lost lateral rectus muscle by tracing the inferior oblique muscle back to its insertion.

Vertical rectus muscles   Unlike the horizontal muscles the vertical rectus muscles have primary (vertical), secondary (horizontal), and tertiary (torsional) actions. Vertical rectus muscles have these secondary and tertiary actions because the muscle is not in line with the visual axis when the eye is in primary position (see Figs. 13-2 and 13-7). In primary position the visual axis angles 23° nasal to the muscle and orbital axis. This causes the vertical rectus muscles to have the secondary action of adduction and tertiary action of torsion (intorsion for the

superior rectus muscle and extorsion for the inferior rectus muscle) (see Fig. 13-7, *A*). However, if the eye is abducted 23°, the muscle and visual axes are in line so the vertical rectus muscles lose their secondary and tertiary functions. In this position, the superior rectus acts purely as an elevator, and the inferior rectus purely as a depressor (see Fig. 13-7, *B*). Abduction past 23° results in return of secondary and tertiary functions. With the eye abducted past 23°, the secondary functions of both vertical rectus muscles changes to abduction and the tertiary functions become intorsion for the superior rectus, and extortion for the inferior rectus muscle (see Fig. 13-7, *C*). Thus the secondary and tertiary functions of the vertical rectus muscles are dependent on the position of the eye.

Superior rectus muscle   The upper division of the oculomotor nerve innervates the superior rectus muscle (Fig. 13-11). It is the major elevator of the eye and its actions include supraduction (primary), adduction (secondary), and an intorsion (tertiary). The superior rectus muscle has connective tissue connections to the overlying levator palpebrae muscle and underlying superior oblique tendon. This anatomic relationship is important because a superior rectus recession will pull the levator muscle posteriorly, causing upper lid retraction and lid fissure widening. A superior rectus resection pulls the upper lid down, resulting in lid fissure narrowing. Lid fissure changes associated with superior rectus surgery can be minimized by surgically removing the fascial connections to the levator muscle.

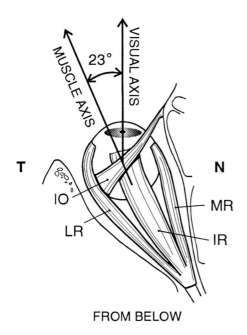

Fig. 13-12   Eye and orbit from below. Note that the inferior oblique underlies the inferior muscle.

Inferior rectus muscle   The inferior rectus muscle is innervated by the lower division of the oculomotor nerve (Fig. 13-12), and it is the principal depressor of the eye. Actions of the inferior rectus muscle include infraduction (primary), adduction (secondary), and extortion (tertiary). The inferior rectus is sandwiched between the inferior oblique below and the sclera above. Fascial connections between the inferior rectus muscle, the inferior oblique, and muscle lower lid retractors (capsulopalpebral fascia) is termed *Lockwood's ligament* (Fig. 13-13). This relationship is important because an inferior rectus muscle recession can result in lower lid retraction with lid fissure widening. Resection results in lid advancement with lid fissure narrowing. Surgical replacement of the lower lid retractors and removal of check ligaments from the inferior rectus can help prevent lid changes. If the inferior rectus is inadvertently disinserted or lost during surgery, these connections will hold the inferior rectus to the inferior oblique and keep it from retracting posteriorly. The surgeon who is in search of a lost inferior rectus muscle can usually find it lying between the inferior oblique and sclera.

Oblique Muscles

Like the vertical rectus muscles, the oblique muscles also have primary, secondary, and tertiary actions, because the muscle axis does not parallel the visual axis when the eye is in primary position. In the case of the oblique muscles, the muscle axis is 51° nasal from the visual axis (Figs. 13-14 and 13-15). Each oblique muscle

courses below its corresponding vertical rectus muscle with the majority of the insertion lying posterior to the equator of the eye (Fig. 13-16). The posterior insertion gives the oblique muscles their seemingly paradoxical vertical functions, with the superior oblique being a depressor and inferior oblique being an elevator.

Superior oblique muscle   The trochlear nerve innervates the superior oblique muscle at its midpoint, from outside of the muscle cone. The superior oblique muscle is in fact, the only eye muscle innervated on the outer surface of the muscle belly. This unique innervation is clinically important, since it explains why a retrobulbar anesthetic block results in akinesia of all the eye muscles except the superior oblique. The primary function of the superior oblique muscle is intorsion, but it also acts as a depressor (secondary) and an abductor (tertiary). Depression and abduction occur as the back of the eye is pulled up and in towards the trochlea.

The superior oblique muscle originates at the orbital apex just above the annulus of Zinn and gradually becomes tendonous at the trochlea. Even though the anatomic origin is at the apex of the orbit, the superior oblique's functional origin is at the trochlea. After passing through the trochlea, the superior oblique tendon turns in a posterior temporal direction to course under the superior rectus muscle and insert on sclera along the temporal border of the superior rectus muscle (Fig. 13-17). This tendon is the longest tendon of the extraocular muscles, measuring 26 mm in length. The tendon insertion fans out broadly under the superior rectus muscle, extending from the temporal pole of the superior rectus muscle to 6.5 mm from the optic nerve. Fibrous bands connect the superior oblique tendon to the superior rectus above and the sclera below. The tendon insertion can be functionally divided into two parts, the anterior one third and the posterior two thirds. When the superior oblique muscle contracts, the posterior fibers act to bring the back of the eye up to the trochlea, which results in depression and abduction of the front of the eye. In contrast to the posterior fibers, the anterior one third of the superior oblique tendon is almost entirely devoted to intorsion. This distinction between the functions of the anterior one third (torsion) and posterior two thirds (depression and abduction) of the superior oblique tendon is important since the surgeon can manipulate these functions surgically to correct specific torsional or vertical/horizontal abnormalities. The *Harada-Ito* procedure, for example, corrects extorsion by tightening the anterior fibers of the superior oblique tendon.

Trochlea-tendon interaction   The trochlea is a cartilaginous U-shaped structure attached to the periosteum that overlies the trochlear *fossa* of the frontal bone in the superior nasal quadrant of the orbit. Trochlea is Latin for pulley and, until recently, it was taught that the superior oblique tendon moves through the trochlea much like a

Fig. 13-13 Relationship between inferior rectus, inferior oblique, lower lid retractors, and Lockwood's ligament. The inferior tarsal muscle (ITM) courses from the posterior border of the tarsus toward the inferior oblique muscle. It then passes between the inferior oblique muscle and the inferior rectus muscle to insert at the capsulopalpebral head (CPH). The CPH extends posteriorly to connect the inferior oblique to the inferior rectus muscle. The capsulopalpebral fascia (CPF) is the anterior extension of the CPH and courses from the inferior oblique anteriorly to the tarsus along with the ITM. Lockwood's ligament consists of anterior fascial attachments that connect the lower lid, inferior rectus, and interior oblique muscles.

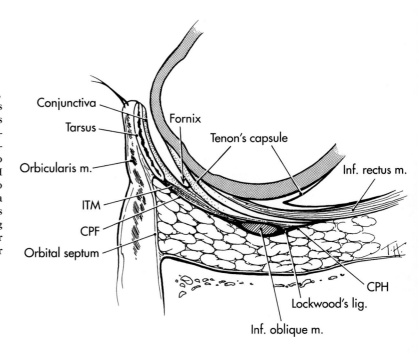

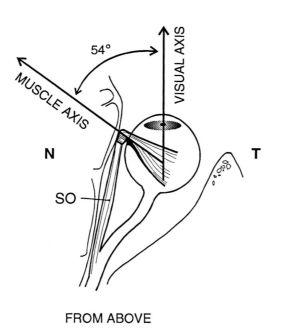

FROM ABOVE

Fig. 13-14 Superior oblique muscle and tendon. Note that the functional muscle axis extends from the trochlea to the superior oblique insertion. The muscle axis is 54° nasal to the visual axis.

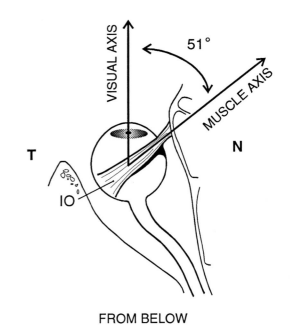

FROM BELOW

Fig. 13-15 Inferior oblique from below. Note that the inferior oblique muscle axis is 51° nasal to the visual axis.

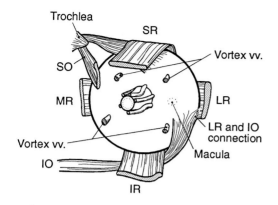

Fig. 13-16 Posterior anatomy of the eye and muscles. Note the proximity of the inferior oblique to the macula and vortex veins. The posterior aspect of the superior oblique insertion is in proximity to the superior temporal vortex vein and is approximately 6 to 8 mm from the optic nerve.

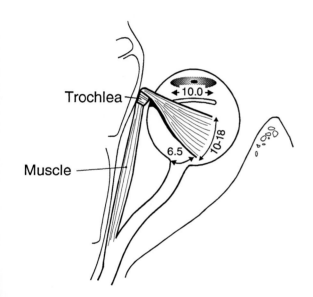

Fig. 13-17 Top view of the superior oblique tendon with the superior rectus muscle reflected. Note the wide insertion of the superior oblique. The anterior one third of the superior oblique tendon is primarily devoted to intorsion, whereas the posterior two thirds of the tendon insertion produces abduction and depression.

rope through a pulley. Anatomic studies have shown that tendon movement is not that simple. Within the trochlea is a connective tissue capsule that unites the tendon to the surrounding trochlea and limits the passage of the tendon through the trochlea. Instead, much of the tendon slackening distal to the trochlea comes from a telescoping elongation of the central tendon (Fig. 13-18). This telescoping elongation of the tendon is due to movement of the central tendon fibers that have scant interfiber connections. This is similar to the telescopic mechanism of your car antenna. Thus the mechanism for

tendon movement is complex, with at least two mechanisms: tendon movement through the trochlea (pulley and a rope), and tendon elongation (telescoping).

Inferior oblique muscle The inferior oblique muscle is innervated by the inferior branch of the third nerve at a point just lateral to the inferior rectus muscle. It is the principal extortor of the eye; however other functions include elevation (secondary) and abduction (tertiary). The inferior oblique muscle originates at the lacrimal fossa located at the anterior aspect of the inferior nasal quadrant of the orbit (see Fig. 13-15). Starting at the lacrimal fossa the inferior oblique muscle courses posterior and temporally underneath the inferior rectus muscle to its insertion, which is close to the macular area and adjacent to the inferior border of the lateral rectus muscle (see Fig. 13-16). The inferior oblique muscle has fascial connections to the lower border of the lateral rectus muscle and to the overlying inferior rectus muscle via Lockwood's ligament (see Fig. 13-13). When the inferior oblique muscle contracts, it pulls the back of the eye down and in toward the insertion at the lacrimal fossa, thus producing elevation, abduction, and extorsion (see Fig. 13-12). Important structures near the inferior oblique insertion includes the macula and inferior temporal vortex vein (see Fig. 13-13). The inferior oblique muscle has essentially no tendon at the insertion and has no anterior ciliary blood supply; thus it does not contribute to the anterior segment circulation.

Extraocular Muscle Fascia

A smooth white connective tissue underlies the conjunctiva and envelops the globe and extraocular muscles. This delicate membrane partitions the orbital contents, isolating the globe and extraocular muscles from the surrounding orbital fat. Because of the elasticity of this subconjunctival fascia, the eye is free to rotate with minimal friction. The general term for the connective tissue is *Tenon's capsule*. Even though Tenon's capsule is a continuous membrane, it is clinically useful to subdivide it into the categories listed in Box 13-1.

The *intermuscular septum* lies sandwiched between the conjunctiva and sclera, spanning between the rectus muscles (Fig. 13-19). During strabismus surgery, intermuscular septum can be identified as the white membrane on each side of the rectus muscles. When elevated with muscle hooks, the intermuscular septum takes on the appearance of the wings of a manta ray (Fig. 13-20).

Posterior Tenon's capsule lines the orbital fat where it interfaces with the globe and functions to separate orbital fat from the sclera (Fig. 13-21). Just anterior to the equator of the eye, the four rectus muscles penetrate Tenon's capsule and become surrounded by intraconal and extraconal orbital fat (see Fig. 13-21). At this juncture, Tenon's capsule unites with the capsule of the rec-

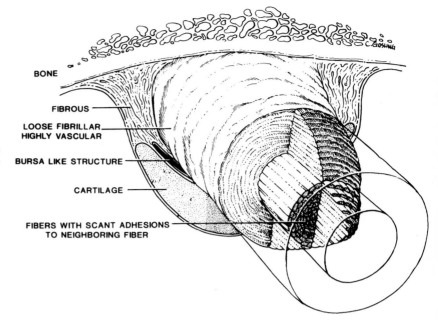

Fig. 13-18   Anatomy of the trochlea. (From Helveston EM, Meriam WW, Ellis FD, et al: *Ophthalmology* 89:124-133, 1982.)

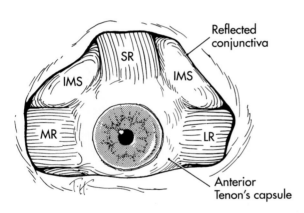

Fig. 13-19   View of anterior ocular fascia. Intermuscular septum (IMS) is the connective tissue that spans between the rectus muscles underneath the conjunctiva. Anterior Tenon's is that tissue anterior to the rectus muscle insertions. The anterior Tenon's fuses with the conjunctiva at 3 mm posterior to the limbus.

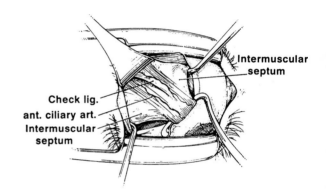

Fig. 13-20   View of lateral rectus muscle hooked by a large hook. Intermuscular septum is seen on either side of the lateral rectus muscle and the check ligaments overlie the lateral rectus muscle and connect muscle to overlying conjunctiva. (From Wright KW: *Color atlas of ophthalmic surgery: strabismus*, Philadelphia, 1991, JB Lippincott.)

Box 13-1   Categories of Tenon's Capsule
1. Intermuscular septum
2. Anterior Tenon's capsule
3. Posterior Tenon's capsule
4. Check ligaments
5. Muscle sleeve

tus muscle to form a "muscle sleeve." The muscle sleeve is an important surgical landmark when looking for a "lost" rectus muscle. A lost muscle is a rectus muscle that has become completely detached from the globe because of accidental trauma or following surgery involving

the eye muscles. Once lost, the muscle will slip posteriorly behind the opening of the muscle sleeve to be surrounded by intraconal and extraconal orbital fat. To find a lost muscle, the surgeon must first find the muscle sleeve, then carefully open the sleeve to retrieve the muscle.

Anterior Tenon's capsule is the subconjunctival membrane anterior to the muscle insertions. It proceeds forward with intermuscular septum and fuses with the conjunctiva at 2 to 3 mm posterior to the corneal limbus (see Figs. 13-19 and 13-21). When suturing a muscle during strabismus surgery, it is important to clear anterior Tenon's capsule off of the tendon insertion to avoid the complication of a "slipped muscle." If anterior Tenon's capsule is left on the tendon, the surgeon may inadvertently

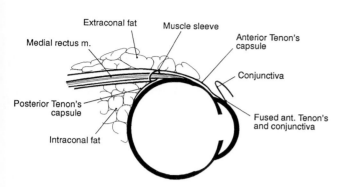

Fig. 13-21   Cross-section of eye and medial rectus muscle showing fascial relationships. Note that the muscle penetrates posterior Tenon's capsule and the capsule at this point forms a muscle sleeve. Intraconal and extraconal fat are isolated from globe by Tenon's capsule.

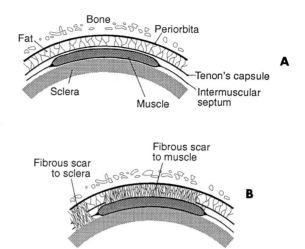

Fig. 13-22   Fat adherence syndrome. **A,** Normal anatomy with orbital bone, periorbita, extraconal fat, muscle, and intramuscular septum. Note that the fat is isolated from muscle and sclera by intact Tenon's capsule and intermuscular septum. **B,** Violation of Tenon's capsule with fat adherence to the globe and muscle. (From Wright KW: *Ophthalmology* 93:411-415, 1986.)

secure anterior Tenon's capsule instead of the tendon fibers. The surgeon then removes the unsecured muscle and allows it to slip posteriorly while anterior Tenon's capsule is placed at the intended recession site. A slipped muscle is a frequent cause of unexpected overcorrection after recession procedures. Remember that some slipped muscles involve only part of the muscle and can present as a mild overcorrection with relatively good muscle function.

Together, posterior Tenon's capsule, anterior Tenon's capsule, and muscle sleeves are very important structures since they are the barriers that keep orbital fat from the globe and extraocular muscles. If posterior Tenon's capsule or muscle sleeve is traumatically violated, "fat adherence" can occur. The orbital fat prolapses through the torn Tenon's capsule and scars to the sclera or an extraocular muscle (Fig. 13-22). Scarring of orbital fat produces a restrictive band that extends from the periosteum to the globe. As the scar contracts over weeks to several months, the scar pulls the eye, producing a restrictive strabismus associated with limitation of eye movements. Fat adherence can occur as a complication of almost any extraocular surgery (e.g., strabismus surgery, retina surgery) or periocular trauma. Extreme care must be taken when operating in the area of orbital fat that starts 10 mm posterior to the limbus, since once fat adherence occurs it is almost impossible to correct. Surgically induced fat adherence can usually be avoided if the surgeon carefully dissects close to muscle belly or sclera, thus preserving the integrity of the overlying posterior Tenon's capsule and muscle sleeve.

Check ligaments are fine falciform webs that overlie the rectus muscles and join the muscle capsule with over-

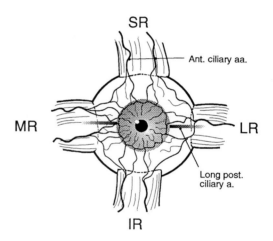

Fig. 13-23   Circulation of the anterior segment with the rectus muscle supplying the anterior ciliary arteries and the deep long posterior arteries are also shown. (From Wright KW: *Color atlas of ophthalmic surgery:strabismus,* Philadelphia, 1991, JB Lippincott.)

lying bulbar conjunctiva (see Fig. 13-20). In the case of the superior and inferior rectus muscles, check ligaments also connect to the levator muscle and lower lid retractors respectively. A recession or resection of vertical rectus muscles requires removal of these ligaments to avoid lid fissure changes after surgery.

Vascular Supply to the Anterior Segment

The anterior ciliary arteries, conjunctival vessels and the long posterior ciliary arteries (Fig. 13-23) supply the anterior segment and iris. Approximately 50% of the anterior segment circulation comes from the long posterior ciliary arteries and 50% from the anterior ciliary arteries. The conjunctival vessels also contribute to anterior segment circulation. Anterior ciliary arteries and the conjunctival vessels merge at the limbus to form the episcleral limbal plexus. These vessels in turn connect with the major arterial circle of the iris that is also fed by the two long posterior ciliary arteries. The superior rectus, inferior rectus, and medial muscles have at least two anterior ciliary arteries and are major contributors to the anterior segment circulation. The lateral rectus has a single anterior ciliary artery and, of the four recti muscles, the lateral rectus contributes least to the anterior segment circulation. The oblique muscles do not have anterior ciliary arteries and they do not contribute to the anterior segment circulation.

Iris angiograms can be used to assess anterior segment circulation in blue-eyed patients. Removal of a vertical rectus muscle in older adults will cause hypoperfusion in that area that relates to the vascular input. Infants and children do not typically show hypoperfusion even when multiple rectus muscles are removed. Removal of a rectus muscle during strabismus surgery will permanently interfere with vascular supply of the anterior ciliary arteries unless the surgery is performed specifically to maintain anterior segment circulation. Special strabismus surgeries have been devised and attempt to maintain anterior segment circulation despite manipulations of the muscle position. Two vessel-sparing procedures include dissecting the anterior ciliary vessels of the anterior muscle before recessing the muscle and a muscle tuck that leaves the vessels intact.

Anterior segment ischemia can be a consequence of strabismus surgery, most often after a three- or four-muscle procedure. This is a rare occurrence since collateral circulation from the long posterior ciliary arteries usually can maintain adequate perfusion to the anterior segment even when three or four rectus muscles have been removed. Factors that predispose to anterior segment ischemia include arteriosclerosis, hyperviscosity of the blood, and scleral encircling elements (e.g., 360° retinal buckle), which compromise the long posterior ciliary arteries. Older patients have a higher likelihood for developing anterior segment ischemia, whereas infants and children are generally protected from anterior segment ischemia. Anterior segment ischemia has even been reported after removing as few as two rectus muscles in high-risk patients. However, it is important to remember that disruption of anterior ciliary arteries associated with strabismus surgery is permanent and that anterior segment ischemia can occur years later since the collateral circulation diminishes with age. Anterior segment ischemia may occur decades after strabismus surgery.

PHYSIOLOGY OF EYE MOVEMENTS

Muscle Physiology

Like other skeletal muscles, extraocular muscles are made up of striated muscle fibers that on electromicroscopy show the typical banding pattern of sarcomeres with overlapping bands of actin and myosin. Also like other muscles, the strength of an extraocular muscle's contraction is dependent on the number of motor units activated (recruitment) and the frequency of muscle fiber stimulation. Extraocular muscles, however, have some interesting anatomic and physiologic differences from other skeletal muscles. Extraocular muscle fibers are considerably smaller and contract more than 10 times faster than other skeletal muscle. These muscle fibers are innervated at a high nerve fiber to muscle fiber ratio (almost 1:1), whereas other skeletal muscle can have up to 100 muscle fibers for every nerve fiber. This rich innervation and fast muscle reaction time may contribute to the precision, accuracy, and control of eye movements. Another feature of extraocular muscles is the presence of two distinct muscle types. The fast or *twitch fibers* are innervated by a single large motor neuron with "en plaque" neuromuscular junctions, and the slow or *tonic fibers* are innervated by multiple small diameter motor nerves with "en grappe" neuromuscular endings. Early experiments identified a functional distinction between these two fibers, whereby the fast twitch fibers were responsible for saccadic eye (fast) movements, and the slow tonic fibers caused smooth pursuit movements and static muscle tone to hold and maintain eye position (see the following discussion for saccades and smooth pursuit). Despite the attractiveness of this simple explanation that ties morphologic and physiologic properties of two types of muscle fibers, further studies have shown there are at least five different types of muscle fibers, the characteristics of which range from a classic fast twitch fiber to the slow tonic fiber. Additionally, electromyographic studies have shown that the singly innervated fast muscle fibers play a supportive role in tonic control of eye position and pursuit eye movements. These more recent studies point out the complexity of extraocular muscle physiology and the overlapping functions of the various fibers. Even so, the principle that fast twitch fibers produce saccadic movements and slow tonic muscle fibers produce smooth pursuit and tonic control of eye position still generally hold.

Within extraocular muscle tissue are muscle spindle cells. Spindle cells are most dense in the area of the muscle tendon junction. The exact role of the muscle spindles is unknown, but they may involve proprioception and provide feedback to motor centers in the brain regarding muscle tone. The presence of muscle spindles probably explains why some patients who have strabismus surgery of the fixing eye experience transient spatial disorientation.

Smooth Pursuit and Saccadic Movements

Smooth pursuit eye movements are generated in the occipital parietal cortex with the right cortex controlling movements to the right and left cortex movements to the left. In humans, smooth pursuit first occurs at 4 to 6 weeks of age. These are slow, accurate eye movements, which require good central foveal fixation and visual feedback. Accurate smooth pursuit can occur at velocities up to 30 degrees per second. Clinically, central fixation and smooth pursuit is used as an indication of good vision in preverbal children. *Saccadic movements* are rapid refixation eye movements that quickly move the eye to place a target on the fovea. These fast correctional eye movements occur as early as the first week of age and are the first eye movements of the newborn. Saccadic movements are so fast that there is no time for visual feedback to adjust the movement, once it starts. It is thought that the amplitude of a saccadic movement is preprogrammed based on the degree of retinal eccentricity of the target. That is why saccadic movements are termed *ballistic*. The velocity of saccadic eye movements range from 200 to 700 degrees per second and last from 50 to 100 milliseconds. Vision during a saccadic eye movement is suspended or suppressed. Some have used the term *saccadic omission* because the process of eliminating vision during a saccade may be a combination of visual masking and cortical suppression. A tremendous force is required to produce a saccadic eye movement; therefore the presence of saccadic eye movements indi-

cates "good" muscle function. When evaluating a patient with limited ductions, the presence of a normal saccadic eye movement to the field of limited ductions indicates good agonist muscle function and the presence of a restriction rather than a muscle paresis. The OKN drum is useful for clinically accessing saccades and smooth pursuit eye movements. The fast, jerk movement is a saccade, and the slow following movement is smooth pursuit (as long as the drum turns slowly).

Sherrington's Law (Monocular Agonist and Antagonist Muscles)

Monocular rotations result from muscle contraction that pulls the scleral insertion site towards the muscle's origin while the opposing muscle simultaneously relaxes. The contracting muscle is referred to as the *agonist* and the relaxing muscle the *antagonist*. Box 13-2 lists agonist/antagonist pairs for the primary function of the muscle. This relationship between agonist and antagonist muscles of one eye is referred to as "Sherrington's law of reciprocal innervation."

Sherrington's law can be demonstrated by using *electromyography (EMG)*. The EMG measures electrical potential changes within a muscle as the muscle fibers contract and indicates the degree of overall neuromuscular activity. A needle is placed in the muscle (extracellularly) to measure electrical activity from the muscle, and this activity is amplified and then recorded. Fig. 13-24 shows results of the EMG for agonist and antagonist muscles demonstrating Sherrington's law. Needle electrodes are placed in the medial and lateral rectus muscles. At the beginning of the EMG tracing there is low-amplitude tonic activity that maintains the eye position in primary position. As the eye is adducted, the medial rectus contracts resulting in increasing EMG activity, while the lateral rectus muscle simultaneously relaxes and EMG activity is inhibited. At the end of the tracing both muscles show tonic activity to maintain eye position. In patients with motor neuron misdirection syndromes, such as Duane's retraction syndrome, Sherrington's law is violated. In *Duane's syndrome* the lateral rectus muscle is

---

Box 13-2 Agonist-Antagonist Pairs
Medial Rectus   —Lateral Rectus
Superior Rectus —Inferior Rectus
Superior Oblique—Inferior Oblique

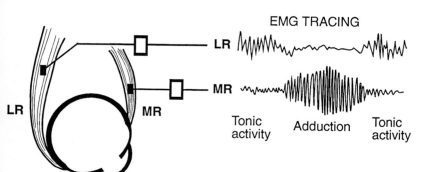

Fig. 13-24 Electromyographic (EMG) tracing from the lateral rectus muscle (LR) and medial rectus muscle (MR). Note that when the eye adducts, the medial rectus muscle increases EMG activity as the muscle contracts and EMG activity from the lateral rectus muscle diminishes as the antagonist lateral relaxes.

Table 13-2   Synergists

Duction	Primary mover	Secondary mover
Supraduction	Superior rectus	Inferior oblique
Infraduction	Inferior rectus	Superior oblique
Adduction	Medial rectus	Superior rectus/ inferior rectus
Abduction	Lateral rectus	Superior oblique/ inferior oblique
Extorsion	Inferior oblique	Inferior rectus
Intorsion	Superior oblique	Superior rectus

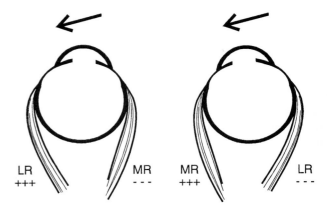

Fig. 13-25   Hering's Law of Yoke Muscles. Diagram shows version movements to the left. As the left lateral rectus (LR) contracts (+++), the contralateral medial rectus (MR) simultaneously contracts (+++). Also note that the left medial rectus relaxes (–––) and the right lateral rectus also relaxes (–––).

aberrantly innervated by a branch of the medial rectus nerve. When the patient adducts the eye, instead of the medial rectus contracting and the lateral rectus relaxing, both the medial and lateral rectus muscles contract simultaneously. It should be remembered that Sherrington's law of reciprocal innervation refers strictly to a monocular eye movements, as does the term *ductions*.

In contrast to agonist-antagonist muscles, *synergist muscles* act to move the eye in the same direction. In other words, synergist muscles have common actions. For example, the superior oblique and the inferior rectus muscles, both act as depressors; therefore they are synergists for infraduction. These muscles are not, however, synergists for horizontal or torsional rotations since the inferior rectus muscle is an adductor and extortor, whereas the superior oblique is an abductor and intortor. Table 13-2 lists synergist muscles for various duction movements. Note that synergist muscles relate to monocular rotations, not to be confused with yoke muscles that cause binocular eye movements (see yoke muscles in the following section).

Hering's Law (Binocular-yoke Muscles)

Normally, the two eyes move together in concert. When the two eyes move together in the same direction, this is termed *version* movement. Coordinated binocular eye movements require symmetrical innervation of each eye. When one looks to the left, the two agonist muscles (i.e., left lateral rectus and right medial rectus) simultaneously contract, as the two antagonist muscles (i.e., left medial and right lateral) relax (Fig. 13-25). The paired agonist and antagonist muscles from each eye are referred to as "yoke muscles." Fig. 13-26 shows the yoke agonist muscles responsible for various fields of gaze. Hering's law relates to the teamed eye movements of both eyes and states that yoke muscles receive equal innervation from the brain. In most situations the term *yoke muscles* refers to yoke agonist muscles as shown in Fig. 13-26.

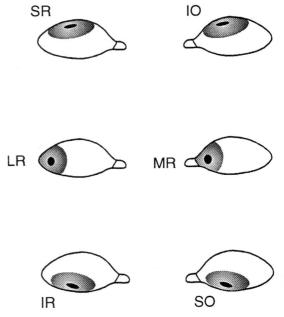

Fig. 13-26   Yoke muscles are shown for specific field of gaze. *Top* shows gaze up and to the side with yoke muscles being the superior rectus and inferior oblique; *middle*, straight-side gaze with the yokes being lateral rectus, medial rectus; and *bottom*, showing side gaze and down with yoke muscles being inferior rectus and superior oblique.

Version eye movements can be classified as follows: *dextroversion* for right gaze, *levoversion* for left gaze, *supraversion* for up gaze, and *infraversion* for down gaze (Fig. 13-27). In contrast to ductions, versions are performed with both eyes open and compares how well the eyes move in synchrony. Versions will identify a subtle restriction or paresis and oblique muscle overaction that result in asymmetrical eye movements.

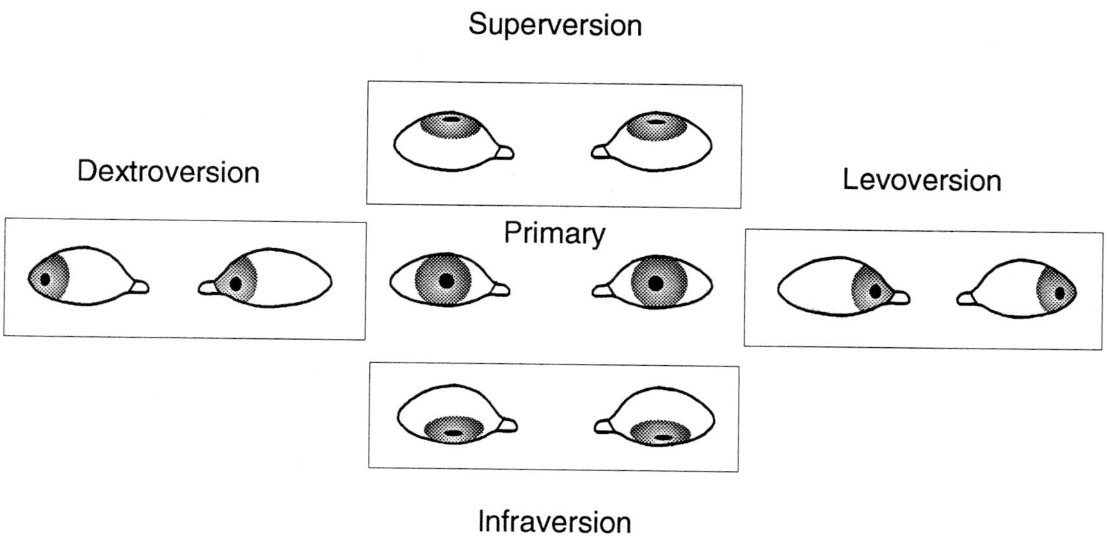

Superversion

Dextroversion

Primary

Levoversion

Infraversion

Fig. 13-27 Normal versions from primary position to right gaze (dextroversion), left gaze (levoversion), up gaze (supraversion), and down gaze (infraversion).

Remember, Hering's law relates to yoke muscles and binocular eye movements (versions), whereas Sherrington's law explains agonist-antagonist relationships and monocular eye movements (ductions).

Oculomotor Reflexes

Two important oculomotor reflexes are the vestibulo-ocular reflex (VOR) and optokinetic nystagmus (OKN). The *vestibulo-ocular* reflex functions to keep the eyes steady when the head moves. Vestibular stimulation, induced by turning the head, results in a compensatory movement of the eyes to maintain the position of gaze. If the head is rapidly turned to the left the eyes move to the right with the same velocity. A similar reflex, the *orthostatic reflex,* is responsible for keeping the torsionally aligned when the head is tilted. This reflex is the basis of the Bielschowsky head tilt test for vertical muscle palsies. *Optokinetic nystagmus* is a visually mediated reflex consisting of smooth pursuit alternating with saccadic refixation as a series of objects cross the visual field. The eyes follow in response to full-field movement of the environment with smooth pursuit, then a saccadic movement in the opposite direction to refixate is made. The most commonly used stimuli to produce OKN are black and white stripes that are presented on a rotating drum or moving tape. The best OKN stimuli fill the visual field.

Physiology of Strabismus Surgery

When a rectus muscle contracts it produces a force that rotates the globe. The rotational force is proportional to the force of the contracting muscle, times the rotational leverage or length of the moment arm.

Rotational force = Muscle force × Length of moment arm

The amount innervational activity and the muscle tension according to Starling's length-tension curve determine muscle force. The length-tension curve dictates that the more a muscle is stretched the more force it can generate, whereas the more it is slackened the weaker it becomes. The *moment arm* is a tangent from the posterior point of muscle-scleral contact to the center of the eye (Fig. 13-28). The longer the moment arm, the greater the rotational force. Because the rectus muscles insert several millimeters anterior to the equator, there is an *arc of muscle-scleral contact.* This arc of contact persists even with extreme ocular rotations and ensures that the length of the moment arm will remain constant throughout all ocular rotations.

Rectus muscle recession A rectus muscle recession is the most common strabismus surgery and consists of moving the muscle insertion posteriorly, thus slackening the muscle (Fig. 13-29). Since muscle force is determined by the amount of muscle tension according to *Starling's length-tension curve,* a recession weakens the muscle force by slackening the muscle. The slack that is produced by a recession increases as the eye rotates toward the recessed muscle. Thus a recession weakens the muscle most in the field of action of the muscle. For example, a recession of the right medial rectus will weaken the medial rectus more in left gaze. This effect of the recession can be used to correct incomitant strabismus.

The muscle length-tension curve does not follow a linear pattern, since the more a muscle is slackened, the greater the weakening effect of further slackening. For example, according to standard surgical charts a medial rectus recession of 3.0 to 5.5 mm yields only 5 prism diopters of esotropia correction for each 0.5 mm of recession, although recessions over 5.5 mm result in 10 prism diopters change per 0.5 mm of recession. The surgeon must be particularly careful when performing large rectus muscle recessions since even small measurement errors may result in significant overcorrections or undercorrections. Beisner demonstrated that the "weakening" effect of large rectus muscle recessions is caused by producing muscle slack, not because of a reduction of the length of the moment arm. The long arc of contact of the anterior to the equator of the globe of the rectus muscles, allows large recessions without significantly changing the moment arm. This is why many experts feel it is preferable to measure a recession from the insertion site rather than an limbus, since measurement from the insertion quantitates the amount of muscle slack produced.

Faden operation *Faden,* German for suture, is an operation designed to weaken a muscle by reducing the moment arm without significantly changing the muscle slack. The Faden operation consists of suturing the mus-

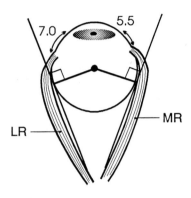

Fig. 13-28 Medial rectus and lateral rectus muscles showing the moment arm as the tangent of the posterior point where the muscle contacts the sclera to the center of the eye.

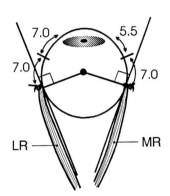

Fig. 13-29 Position of the medial and latera rectus muscle after a 7-mm recession. Note that in primary position, the moment arm (*m*) has not changed. Note the major effect of a recession is on the length tension and creating slack rather than changing the moment arm.

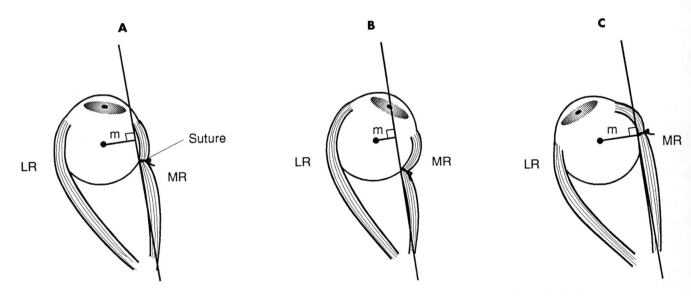

Fig. 13-30 Effect of Faden operation on moment arm (*m*). **A,** In primary position, the Faden operation does not change the moment arm. **B,** With the eye turned towards the Faden muscle (medial rectus, *MR*), the Faden prevents the muscle from unraveling and the arc of contact persists because of the suture holding the muscle against the sclera. Note that the moment arm is diminished. **C,** The eye looking away from the Fadened muscle shows arc of contact in place and no effect on the moment arm.

cle to the sclera at or slightly behind the equator of the eye (Fig. 13-30). In primary position the Faden has essentially no weakening effect since there is no slackening of muscle and no change in the length of the moment arm (see Fig. 13-30, *A*). However, when the eye rotates to the side of the Fadened muscle the arc of contact persists rather than unraveling (see Fig. 13-30, *B*). The muscle now acts to pull the eye straight back posteriorly rather than producing rotational force since the moment arm has significantly shortened. Thus, like a recession, the Faden operation weakens the muscle in the field of action of the muscle without, however, significantly altering primary position. Note that with the eye rotated in the opposite direction to the Fadened muscle, there is no change in the length of the moment arm (see Fig. 13-30, *C*). Practically speaking, the Faden operation has a minimal weakening effect by itself because of the long arc of contact of the rectus muscles. The medial rectus muscle has the shortest arc of contact and it is the only muscle that is significantly affected by the Faden operation. There are relatively few indications for a Faden operation, but it can be used on the medial rectus muscle to correct incommitance (e.g., incommitance associated with a partial sixth nerve paresis). When a Faden operation is performed it is usually combined with a muscle recession.

Resection Resections remove a segment of the anterior muscle to tighten the muscle but do not truly strengthen the muscle. This effect also can be accomplished by tucking the muscle. A resection has its greatest effect when the eye rotates away from the resected muscle, since this causes the resected muscle to become even tighter. For example, a resection of the right lateral rectus muscle will limit the right eye from adducting and have its greatest effect in left gaze. A recession and resection are often used together to correct strabismus— the *recession/resection procedure (R&R)*. A recession/resection tends to limit ductions and induce incommitance since it weakens the antagonist and tightens the antagonist. Bilateral symmetrical surgical procedures (e.g., *bilateral recessions*) produce less limitation of ductions and induce less incommitance.

Rectus muscle transposition Transposing a rectus muscle insertion up or down will change the muscle function, with the transposed muscle taking on some of the function of the muscle it is moved toward. For example, if a horizontal rectus muscle insertion is moved up towards the superior rectus muscle, the horizontal muscle becomes an elevator in addition to the horizontal function. Supraplacing a horizontal rectus insertion will induce a hyperdeviation, whereas infraplacement causes a hypodeviation. Vertically displacing the medial and lateral rectus muscle insertion can be used to correct small vertical deviations.

Transpositions can be used to correct strabismus caused by a muscle palsy. A sixth nerve palsy can be treated by transposing the vertical rectus muscle insertions toward the lateral rectus muscle (i.e., superior rectus moves down, inferior rectus moves up). This operation will provide lateral muscle force to help correct for the lateral rectus palsy (see Chapter 19).

> ► **MAJOR POINTS** ◄
>
> Large rectus muscle resections can result in relative enophthalmos and lid fissure narrowing as the tightened rectus muscles pull the eye back into the orbit, whereas recessions reduce muscle tension and tend to cause mild proptosis producing lid fissure widening.
>
> The four rectus muscles originate at the annulus of Zinn, are 40 mm long, insert to form the spiral of Tillaux around the corneal limbus; the medial rectus is closest to the limbus (5.5 mm), inferior rectus next (6.5 mm), the lateral rectus next (7.0 mm), and superior rectus is the furthest from the limbus (8.0 mm).
>
> The superior oblique muscle is the only muscle that is innervated outside the muscle cone and therefore is difficult to anesthetize with a retrobulbar block.
>
> The superior oblique has the longest tendon (26 mm) and the functional insertion is the trochlea, whereas the inferior oblique has the shortest tendon.
>
> Fascial connections between the inferior rectus muscle, the inferior oblique, and muscle lower lid retractors (capsulopalpebral fascia) is termed *Lockwood's ligament.*
>
> Each oblique muscle courses below its corresponding vertical rectus muscle with the majority of the insertion lying posterior to the equator of the eye.
>
> Removal of a rectus muscle during strabismus surgery will permanently interfere with vascular supply of the anterior ciliary arteries, and if three or four rectus muscles are removed anterior segment ischemia may occur.
>
> Sherrington's law of reciprocal innervation relates to the relationship between agonist and antagonist muscles of one eye.
>
> Hering's law relates to binocular eye movements and states that yoke agonist muscles receive equal innervation from the brain.
>
> Since muscle force is determined by the amount of muscle tension according to *Starling's length-tension curve,* a recession weakens the muscle force by slackening the muscle.
>
> The Faden operation sutures the muscle to the sclera behind the equator and is designed to weaken a muscle by reducing the moment arm without significantly changing muscle slack.
>
> A resection is removing a segment of the anterior muscle to tighten the muscle, but it does not truly strengthen the muscle.

SUGGESTED READINGS

Beisner DH: Reduction of ocular torque by medial rectus recession, *Arch Ophthalmol* 85:13, 1971.

Hawes MJ, Dortzbach RK: The microscopic anatomy of the lower eyelid retractors, *Arch Ophthalmol* 100(8):1313-1318, 1982.

Hayreh SS, Scott WE: Fluorescein iris angiography, *Arch Ophthalmol* 96:1390-1400, 1978.

Helveston EM, Merriam WW, Ellis FD, et al: The trochlea: a study of the anatomy and physiology, *Ophthalmology* 89:124-133, 1982.

Morrison JC, van Buskirk EM: Anterior collateral circulation in the primate eye, *Ophthalmology* 90:707-715, 1983.

McKeown CA, Lambert HM, et al: Preservation of the anterior ciliary vessels during extraocular muscle surgery, *Ophthalmology* 96:498-507, 1989.

Plager DA, Parks MM: Recognition and repair of the "lost" rectus muscle, *Ophthalmology* 97:131, 1990.

Saunders RA, Phillips MS: Anterior segment ischemia after three rectus muscle surgery, *Ophthalmology* 95:533-537, 1988.

Wright KW, Lanier AB: Effect of a modified rectus tuck on anterior segment circulation in monkeys, *J Pediatr Ophthalmol Strabis* 28:77-81, 1991.

Wright KW: *Color atlas of ophthalmic surgery: strabismus,* Philadelphia, 1991, JP Lippincott.

Wright KW: The fat adherence syndrome and strabismus after retinal surgery, *Ophthalmology* 93:411-415, 1986.

CHAPTER 14

Motor Fusion and Basics of Strabismus

Normally, both eyes are aligned on the same object of regard, so the retinal images fall appropriately on each fovea; this normal alignment is called *orthotropia* (Fig. 14-1). Bifoveal stimulation by the target of regard permits cortical processing that results in the merging of images from each eye into a single binocular picture with stereopsis or depth perception. This chapter discusses motor fusion that locks the two eyes together and provides an introduction to motor aspects of strabismus.

MOTOR FUSION

The cortical merging of the two images from each eye is termed *binocular fusion* or just *fusion*. Cortical binocular fusion controls eye alignment to lock the two eyes on a visual target through a feedback mechanism called motor fusion. Small tendencies for the eyes to drift are controlled by motor fusion. Motor fusion also keeps the eyes aligned on objects as they move close or move away. These correctional movements to maintain fusion and proper alignment are called vergence movements. The strength of vergence movements are termed *vergence amplitudes* and can be measured by prisms (see the following discussion on measuring fusional vergence amplitudes).

Unlike version movements where yoke muscles from both eyes move in the same direction to follow an object moving on a horizontal or vertical plane (Chapter 13); vergence eye movements are disjunctive, since the eyes move in opposite directions to keep the eyes aligned on objects moving towards or away from us. There are three types of vergence eye movements, two are in the horizontal plane for following objects as they move through depth, convergence and divergence, and one vertical vergence that keeps the eyes vertically aligned (Fig. 14-2).

Convergence

Convergence is characterized by both eyes moving towards the midline to follow an approaching target from distance to near (see Fig. 14-2, *A*). You can experience convergence by fixating on a pencil at arm length and slowly bring the pencil to your nose. As the pencil ap-

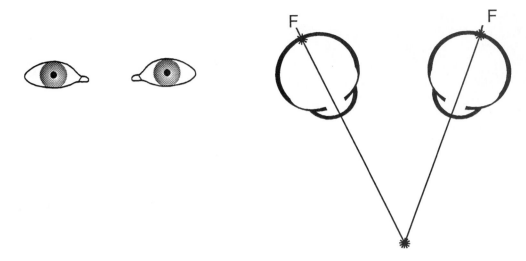

Fig. 14-1   Normal eye alignment with image falling on both foveae.

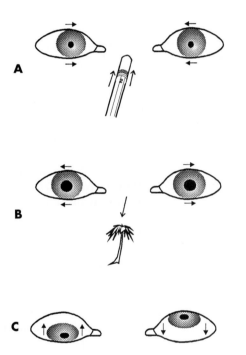

Fig. 14-2   Vergence. **A,** Convergence of the eyes as the pencil approaches from the distance. **B,** Divergence as the patient changes fixation from a near target to a distance target. **C,** Vertical vergence as the patient vertically aligns the eyes to compensate for vertical phoria or an induced deviation produced by a vertical prism.

proaches your nose, the eyes converge to hold alignment on the pencil.

Convergence is by far the strongest of the vergence movement with fusional convergence amplitudes of 25 to 35 PD. Fusional convergence can be strengthened by convergence exercises to control some forms of exotropia. There are at least five convergence mechanisms; fusional convergence, tonic fusional convergence, accommodative convergence, voluntary convergence, and proximal or instrument convergence.

Fusional convergence   Fusional convergence is based on binocular vision, and is stimulated by feedback from the two retinal images. It is the binocular fusion mechanism that keeps the eyes locked together on an approaching object. Occluding or severely blurring the image of one eye will disrupt the binocular visual input and break fusional convergence.

After monocular occlusion, a type of fusional convergence persists called tonic fusional convergence. This is a form of proprioceptive eye position control that keeps the eyes converged even after one eye is occluded. Tonic fusional convergence dissipates with prolonged monocular occlusion. Patching one eye for 30 to 60 minutes eliminates most tonic fusional convergence.

Accommodative convergence   When an object approaches from distance to near, the images falling on the retina are displaced temporally, blur, and enlarge. These retinal image changes stimulate the near reflex. The *near reflex* includes accommodation, convergence, and pupillary miosis. The ciliary muscles contract to increase the lens power to focus at near (*accommodation*), contraction of both medial rectus muscles occurs to keep the eyes aligned on the approaching target (*convergence*), and the pupil constricts to increase the depth of focus (*miosis*). The synkinetic reflex of accommodation and convergence is termed *accommodative convergence*. In contradistinction to fusional convergence, accommodative convergence is not dependent on binocular vision and occurs even if one eye is occluded. Patients with one blind eye still show convergence of the eyes when accommodating on near objects. Accommodation is one of the main driving forces of convergence. For any individual, a specific amount of accommodation will result in a specific amount of convergence. The quantitative relationship between the amount of convergence associated with an amount of accommodation is referred to as the *accommodative convergence/accommodation ratio (AC/A ratio)*. Methods for measuring the AC/A ratio are described in the following discussion.

Voluntary convergence This is convergence that is voluntarily invoked. Comedians use this to cross their eyes and patients will use voluntary convergence to produce convergence nystagmus.

Proximal or instrument convergence This type of convergence is induced by a psychologic awareness of an object at near, or when one views through an instrument such as a microscope. It is important to note that multiple types of convergence mechanisms act together to maintain alignment as an object approaches from the distance to near.

Divergence

Divergence is an outward or temporally directed movement of both eyes that occurs as the patient follows an object moving form near to distance (see Fig. 14-2, *B*). Patients with an esophoria use divergence to hold proper eye alignment. Divergence is relatively weak with fusional divergence amplitudes of 6 to 8 PD. Divergence amplitudes are difficult to improve with eye muscle exercises; therefore exercises are not usually prescribed to treat esotropia.

Vertical Vergence

Vertical vergence is not used to follow moving objects but to maintain vertical alignment. Vertical vergence consists of depression of one eye with elevation of the fellow eye. It is the weakest of the three vergence movements and normally measures only 2 to 3 PD (see Fig. 14-2, *C*). However, patients with congenital superior oblique paresis can develop large vertical vergence and fuse hyperphorias of 20 PD or greater.

Cyclovergence is characterized by slight intorsion of both eyes or extorsion of both eyes to correct for torsional drift. Cyclovergence is difficult to demonstrate even in a laboratory setting and it probably does not exist.

STRABISMUS

Strabismus is misalignment of the eyes, with the fovea of one eye is aligned with the fixation target and the fovea of the fellow eye off the target. As one eye fixates on a target, the fellow eye points in another direction, causing the image from the deviated eye to fall on peripheral retina (Fig. 14-3).

Patients with a manifest strabismus fixate with one eye at a time, so there is a fixing eye looking at the target, and a deviating eye. Note that according to Herring's law of yoke muscles, if the deviated eye comes to primary position to pick up fixation, the fellow eye moves off fixation and deviates (see Fig. 14-3). Strabismic patients may alternate fixation or show strong fixation preference. Another term for strabismus is *squint*. This term comes from the fact that strabismic patients often close one eye or squint to block out one image.

Phoria Versus Tropia

The term or suffix *tropia* is short for *heterotropia* and means the strabismus is manifest and the eyes are misaligned. In contrast a *phoria* (short for heterophoria) is a latent deviation where there is an underlying tendency for the eyes to drift apart, yet the eyes are held in alignment by motor fusion. A phoria can be disclosed by disrupting fusion, by either occluding one eye or severely blurring the image of one eye (Fig. 14-4). If a phoria is present it indicates the patient has motor fusion.

The majority of the normal population will have a small phoria, but maintain alignment through motor fusion. The term *intermittent tropia* refers to a large phoria that is so difficult to control with motor fusion, and fusion will at times spontaneously break, allowing the latent deviation to become manifest. A phoria may become manifest into a tropia when the central nervous system is globally depressed, such as when a patient is tired or sick. Central nervous system depressants also diminish motor fusion, and patients with phorias often manifest their deviations after imbibing alcoholic beverages or taking sedatives.

Esotropia, Exotropia, and Hypertropia

Strabismus can be horizontal, vertical, torsional, or any combination of these three. The term *esotropia (ET)* refers to an in-turning strabismus, with the image in the deviated eye falling nasal to the fovea (see Fig. 14-3), and *exotropia (XT)* means the eye turns out and the image falls temporal to the fovea (Fig. 14-5). A *hypertropia (HT)* refers to one eye being higher than the other, with the image falling superior to the fovea in the deviated eye (Fig. 14-6). Note that a left hypertropia is the same deviation as a right hypotropia in Fig. 14-6, and the direction of the deviation is determined by which eye is fixing. By convention, we usually refer to vertical deviations as a right or left hypertropia, rather than hypotropia, unless there is an obvious restriction or paresis that keeps one eye in a hypotropic position. Phorias are termed *esophoria (E), exophoria (X),* or *hyperphoria (H)*. Fusional convergence acts to control an exophoria, divergence controls an esotropia, and vertical vergence

OD Fixing

OS Fixing

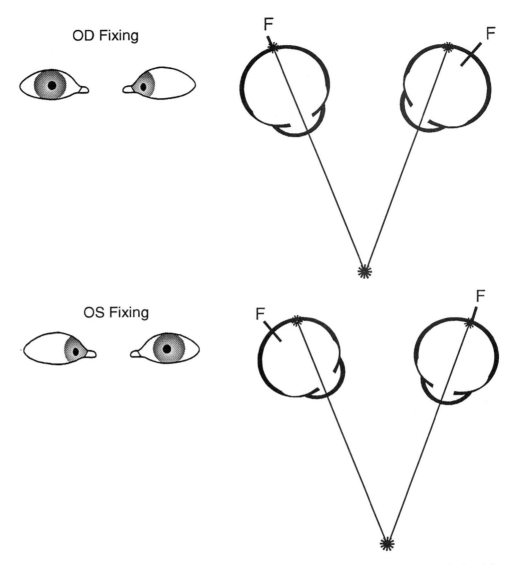

Fig. 14-3   Alternating esotropia. *Top,* right eye is fixing and the image is aligned with the right fovea while the image falls nasal to the left fovea since the left eye is deviated. *Bottom,* left eye fixing with the image falling on the left fovea and the image falling nasal to the right fovea since the right eye is deviated.

controls a hyperphoria. Cyclotropia refers to a torsional misalignment around the Y-axis of Fick. *Excyclotropia* (extorsion) is a temporal rotation of the 12 o'clock position and *incyclotropia* (intorsion) means a nasal rotation of the 12 o'clock position of one eye relative to the follow eye. Clinically, we do not find cyclophorias since there is no cyclovergence to control torsional deviations.

Comitant Versus Incomitant Strabismus

All strabismus can be classified into two broad categories, comitant strabismus and incomitant strabismus. Comitant strabismus is present when the deviation measures the same in all fields of gaze. Most types of con-

genital and childhood strabismus are comitant. With comitant strabismus, both eyes move together equally well and there is no significant restriction or paresis. Comitant strabismus is usually a "good" sign and indicates that the strabismus is not secondary to a neurologic problem. Occasionally, however, acquired neurologic disease processes such as early-onset myasthenia gravis, chronic progressive external ophthalmoplegia (CPEO) or even Arnold-Chiari syndrome can present as a clinically comitant strabismus.

Incomitant strabismus means the deviation changes depending on the field of gaze. Incomitance is caused by a limitation of ocular rotations resulting from ocular *restriction* or extraocular muscle *paresis.* Causes of ocular

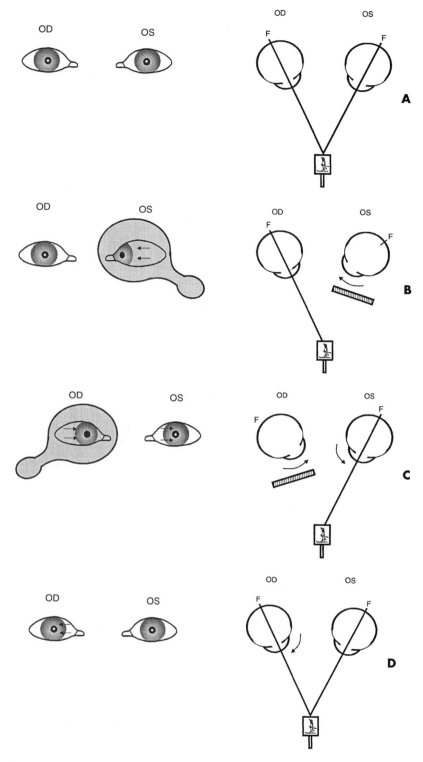

Fig. 14-4   Alternate cover test in a patient with an esophoria. **A,** Eyes are straight; the patient has a tendency to cross (esophoria), but fusional divergence maintains proper alignment. **B,** Left eye is covered, dissociating fusion and allowing the left eye to manifest the esophoria. Note that the left eye turns in under the cover. **C,** The cover is quickly shifted from the left eye to the right eye without allowing binocular fusion. Now the left eye moves out as the right eye turns in under the cover. **D,** The cover is removed and the right eye moves out by fusional divergence to allow patient to regain binocular fusion.

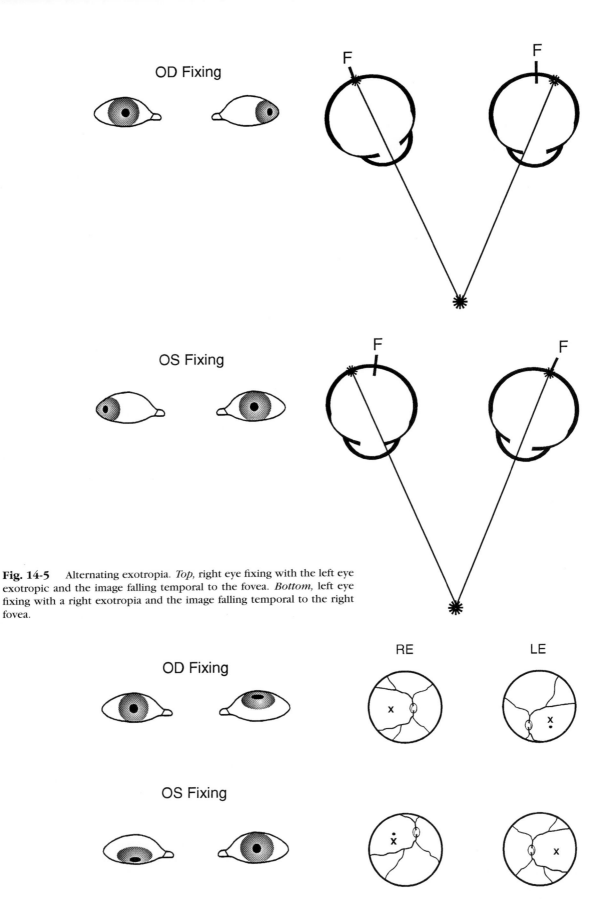

OD Fixing

OS Fixing

Fig. 14-5 Alternating exotropia. *Top,* right eye fixing with the left eye exotropic and the image falling temporal to the fovea. *Bottom,* left eye fixing with a right exotropia and the image falling temporal to the right fovea.

OD Fixing

OS Fixing

RE   LE

Fig. 14-6 Alternating left hypertropia. *Top left,* right eye fixing and left hypertropia. *Top right,* retinal image (x) falling on the fovea (•) of right eye; however, the left fovea is rotated down (left hypertropia) so the retinal image (x) is located above the fovea (•). *Bottom,* left eye fixing with right eye turned down. Now the retinal image (x) falls below the right fovea (•), which is rotated up (right hypertropia).

restriction include a tight or stiff muscle (thyroid myopathy), or periocular adhesions to the eye and or extraocular muscle. Extraocular muscle paresis can be caused by a lack of innervation (i.e., third, sixth, or fourth nerve paresis), traumatic muscle damage, an over-recessed or lost muscle, or neuromuscular junction disease such as myasthenia gravis.

Fig. 14-7 shows an example of an incomitant esotropia secondary to limited abduction of the left eye. When the patient in Fig. 14-7 looks to the left, the left eye cannot fully abduct; thus the right eye over-shoots, creating an ET that increases in left gaze (Herring's law of yoke muscles). In this example the limited abduction could be caused by either *restriction* (e.g., a tight left medial rectus muscle or a nasal fat adherence scar to the globe) or *paresis* (e.g., left sixth nerve palsy or left slipped lateral rectus muscle). Methods for diagnosing restriction and paresis are presented in the following discussion.

Restriction and paresis are not the only reasons for incomitance. Primary overaction of oblique muscles can also cause incomitance. However, what we clinically refer to as primary muscle overaction may actually represent a previous paresis of the antagonist and secondary overaction of the agonist muscle.

EVALUATING STRABISMUS

Ductions and Versions

Ductions test single eye movements and are examined with one eye occluded, whereas versions test binocular eye movements and show how well the eyes move in synchrony. Fig. 14-8 shows both normal and various degrees of limited abduction. This is a scale of 0 to -4, with -1 limitation meaning slight limitation and -4 indicating severe limitation, with the inability of the eye to move past midline. This scale can be used to quantitate horizontal and vertical ductions. Note that limitation of ductions by itself does not indicate the cause of the limited eye movement, and the terms *restriction* and *paresis* should be used only when the specific etiology is known. Often the term *restriction* is misused to indicate limited eye movements, but the more general term *limitation* is more appropriate if the cause is unknown.

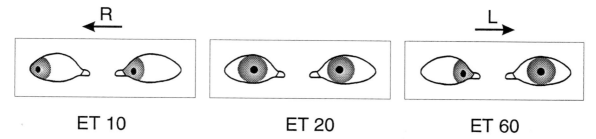

Fig. 14-7   Diagram of left lateral rectus paresis. In primary position, there is a moderate esotropia. In right gaze the esotropia diminishes, and in left gaze the esotropia increases as the right eye fully adducts, but the left eye cannot abduct. A tight left medial rectus muscle would give a similar pattern of incomitance.

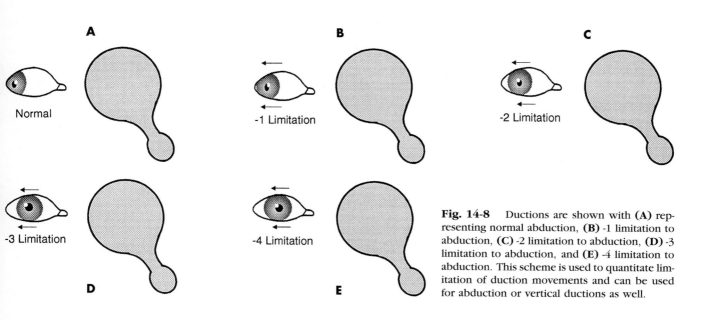

Fig. 14-8   Ductions are shown with (**A**) representing normal abduction, (**B**) -1 limitation to abduction, (**C**) -2 limitation to abduction, (**D**) -3 limitation to abduction, and (**E**) -4 limitation to abduction. This scheme is used to quantitate limitation of duction movements and can be used for abduction or vertical ductions as well.

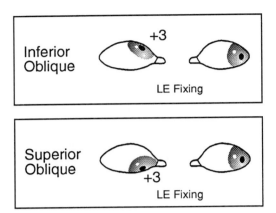

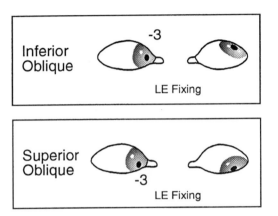

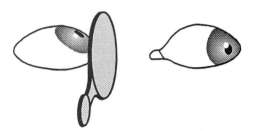

Fig. 14-9   Versions showing oblique overaction. The upper drawing shows right inferior oblique overaction +3, while the lower drawing shows superior oblique overaction +3 left eye.

Fig. 14-10   Versions showing underaction of the oblique muscle. Upper drawing shows -3 underaction of the right inferior oblique; lower drawing shows -3 underaction of the right superior oblique.

Fig. 14-11   An occluder over the right eye to ensure that the patient fixates left eye. When patient is fixing left eye it allows the inferior oblique overaction to become obvious and manifest. If the patient were to fix with the right eye; however, the examiner would not see the upshoot associated with inferior oblique overaction.

Abnormal versions can be noted on a 0 to 4 scale of +4 to 0 to -4 with 0 indicating normal and +4 indicating maximum overaction (Fig. 14-9), whereas -4 indicates most severe underaction (Fig. 14-10). It is important to remember that when evaluating for oblique dysfunction, make sure the abducting eye is fixing so the adducting eye is free to manifest the oblique dysfunction. This can be accomplished by partially occluding the adducting eye (with your thumb or occluder) and looking around the occluder to see if the eye manifests the oblique dysfunction (Fig. 14-11).

Prisms and Strabismus

Prisms are important tools for the diagnosis and treatment of strabismus since they are used to measure and neutralize ocular deviations. A prism bends light toward the base of the prism. The power of a prism to bend light is measured in *prism diopters (PD)*. One prism diopter

will shift light 1 centimeter at a distance of 1 meter or a displacement of approximately ½ degree. A 20 PD esotropia would mean the eye turns in approximately 10 degrees.

When a prism is placed in front of one eye, it moves the image off the fovea causing a perceived image "jump." The retinal image will shift toward the base of the prism, but the perceived image jump is in the opposite direction, toward the apex of the prism. This is because the retinal images are reversed; right/left and up/down (Fig. 14-12, *A* and *B*). To refixate on the shifted image the eye will move in the direction of the prism's apex, thus aligning the fovea with the new image location (Fig. 14-12, *C*).

Prism neutralization of a deviation   Prisms can be used to optically neutralize or correct strabismus. Neutralization occurs when enough prism is placed in front of the eye so the two foveae are aligned on the same object of regard. For example, when the appropriate amount of base-out prism (prism held horizontally with the apex directed toward the nose) is placed in front of the deviated eye of a patient with esotropia, the retinal image shifts temporally onto the fovea (Fig. 14-13).

The rule for neutralizing a deviation is to orient the prism so the apex is in the direction of the deviation. For esotropia, the apex is directed nasally, for exotropia the apex is directed temporally, and for hypertropia the apex is directed towards the hypertropic eye. The prism can also be placed in front of the fixing eye (straight eye) to neutralize the deviation (Fig. 14-14). When a base-out prism is placed in front of the fixing eye, both eyes move in the same direction as the apex of the prism, and both foveae shift into alignment (see Fig. 14-14, *B* and *C*).

Prism-induced strabismus   A prism can be used to induce strabismus. Place a prism in front of one eye and orient the prism in the opposite direction for neutralizing

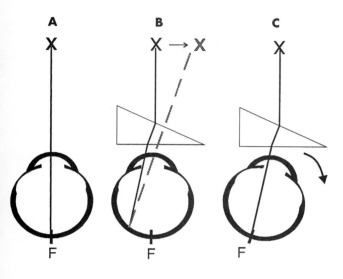

Fig. 14-12   The effect of a prism over one eye. **A,** Patient fixates on the X. **B,** A prism is introduced and the image is displaced towards the base of the prism and off the fovea. Note that the patient will perceive the image to jump in the direction of the apex of the prism. **C,** Patient refixates to place the image on the fovea by rotating the eye towards the apex of the prism. Note that when a prism is introduced, the patient will always refixate by rotating the eye in the direction of the apex of the prism.

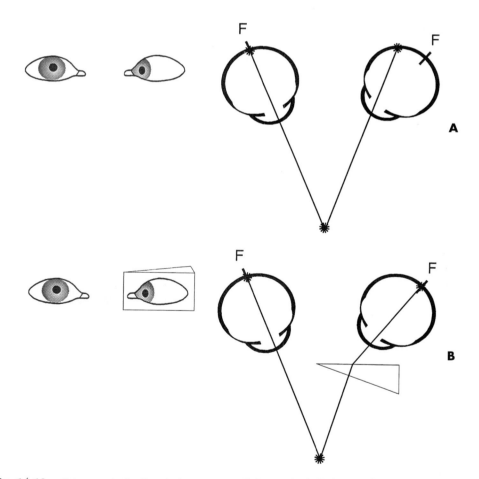

Fig. 14-13   Prism neutralization (prism over nonfixing eye). **A,** Patient with an esotropia. **B,** A prism is introduced base-out to direct the image onto the fovea of the left eye, thus correcting or neutralizing the deviation.

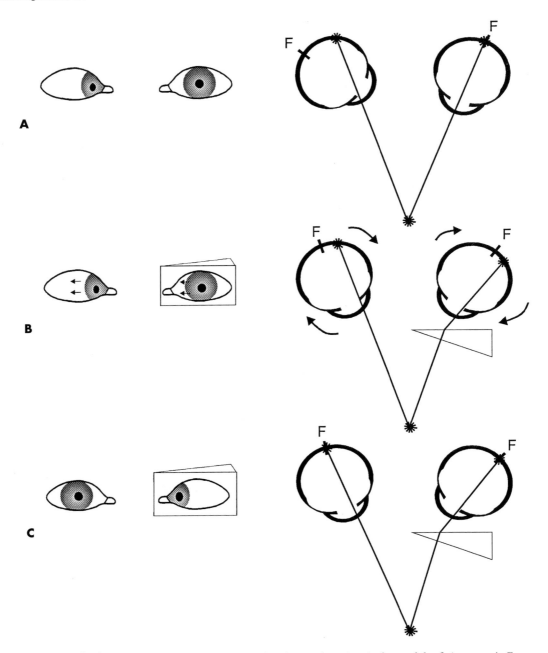

Fig. 14-14 Neutralization of an esotropia by placing the prism in front of the fixing eye. **A,** Esotropia with left eye fixing. **B,** Prism is placed in front of the fixing eye (left eye), which displaces the image off the fovea of the left eye. The left eye rotates to refixate to the image and, because of Herring's law, both eyes rotate in the direction of the apex of the prism. **C,** Deviation is neutralized, since images are on both foveae. The left eye has deviated nasally to put the image on the fovea and, because of Herring's law, the right eye moved temporally and the fovea is in alignment with the fixation target.

the deviation. For example, to induce an esotropia orient the prism base-in just the opposite of the way you would neutralize an esotropia. A base-in prism induces esotropia since the retinal image is displaced nasal to the fovea, and the eye must turn out to refixate (eso-shift) (Fig. 14-15). Likewise, a base-out prism neutralizes an esotropia but induces an exotropia, and a base-down prism

right eye neutralizes a right hypertropia but induces a left hypertropia (or right hypotropia).

Prism-induced vergence Normal subjects with binocular fusion will see double when a prism is placed in front of one eye to induce strabismus. However, if the prism is relatively small, the patient's motor fusion or vergence eye movements will realign the eyes to keep

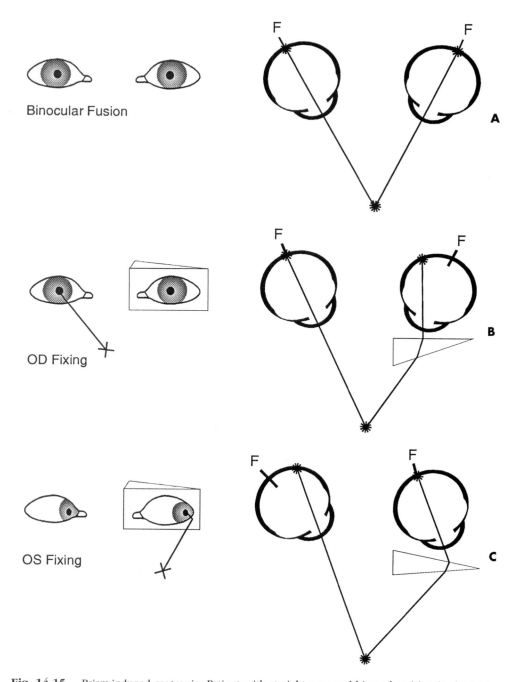

Fig. 14-15   Prism-induced esotropia. Patient with straight eyes and binocular vision is given an esotropia by placing a base-in prism over one eye. **A,** Patient orthotropic with images falling on both foveae. **B,** Base-in prism is placed before the left eye, causing the image to move nasally off the fovea. Patient is fixing with right eye. **C,** Patient now refixates with the left eye, viewing through the base-in prism. Left eye moves temporally to place the image on the fovea and, because of Herring's law, the right eye moves nasally and the right retinal image is displaced nasally off the fovea.

the images appropriately on the foveae (Fig. 14-16). Thus the prism will causes diplopia for a second or two until fusional vergence realigns the eyes so retinal images fall directly on each fovea (see Fig. 14-16, *C* and *D*). The key aspect of a vergence movement is the correctional fusion movement of the eye without the prism (see Fig. 14-16,

C). A base-out prism induces an exo-deviation and evokes fusional convergence, a base-in prism induces an eso-deviation and causes fusional divergence, and a base-up or base-down prism will evoke vertical fusional vergence. If the patient is not able to fuse a prism-induced strabismus, there will be no fusional corrective

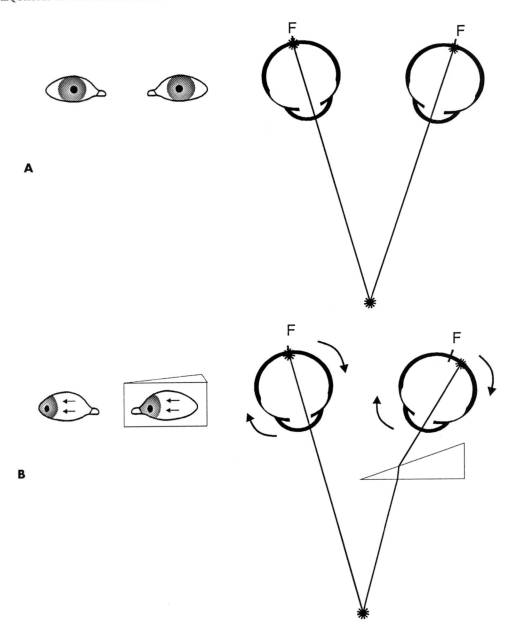

Fig. 14-16   Four steps of prism convergence. **A,** Eyes are well aligned in a patient with good fusional convergence. **B,** Exophoria is created by introducing a base-out prism in front of the left eye, causing a version movement of both eyes to the right.

movement of the eye without the prism and both eyes shift in the same direction (compare Figs. 14-16, *D* and 14-15, *C*).

Measuring fusion vergence amplitudes   Fusion vergence amplitudes are the amount of deviation that can be fused. It is measured by inducing a progressively larger deviation until fusion breaks. Start by inducing a small deviation with a prism that can be easily fused, and increase the size of the prism until the fusion breaks. A

deviation can be induced by progressively increasing prisms (usually by a prism bar) over one eye, or with the amblyoscope by moving the arms off parallel. Because our normal vertical vergence amplitudes are small, even small vertical misalignments are difficult to control by motor fusion; however, our innate fusional convergence is quite strong. The maximum base-out prism that can be fused is around 30 PD (convergence), maximum base-in prism that can be fused is 6 to 10 PD (divergence), and

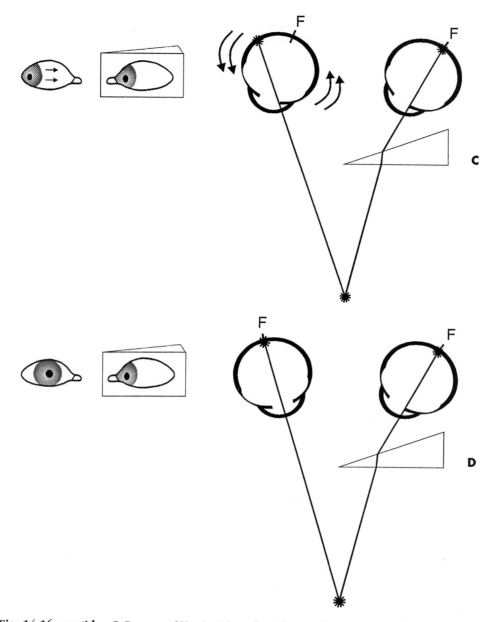

Fig. 14-16, cont'd   **C,** Because of Herring's law, the right eye also rotates and the image is now off the right fovea. To compensate for this, patient exercised fusional convergence and the right eye rotates nasally to put the image on the fovea. This is a vergence movement in distinction to the version movement shown in *B.* **D,** Patient is once again fusing, using fusional convergence to maintain eye alignment on the fixation target. Note that the eye behind the prism is deviated nasally. The base-out prism induces an exophoria, even though the eye behind the prism is nasally deviated and looks esotropic.

the maximal vertical prism that can be fused is usually 2 to 3 PD (vertical vergence). Table 14-1 shows normal fusion vergence amplitudes. In certain conditions divergence and vertical vergence fusional amplitudes can be quite large. Patients with congenital superior oblique palsy, for example, can have vertical fusion vergence amplitudes up to 25 to 30 PD.

MEASURING THE ANGLE OF STRABISMUS

The methods for measuring the angle of strabismus have been divided into the following categories: light reflex tests, cover tests, and subjective tests. Light reflex

Table 14-1   Fusion vergence amplitudes

	Distance (6 meters)	Near (⅓ meter)
Convergence (Base-out prism)	20 to 25 PD	30 to 35 PD
Divergence (Base-in prism)	6 to 8 PD	8 to 10 PD
Vertical Vergence (Vertical prism)	2 to 3 PD	2 to 3 PD

tests provide an estimate of the size of strabismus and are usually used on uncooperative patients such as young children and infants. These tests, however, are not as precise as the other tests such as the cover tests. The Lancaster red/green test requires the patient's subjective response and is useful in adult patients with diplopia and incomitant deviations.

When measuring any deviation, it is critical to keep the patient's attention and be sure the patient is appropriately accommodating on the fixation target. Accurate measurements cannot be obtained, if the patient is gazing around the room or day dreaming and not accommodating on the fixation target. To obtain accurate strabismus measurements, be sure to use an accommodative fixation target. An accommodative target is a target that has fine detail, which requires accurate accommodation to be seen. A penlight, for example, is the antithesis of an accommodative target since there is no fine detail, and accommodation is not required to see the light. One of the best accommodative targets for adults in the distance or near, is Snellen letters at a size close to visual threshold. By having the patient read the letters, the examiner knows that the patient is accommodating on the fixation target. For young children small detailed toys or small pictures with fine detail can be used at near and a cartoon movie or animated toys in the distance.

Light Reflex Tests

Hirschberg test

The Hirschberg test or corneal light reflex test, assesses eye alignment by the location of the corneal light reflex within the pupil. The term *corneal light reflex* is a misnomer, since it is not a reflex off the cornea. What we perceive as the light reflex is actually the first Purkinje image, which is a virtual image, located behind the pupil. The Hirschberg test should be performed by holding a light source (muscle light or penlight) in front of one of the examiner's eyes and directing the light into the patient's eyes. Have the patient look at the light, then assess the location of the light reflex in each eye. Hirschberg

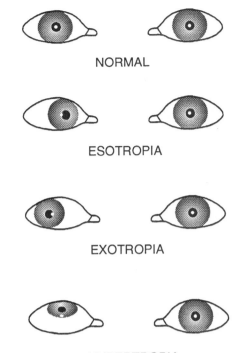

Fig. 14-17   Hirschberg test with the top drawing showing normal reflexes centered. Second drawing shows esotropia right eye with the light reflex deviated temporally. Third drawing shows exotropia with the light reflex deviated nasally. Bottom drawing shows right hypertropia with the light reflex deviated inferiorly.

testing is only valid if the patient fixes on the light source. The examiner must view the light reflexes from behind the light source; therefore for practical purposes, the Hirschberg test can only be performed at near. An accommodative fixation target can be placed next to the light source to attract the patient's attention and provide an accommodative target.

With normal orthotropic alignment, the light reflexes are slightly decentered nasally, but they are symmetrically located within each pupil. Slight symmetric nasal displacement is normal and it is caused by "physiologic" positive angle kappa (see angle kappa in the following section). Asymmetric displacement of the light reflex, however, indicates a possible tropia or asymmetric angle kappa. An asymmetric angle kappa can be distinguished from a tropia by the cover-uncover test (see the following discussion). Temporal displacement of the light reflex indicates esotropia, nasal displacement exotropia, and inferior displacement hypertropia (Fig. 14-17). The clinician can estimate the size of an ocular deviation by the amount of light reflex displacement. Temporal displacement of the light reflex to the pupillary margin indicates an esotropia of 15° (ET 30 PD), displacement to the temporal mid iris indicates esotropia 30° (ET 60 PD) and temporal displacement to the limbus indicates an esotro-

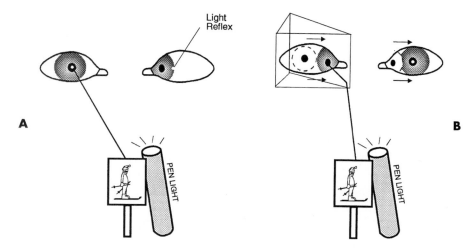

Fig. 14-18   Krimsky test in a patient with esotropia. Note in **A** that the light reflex is deviated temporally in the esotropic left eye. In **B** a base-out prism is presented in front of the right eye, which is fixing. The patient continues to fixate with the right eye, but the right eye turns to pick up fixation and the left eye, because of Herring's law, moves temporally. The left eye is now centered and the right eye is turned in; however, the light reflex would be centered in both eyes. This is the neutralization point and the amount of prism needed to achieve the neutralization point measures the angle of deviation.

pia of 40° (ET 80 PD). Another way to estimate the angle of deviation is to multiply the millimeters of light displacement by 15 PD to give the deviation in prism diopters. Thus 2 mm of nasal displacement of the reflex from its normal location when monocularly viewing indicates an exotropia of 30 PD. These are relatively gross estimates and as a rule are not used to determine amount of surgery.

Krimsky test   The Krimsky test is a modification of the Hirschberg test that allows for better quantitation of a deviation through the use of a prism (Fig. 14-18). A prism is placed in front of one eye, with the base oriented appropriately to neutralize the deviation (esotropia, base-out; exotropia, base-in; and hypertropia, base down). A penlight is then directed into both eyes as described for the Hirschberg test and the patient fixates on an accommodative target juxtaposed to the penlight. The prism is increased or decreased until the reflex from each eye becomes symmetrically centered in the pupil.

Bruckner reflex test   The Bruckner reflex test is performed by using the direct ophthalmoscope to obtain a red reflex from both eyes simultaneously. Make sure that the patient is looking at the light during the Bruckner test. If the patient looks to peripheral targets, the test is invalid. In patients with strabismus, the Bruckner test usually shows asymmetric reflexes with a brighter reflex coming from the deviated eye. This will identify any pathologic conditions that changes the normal red reflex, including anisometropia; gross retinal pathology; large retinal detachment; and corneal, lenticular, or vitreous opacities (Fig. 14-19). This is a screening test and does not determine the size of a strabismus.

Angle Kappa

If the fovea is not exactly centered in the posterior pole of the eye, then when the eye fixates on a target the cornea will not be exactly aligned with the target. This monocular misalignment because the fovea is off center is called the angle kappa. The angle kappa is the angle between the line of sight and the corneal/pupillary axis (Fig. 14-20).

A *positive angle kappa* is associated with a temporal displacement of the fovea, and an out-turning or temporal orientation of the fixing eye. Normally, we all have a small *physiologic positive angle kappa* with the fovea positioned slightly temporal to center, and the eye directed slightly temporal to the fixation target. This is why we normally see the Hirschberg light reflex to be slightly decentered nasally, since the eye is pointing slightly temporal to the light source (see Hirschberg test in the previous section). Large pathologic positive angle kappas occur in diseases that displace or pull the macula temporally, such as retinopathy of prematurity and *Toxocara canis* (Fig. 14-21). With a pathological positive angle kappa, the eye must turn out to place the target image on the fovea, which causes a nasal displacement of the light reflex. A *negative angle kappa* is caused by nasal displacement of the fovea towards the optic nerve. This results in an in-turning of the eye and a temporal shift of the light reflex. Nasal macular displacement can be secondary to a retinal scar located between the fovea and optic nerve or can occur congenitally without a specific etiology.

Fig. 14-21 shows a patient with a positive angle Kappa

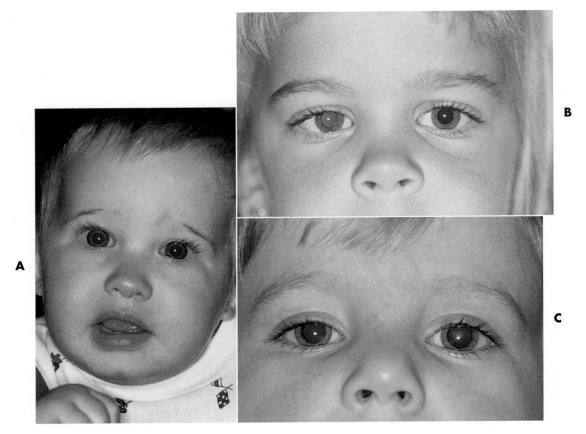

Fig. 14-19   Bruckner test (red reflexes). **A,** Eyes are straight and the Bruckner red reflexes are symmetric. **B,** Patient with a small right esotropia. Note that the reflex is brighter in the deviated right eye. In patients with strabismus, the deviated eye shows a brighter reflex. **C,** Patient with a cataract left eye. Note that the reflex is dull left eye secondary to the lens opacity. See color plate.

Fig. 14-20   Positive and negative angle kappa are depicted. *Left,* the eye turns out to pick up fixation under monocular viewing conditions since the fovea (*F*) is displaced temporally. Note that the line of sight differs from the corneal pupillary axis. *Right,* the eye deviates nasally to pick up fixation since the fovea is displaced nasally close to the optic nerve. Again, the line of sight is not parallel with the corneal pupillary axis.

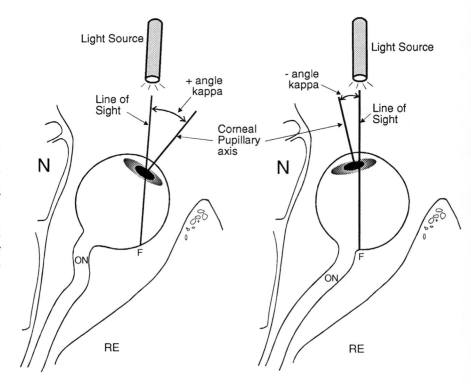

Positive Angle Kappa   **Negative Angle Kappa**

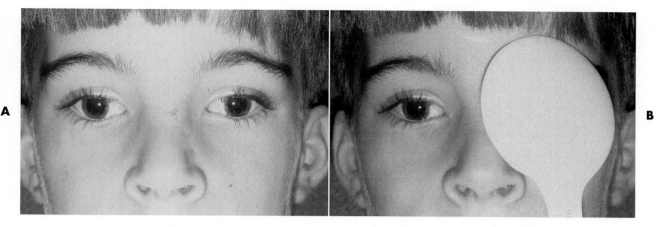

Fig. 14-21   Clinical photograph of a patient with retinopathy of prematurity who has both foveae dragged temporally. **A,** Patient appears exotropic; however, both eyes are exotropic, unlike true exotropia where the fixing eye is straight and the nonfixing eye is deviated. This patient has a positive angle kappa and is actually fusing with both eyes deviated temporally to align the foveae. **B,** There is no ocular shift when the left eye is covered.

secondary to a dragged macula caused by retinopathy of prematurity. This patient appears to have misalignment of the eyes (exotropia), but actually is orthotropic since both foveae are aligned on the fixation target. When the left eye is covered, the right eye remains deviated laterally since this is the position necessary for foveal fixation. Remember angle kappa relates to the eye position during monocular viewing and is associated with central fixation by the displaced fovea.

Cover Tests

Cover-uncover test

The cover-uncover test is designed to detect the presence of a tropia, without dissociating an existing phoria. The test is performed by very briefly covering and then uncovering one eye, while observing the fellow eye for a tropia shift since the eye picks up fixation. If there is no shift, then several seconds later cover and uncover the opposite eye. If there is no shift of either eye after performing the cover-uncover test for each eye, then there is no manifest tropia and the eyes are straight, that is, orthotropia. If briefly covering one eye produces a refixation shift, then a manifest tropia is present. A nasal to temporal ocular shift indicates esotropia, a temporal to nasal ocular shift indicates exotropia, and a downward ocular shift indicates a hypertropia (Fig. 14-22). Note that no shift to cover-uncover testing means there is no tropia, but it does not rule out the possibility of an underlying phoria. A phoria is detected by following the cover-uncover test with the alternate cover testing (see the following).

When performing the cover-uncover test be sure to have the patient fixate on an accommodative target to control fixation. Cover the fixing eye for 1 to 2 seconds, just long enough to see if there is a shift of the uncovered

eye to midline. The cover-uncover test can be dissociating and therefore may manifest an underlying phoria if the test is performed too slowly. Prolonged occlusion of one eye for even several seconds will disrupt fusion and the patient will manifest a phoria that may erroneously be called a tropia because it is associated with the cover test. Remember to briefly cover one eye for only one or two seconds, and to remove the cover for several seconds before covering the fellow eye to allow reestablishment of fusion.

Alternate cover testing   The alternate cover test is used to dissociate binocular fusion to determine the full deviation, including any latent phoria. The test is performed by alternately occluding each eye, and then observing for a refixation shift of the uncovered eye to midline (see Fig. 14-4). In contrast to the cover-uncover test, during alternate cover testing it is important to hold the occluder over one eye for several seconds to dissociate fusion, and then to rapidly move the occluder to the fellow eye making sure one eye is always occluded. Refixation shifts of the eyes to alternate cover testing are interpreted as for cover-uncover testing.

Interpreting responses to cover tests   No shift to alternate cover testing indicates orthophoria. A refixation shift to alternate cover testing indicates a strabismus is present, either a tropia, or a phoria. Patients with a phoria have straight eyes, with no shift to cover-uncover testing, but show a shift to the alternate cover testing. Patients with a tropia show a shift to both on cover-uncover testing and alternate cover testing.

Patients with a small angle tropia <10 PD may have peripheral fusion and this is called the *monofixation syndrome* (also see Chapter 15). Monofixators have both a phoria and a tropia, and therefore demonstrate a small shift to cover-uncover testing and a larger shift to alter-

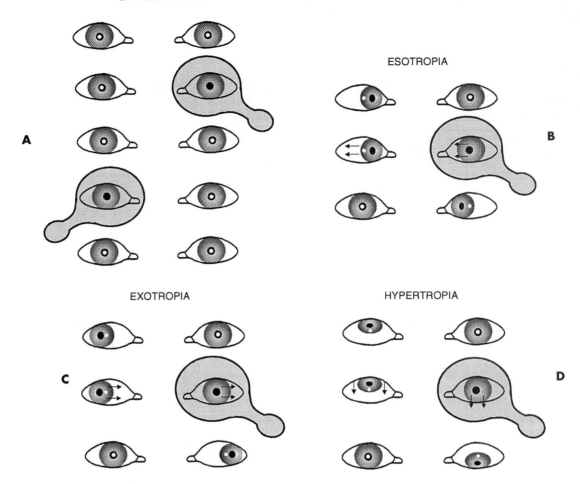

Fig. 14-22   Cover-uncover test on patients with orthophoria, esotropia, exotropia, and hypertropia. **A,** Orthophoria. Note that when left eye is covered, there is no movement. The cover is then removed to allow for binocular fusion, and then the right eye is covered; again there is no movement. **B,** Esotropia. Left eye is fixing, and when left eye is covered the right eye moves out to pick up fixation. This outward movement indicates that the right eye is esotropic. **C,** Exotropia. Left eye is fixing and when left eye is covered, the right eye turns in to pick up fixation. The inward movement of the right eye indicates a right exotropia. **D,** Right hypertropia. Left eye is fixing. Covering the left eye causes the right eye to come down to pick up fixation. Movement of the right eye indicates a right hypertropia.

nate cover testing. Cover-uncover testing discloses the small tropia and alternate cover testing breaks down the phoria to show the full deviation, tropia plus phoria. Patients with a pure tropia and no phoria show the same shift to cover-uncover testing and alternate cover testing. Comparing cover-uncover testing to alternate cover testing is a good way to diagnose the monofixation syndrome, even in children who are too young to cooperate with sensory testing. Remember, the presence of a phoria is an indication of binocular fusion. Table 14-2 shows the clinical findings of phorias, tropias, and monofixation syndrome.

Prism-Alternate cover test   The prism-alternate cover test measures the size of the strabismus including

any latent phoria. A prism is placed over one eye oriented to neutralize the deviation. Alternate cover testing is then performed with the prism in place. If there is a residual refixation shift, the prism is changed (either increased or decreased) to neutralize the deviation (Fig. 14-23). When changing prisms, be sure to always keep one eye covered to maintain binocular dissociation. Also be sure not to stack prisms of the same orientation (horizontal over horizontal or vertical over vertical) to increase the prism power. It is acceptable to stack horizontal over vertical, but stacking prisms of the same orientation results in underestimation of the angle size.

Cardinal positions of gaze   There are nine cardinal positions of gaze; however, in most clinical situations,

Table 14-2 Interpreting cover tests

	Corneal light reflex	Cover-uncover	Alternate cover	Binocular fusion
ORTHOTROPIA	Symmetric	No shift	No shift	Yes
PHORIA	Symmetric	No shift	Shift	Yes
TROPIA >10 PD	Eccentric reflex	Shift	Shift	No
MONOFIXATION <10 PD	Small deviation usually esotropia	Small shift	Larger shift	Yes

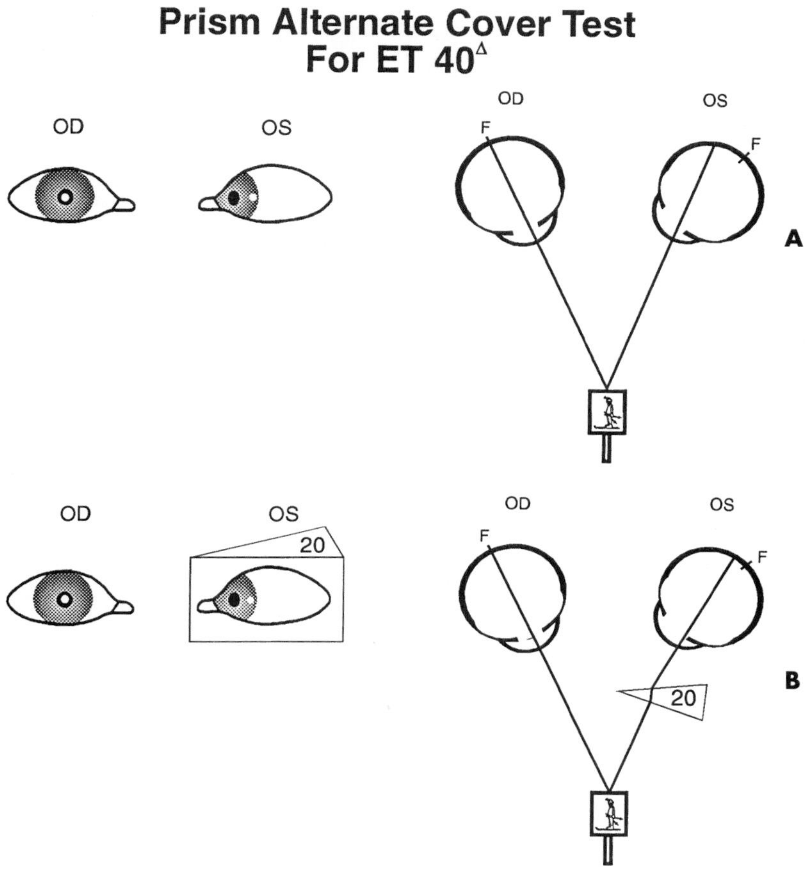

Prism Alternate Cover Test
For ET 40$^\Delta$

Fig. 14-23   Prism alternate cover test to measure esotropia. **A,** Left eye is esotropic, right eye fixing. **B,** Base-out prism is placed before the deviated left eye and the retinal image moves closer to fovea, but the deviation is still undercorrected.   *Continued*

measuring the deviation by alternate prism cover test in 5 positions (primary position, up gaze, down gaze, and right and left gaze) is sufficient. Distance measurements are used, and different positions of gaze are achieved by moving the patient's head. Measurements in the cardinal positions of gaze are very helpful in identifying and quantifying incomitance. Box 14-1 lists causes of variable strabismus measurements.

Simultaneous prism cover test   This special cover test is used to measure the tropia component of patients with a small tropia and a larger phoria (i.e., monofixation

syndrome). The idea is to measure only the tropia without dissociating the phoria. Only use it for patients with a small angle tropia <10 PD since larger tropias do not permit fusion and therefore do not have an associated phoria. The simultaneous prism cover test is performed by first estimating the size of the tropia by corneal light reflex testing. A prism approximately the size of the tropia is placed in front of the nonfixing eye (i.e., deviated eye) to neutralize the tropia and the fixing eye is simultaneously covered by an occluder (Fig. 14-24). If the prism neutralizes the tropia, the fixing eye will stay in its

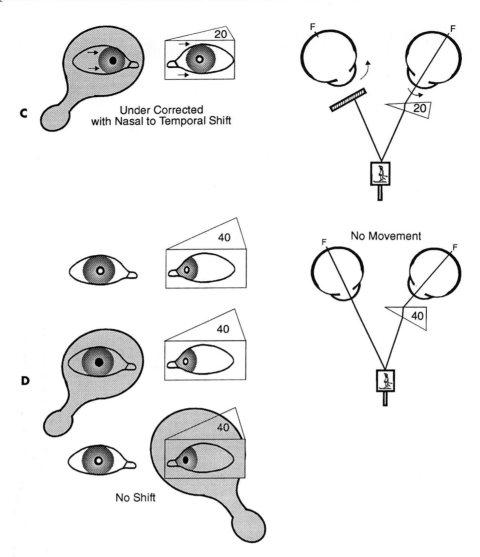

Fig. 14-23, cont'd **C,** Alternate cover testing is performed, first covering right eye then left eye. Because the prism undercorrects the deviation there is an outward shift of the uncovered eye. **D,** Larger prism (40 PD) is placed in front of the left eye and alternate cover testing now reveals no shift in eye position since the deviation is completely neutralized.

deviated position and there will be no refixation shift. If the deviated eye shows a refixation movement, then a residual deviation is present. The prism and occluder are withdrawn from the eyes and after several seconds, a different prism is presented to the deviated eye since the fixing eye is simultaneously covered. It is important to allow several seconds to elapse before repeating the test so the patient can regain binocular fusion and control the phoria. This process is repeated until there is no shift of the deviated eye when the fixing eye is covered. For patients with the monofixation syndrome, the amount of tropia can be measured with simultaneous prism cover testing and the alternate prism cover test can be used to measure the total angle, tropia plus phoria. The notation

in the clinic chart for a typical monofixator with a small angle esophoria-tropia would read: ET 6PD—E 15 PD.

Primary and Secondary Deviations

When measuring a comitant strabismus the prism can be placed in front of either eye to neutralize a strabismic deviation. However, when measuring patients with ocular restriction or muscle pareses, the clinician must consider the primary versus the secondary deviation. In accordance with Herring's law, the deviation is smaller when the normal eye fixates (primary deviation), and larger when the eye with limited ductions is fixing (secondary deviation).

Box 14-1 Common Causes for Variable Measurements

1. *Poor control of accommodation.* Important in young children and patients with a high AC/A ratio. Solution: Use targets that require full accommodation to be seen. Targets with small detail close to visual threshold are best.

2. *Variable working distance* (usually at near). Solution: Control working distance to ⅓ of a meter at near, and standardize distance working distance. This is more critical for near measurements. Have a string ⅓ of a meter long to measure the near working distance.

3. *Tonic fusion not suspended.* Usually seen in patients with intermittent exotropia and accommodative esotropia. Solution: Prevent binocular fusion by prolonged occlusion with alternate cover testing. Make sure one eye is always covered when changing prisms (prism bars are helpful).

4. *Physiologic redress fixation movements.* Commonly associated with large-angle strabismus. Even when the deviation is neutralized, there is an overshoot of the refixating eye. Solution: Move occluder away from the patient's face to allow peripheral vision of the occluded eye. Also judge the point of neutralization, since the point when redress movement is equal to the refixation movement. Finally, bracket the deviation by intentionally overcorrecting with too much prism then reduce prism to the best neutralization achieved.

5. *Incomitant deviation* (A- or V-patterns and lateral gaze incomitance). Small changes of face turns, head tilts, or chin elevation or depression during the examination will change the deviation measured, if the deviation is incomitant. Solution: Control the patient's head position for primary position and cardinal fields of gaze. Consistent head positioning is critical if reproducible measurements are to be obtained.

Simultaneous Prism-Cover Test ET10$^\Delta$

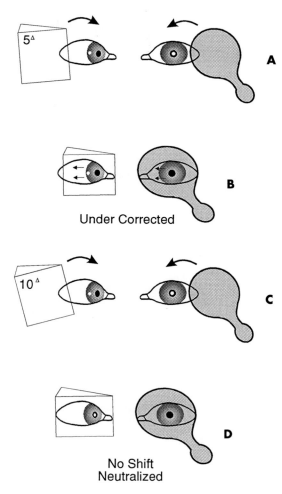

Fig. 14-24 Simultaneous prism cover test for small-angle esotropia. This test is useful for measuring the tropia in patient with a tropia and a phoria (monofixation syndrome). **A,** Right esotropia with left eye fixing. Estimate the deviation, then present a prism over the deviating eye while simultaneously covering the fixing eye. If the prism is sufficient to neutralize the esotropia, the eye behind the prism (in this case the right eye) does not move. **B,** In this case, the 5 diopter prism is too small and the right eye moves out to pick up fixation. **C,** A 10 diopter prism is now used to neutralize the esotropia. In this case the prism neutralizes the esotropia. **D,** The left eye is covered since the 10 diopter prism is placed in front of the right eye. No shift occurs since the 10 diopter prism neutralizes the 10 PD esotropia.

As shown in Fig. 14-25, the *primary deviation* is small because with the nonparetic right eye fixing relatively little innervation (+1) is needed to keep the eye in primary position (see Fig. 14-25, *A*). The paretic eye receives the same +1 innervation and turns in slightly because of the left lateral rectus muscle is slightly weaker than its antagonist, the left medial rectus muscle. The *secondary deviation* is larger because when the paretic eye fixates, the weak left lateral rectus muscle must receive a tremendous amount of innervation (+4) to bring the left eye into primary position (see Fig. 14-25, *B*). Both the paretic left lateral rectus, and its yoke muscle,

the right medial rectus, receive +4 innervation because of Herring's law. This excess drive to the healthy right medial rectus muscle causes a large secondary nasal deviation of the right eye. This same mechanism of primary and secondary deviations also applies to restrictions.

When measuring a deviation with prisms, remember the eye without the prism is considered to be the fixing eye, and the eye looking through the prism is the

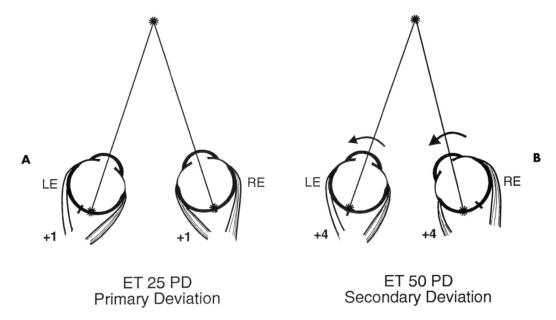

ET 25 PD
Primary Deviation

ET 50 PD
Secondary Deviation

Fig. 14-25 Left lateral rectus paresis showing deviation with the nonparetic eye fixing (primary deviation, *A*) versus deviation with paretic eye fixing (secondary deviation, *B*). **A,** Right eye (nonparetic eye) is fixing with a small left esotropia. **B,** Left eye (paretic eye) is fixing with large secondary right esotropia. Note that the left lateral rectus is paretic and must receive +4 innervation to abduct the eye. A +4 innervation of the yoke muscle (right medial rectus) causes the right eye to dramatically over rotate, thus causing the large secondary deviation.

nonfixing eye, regardless of fixation preference. This is because the eye without the prism must come to primary position to fixate during alternate cover testing (Fig. 14-26). So measure the primary deviation by placing a prism over the eye with limited ductions, and measure the secondary deviation by placing the prism over the normal eye.

Another cause of primary and secondary deviation is uncorrected anisometropia. Uncorrected hypermetropic or myopic anisometropia can cause a different deviation depending on which eye is fixing. This occurs because, if the eyes are not optically corrected, each eye will accommodate a different amount and convergence, which is linked to accommodation, will also vary depending on which eye is fixing. An esotropic patient with uncorrected unilateral hypermetropia will show a greater deviation when the hypermetropic eye fixates. An uncorrected anisometropic myopia on the other hand will show less esotropia with the myopic eye fixing.

Lancaster Red/Green Test

Lancaster red/green test is a fovea-to-fovea test with two fixation targets, one that the examiner controls and one that the patient moves. This test is very useful for measuring incomitant strabismus in patients with diplopia. The fixation targets are red- and green-colored linear streaks of light that are projected on a screen. The pa-

tient wears red/green glasses (usually red over right eye) and holds one light (green light in Fig. 14-27) and the examiner hold the second light (red light in Fig. 14-27). The examiner projects the red light on the screen and the patient is directed to look at the red light. Since the patient's right eye (with the red filter) only sees the examiner's red light, the right eye (fovea) aligns with the examiner's light. The right eye thus becomes the fixing eye and its position is controlled by where the examiner places the red light. Next the patient is directed to aim the green light, on top of the examiner's red light. Since the left eye only sees the green light, wherever he or she points the light indicates the direction of the left fovea. The patient now sees the two lights superimposed since both lights fall on the fovea of each eye. The patient in Fig. 14-27 has a left esotropia, so with the green filter over the left eye, the patient directs the green light to the right of the red light. An orthotropic person will place the lights on top of each other, whereas a patient with a left exotropia will point the green light to the left of the red light. Note the Lancaster red/green test directly shows the examiner where the eyes (foveae) are pointing, which is just the opposite of diplopia tests. The angle of deviation is derived by measuring the amount of separation between the two projected lights on the screen. With the Lancaster red/green test, the eye that sees the examiner's light is the fixing eye, so the examiner can move the target to various positions on the

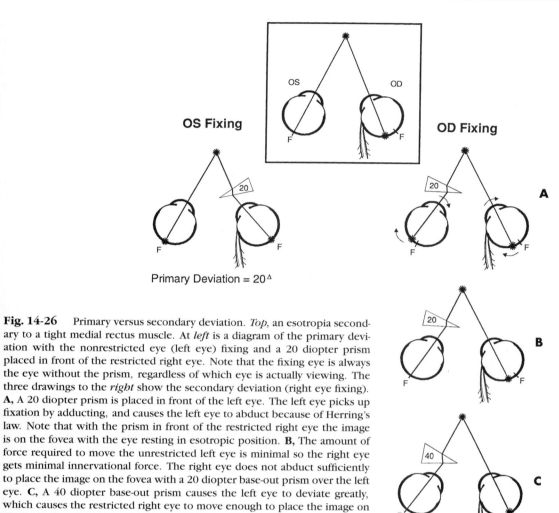

OS Fixing

OD Fixing

Primary Deviation = 20$^\triangle$

A

B

C

Secondary Deviation = 40$^\triangle$

Fig. 14-26   Primary versus secondary deviation. *Top,* an esotropia secondary to a tight medial rectus muscle. At *left* is a diagram of the primary deviation with the nonrestricted eye (left eye) fixing and a 20 diopter prism placed in front of the restricted right eye. Note that the fixing eye is always the eye without the prism, regardless of which eye is actually viewing. The three drawings to the *right* show the secondary deviation (right eye fixing). **A,** A 20 diopter prism is placed in front of the left eye. The left eye picks up fixation by adducting, and causes the left eye to abduct because of Herring's law. Note that with the prism in front of the restricted right eye the image is on the fovea with the eye resting in esotropic position. **B,** The amount of force required to move the unrestricted left eye is minimal so the right eye gets minimal innervational force. The right eye does not abduct sufficiently to place the image on the fovea with a 20 diopter base-out prism over the left eye. **C,** A 40 diopter base-out prism causes the left eye to deviate greatly, which causes the restricted right eye to move enough to place the image on the image on the fovea. Secondary deviation equals 40 PD, whereas the primary deviation is 20 PD. Note that with the prism over the left eye the restricted right eye must come to primary position to fixate.

screen to measure the deviation in eccentric fields of gaze. Primary versus secondary deviations can be measured by the examiner trading lights with the patient. Torsion can also be assessed in various positions of gaze by observing the tilt of the lines on the screen. Nasal displacement of the top of the line indicates intorsion, and temporal displacement of the top of the line indicates extorsion.

Torsion

Objective torsion

In normal patients, the fovea is located between the midpoint and the lower border of the optic nerve. Patients with torsion will have a shift in the position of the fovea relative to the optic disc (Fig. 14-28). With extorsion, the fovea is shifted below the inferior border of the optic disc, whereas intorsion is when the fovea is higher than the midpoint of the optic nerve. Actually, the fovea

is the center of vision and the optic nerve rotates around it. Remember that the indirect ophthalmoscopic view is inverted, so extorsion is seen since the fovea above the upper pole of the disc, and intorsion is when the fovea is below the midpoint of the disc.

Maddox rod test   The Maddox rod can be used for identifying horizontal, vertical, and especially torsional deviations. The Maddox rod has a washboard appearance since it is made up of multiple cylindrical high plus lenses stacked on top of each other. When the patient views a light through the Maddox rod a linear streak of light is seen which is oriented 90 degrees to the cylindrical ribs of the Maddox rod. The single Maddox rod test is performed by placing the Maddox rod over one eye and having the patient view a pen light. The Maddox rod is aligned so the streak is vertical to detect horizontal deviations and so the streak is horizontal for vertical deviations. If the streak of light passes through the pen light the patient is orthophoric. This is one of the most dis-

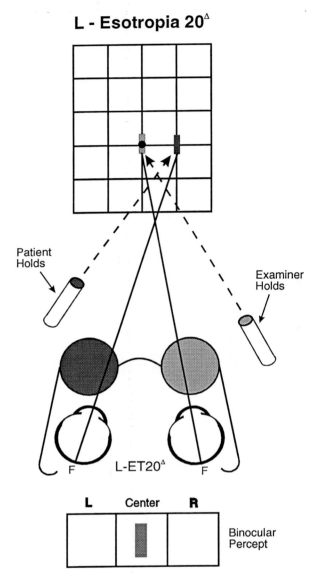

Fig. 14-27 Lancaster red/green test in a patient with NRC, esotropia, and diplopia. This is a fovea-to-fovea test. The patient fixates on the streak of light projected by the examiner. The patient then directs his or her light to align with the examiner's light. Patient perceives a single streak of light since each light falls on the corresponding fovea, even though the streaks are separated.

It can be done with a single lens (single Maddox rod test) or a lens over each eye (double Maddox rod test). With the double Maddox rod test, the patient is asked to make parallel the two streaks of the Maddox rod. If the eyes are straight a prism can be used to induce a deviation either horizontally or vertically to separate the lines of the Maddox rod. Patients without torsion see parallel lines (Fig. 14-29, *A*), those with intorsion see the 12 o'clock position turned nasally (Fig. 14-29, *B*), and those with extorsion see the 12 o'clock position turned temporally (Fig. 14-29, *C*). Note that the Maddox rod test, and most subjective torsion tests for that matter, do not localize the eye with the torsion. They only measure the relative difference in torsion between the two eyes. The examiner often finds a monocular torsion on the subjective Maddox rod testing, but bilateral torsion by objective testing with indirect ophthalmoscopy. This occurs because the eye that the patient perceives to have torsional misalignment depends on which eye is fixing (ocular dominance). The Lancaster red/green test controls which eye is fixing and it therefore can be used to localize torsion. To find the total torsion with the double Maddox rod, add the torsion of the two eyes (Fig. 14-29, *C*).

MEASURING THE AC/A RATIO

To understand the AC/A ratio we must review measurements of accommodation and convergence. Accommodation is the increase in lens power to clearly focus at near. The closer the fixation target, the more accommodation is needed to keep the image focused on the retina. Accommodation is measured in diopters. The number of diopters of accommodation needed to focus at a specific near point is the reciprocal of the fixation distance in meters. For example, if the fixation target is at ⅓ of a meter, then an emmetropic patient has to accommodate 3.00 diopters to put the image in focus, 2.00 diopters at ½ meter, and 1.00 diopter at a meter. Note that a plus 2.00 hypermetrope without correction would have to accommodate 5.00 diopters at ⅓ of a meter (2.00 diopters for the hypermetropia and 3.00 diopters for near fixation).

Convergence keeps the eyes aligned on approaching targets and is linked to accommodation, so as accommodation increases, convergence increases. Additionally, the farther apart the eyes (interpupillary distance), the more convergence is required to keep the eyes aligned at near.

AC/A Ratio

Accommodative convergence to accommodation ratio (AC/A ratio) is the amount of change in convergence for

sociating tests, because the images to each eye are totally different and there are essentially no binocular fusion cues. In fact, the Maddox rod test is so dissociating that it will cause patients with normal bifoveal fusion to manifest their phoria. Because of this, the Maddox rod test, and dissociating tests in general, do not distinguish between phorias and tropias. To make the diagnosis of phoria versus tropia, the examiner must assess the eye alignment objectively before administering this dissociating test.

Maddox rod and torsion The line seen with the Maddox rod can be used to determine subjective torsion.

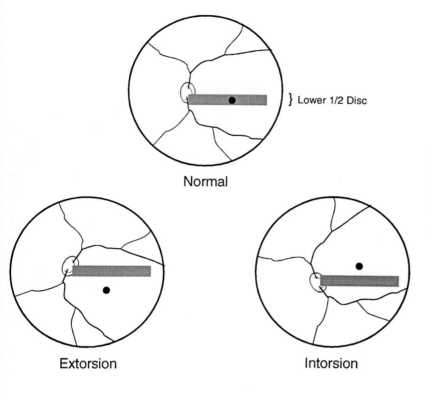

Fig. 14-28   Ocular torsion through the direct view (left eye). *Top*, normal fovea to disc relationship with the fovea located along the lower half of the disc. The lower left drawing shows extorsion with the fovea below the disc. The lower right drawing shows intorsion with the fovea above the upper half of the disc.

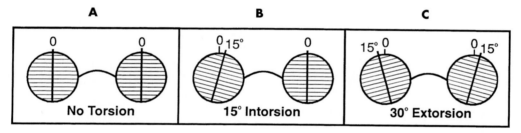

Fig. 14-29   Double Maddox rod test is shown with the patient perceiving the streak of light vertically. **A,** Normal patient with no torsion and the Maddox rods aligned at the 0 position each eye. **B,** Patient with right incyclotorsion 15 degrees with the right Maddox rod turned clockwise. **C,** Patient with bilateral extorsion, 15 degrees each eye. Total extorsion is 30 degrees.

a specific amount of change in accommodation. A high AC/A ratio means the eyes over converge for a given amount of accommodation (esodeviation at near), whereas a low AC/A ratio means there is underconvergence per diopter of accommodation (exodeviation at near).

The three most useful methods for measuring the AC/A ratio are listed in Box 14-2. These are based on changing the patient's accommodation and then measuring the associated change in eye alignment. Accommodation is changed by either changing the fixation distance (heterophoria method, clinical distance-near relationship), or by changing the amount of accommodation needed for a specific fixation distance by introducing various amount of plus and minus spherical lenses (lens gradient method). Most clinicians use either

Box 14-2   Methods for Measuring the AC/A Ratio
Heterophoria method
Clinical distance-near relationship
Lens gradient method

the clinical distance-near relationship, or the lens gradient method. The clinical distance-near relationship provides information about the overall change in convergence when the patient looks from distance to near, including the effects of accommodation and proximal convergence.

When measuring the AC/A ratio with any of these methods, it is important to use accommodative targets, to have the patient wear his or her full optical correction, to use alternate cover testing to measure the deviation, and to control the fixation target distance. By convention, 6 meters (20 feet) is used for distance, and ⅓ meter (14 inches) for near. The *normal AC/A ratio* is approximately 4:1 to 6:1. For calculations of the AC/A ratio, esodeviations are represented as positive numbers and exodeviations as negative numbers.

Heterophoria Method

The heterophoria method compares the distance and near deviations, along with the interpupillary distance, to determine the AC/A ratio. The interpupillary distance is important because the change in accommodation is produced by changing the fixation target distance. The following formula is used to calculate the AC/A ratio by the heterophoria method, with interpupillary distance (IPD) in *centimeters*, distance deviation (D) in prism diopters, near deviation (N) in prism diopters, and accommodation for near (D A) in diopters (fixation at ⅓ meter = 3 diopters). Remember to use centimeters for the interpupillary distance.

$$AC/A = IPD + \frac{N - D}{D A}$$

Example
Distance = ET 31

Near = ET 40 $AC/A = 5 + \frac{(40 - 31)}{3} = +8$ (high AC/A ratio)

Interpupillary distance = 50 mm (5 cm)
Diopters of accommodation at ⅓ m = 3 D

Clinical Distance-Near Relationship

The clinical distance-near relationship is a simple comparison of the deviation in the distance to the deviation at near. The clinician can figure the clinical distance-near relationship by subtracting the distance deviation from the near deviation. A distance-to-near difference within 10 PD is considered normal, whereas those greater than +10 PD are high and those less than -10 PD are low. This clinical distance-near relationship is a simple but very useful method for identifying patients with a high AC/A ratio.

N − D = Clinical distance-near relationship
D = distance deviation viewing target at 6 meters (20 feet)
N = near deviation viewing target at ⅓ meter

Example 1
D = ET 20   AC/A relationship 40 − 20 = **20** (High AC/A)
N = ET 40

Example 2
D = ortho   AC/A relationship −15 − 0 = **−15** (Low AC/A)
N = XT 15

Lens Gradient Method

The lens gradient method determines the AC/A ratio by measuring the change in ocular deviation associated with a specific change in lens-induced accommodation. In this test accommodation is changed by having the patient view an accommodative target through a supplemental plus or minus spherical lens. A plus lens relaxes accommodation; with less accommodation, there is less convergence. A minus lens causes increased accommodation, increased convergence and an eso-shift. The AC/A ratio is calculated by measuring the deviation at a set distance, with and without supplemental spherical lenses, and dividing the difference by the lens power used. Measurements are usually made in the distance to minimize proximal convergence, and a plus 3.00 diopter lens is usually used.

The formula for the gradient method is;

$$AC/A = \frac{\text{Deviation without lens} - \text{Deviation with lens}}{\text{lens in diopters}}$$

Example 1
Deviation without lens = ET 40
Deviation with
+3.00 lens = ET10 $AC/A = \frac{40 - 10}{3} = $ **10 (High AC/A ratio)**

Example 2
Deviation without lens = XT 4
Deviation with
−3.00 lens = ET 14 $AC/A = \frac{-4 - 14}{-3} = $ **6 (Normal)**

Another useful calculation is to estimate the effect of a spectacle lens on a deviation, given an estimated AC/A ratio, as shown in examples 3 and 4.

Example 3
If a child is assumed to have a normal AC/A ratio (5) and an exophoria of 10 PD, what is the effect of increasing the patient's spectacle correction by −2.00 diopters? Since the −2.00 lens increases accommodation by 2.00 diopters, and convergence is increased by a ratio of 5 to 1 (AC/A ratio = 5), the −2.00 lens over correction would result in 10 PD of convergence and orthophoria.

Example 4
A child has a +4.00 refractive error and a 30 PD esotropia. Assuming the AC/A ratio is high normal (6), what will be the effect of the full hypermetropic correction on the deviation? A +4.00 diopter lens will cause 24 PD (AC/A = 6 × +4.00) of divergence and thus the deviation with the +4.00 glasses will be esotropia of 6 PD (30 PD − 24 PD). Prescribing the hypermetropic glasses would have a good chance of correcting the deviation with only a small residual esodeviation.

DIAGNOSING RESTRICTION VERSUS PARESIS

Limitation of ocular rotation is caused by either restriction of eye movement or by a weak muscle. Restriction can be caused by periocular scarring (fat adherence) or a tight muscle (thyroid myopathy or congenital fibrosis syndrome). Muscle weakness can be caused by an innervational abnormality, a slipped or lost muscle, or a primary myopathy. An important step to diagnosing the cause of limited eye movements is to distinguish restriction from paresis. Diagnostic tests for distinguishing restriction versus paresis include, forced duction testing, generated forced duction testing, and saccadic velocity measurement. Restriction and paresis can coexist, especially in cases of long-standing muscle paralysis such as a long-standing sixth nerve palsy. In these cases, the antagonist of the paretic muscle (i.e., the medial rectus muscle in the case of a sixth nerve palsy) contracts and becomes stiff, thus adding a component of restriction to the paralytic condition.

Forced Duction Testing

Forced ductions are indicated if there is evidence of limited ductions. Forced duction testing is somewhat invasive, but it can be performed on most cooperative adults. For patients who will need surgery, forced ductions may be performed at the time of surgery. The technique is to grasp the eye at the limbus, slightly proptose the eye, and then rotate the eye into the field of limited ductions. If the eye is inadvertently pushed posteriorly during testing, the rectus muscles will slacken (even a tight muscle), decreasing the test's sensitivity. When examining awake patients, be sure to ask the patient to look in the direction of the forced ductions to relax the muscle that is being tested. The tightness of oblique muscles can be assessed by a special forced duction test called the exaggerated traction test, which was developed by David Guyton, MD.

Active Force Generation Test

Then active force generation test assesses rectus muscle strength. The eye is anesthetized with topical anesthetic and the eye is grasped at the limbus in the same fashion as forced duction testing. The patient is asked to look into the field of limitation and the eye is held in primary position. The examiner feels the force generated by the muscle and compares this with the fellow nonaffected eye. This test is useful in assessing the amount of muscle function associated with any palsy such as sixth nerve paresis or double elevator palsy.

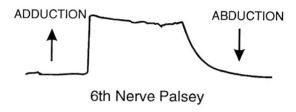

6th Nerve Palsy

Fig. 14-30   Electrooculogram (EOG) of patient with a sixth nerve palsy. *Upward arrow* on the left indicates adduction. Note that the tracing makes a sharp right upturn, showing normal medial rectus function. On the right is abduction (*downward arrows*). Note that the curve is gradual, indicating decreased lateral rectus function.

Saccadic Velocity Measurement

There are various ways to measure saccadic velocities. Clinical estimation is available to all clinicians and is simply the observation of fast eye movements. Fast eye movements can be elicited by having the patient look quickly from side-to-side, or using an OKN drum. An OKN drum is very useful in young children. Patients with rectus palsies will not be able to generate normal saccades. Eye movement velocities can be measured by special equipment such as the electrooculogram (EOG). Fig. 14-30 shows an EOG tracing of a patient with a sixth nerve paresis. The initial part of the tracing shows a vertical spike, indicating the adduction movement; however, the end of the tracing shows a mild slope indicating slow abduction. Clinically, if the patient is able to generate a good saccadic eye movement in the direction of the eye limitation, then the limitation is restrictive, and not secondary to paralysis. Normal saccadic velocity depends on the size of the saccade with large eye movements having higher peak velocities. Normal saccadic velocities range from 200 to 700 degrees per second.

Restriction

Forced duction testing is probably the most useful test for identifying restriction. If the eye cannot be easily rotated into the field of limited ductions then a restriction is present. Another sign of restriction is the "dog on a leash" eye movement. A patient with restrictive strabismus and good muscle function will show a normal saccadic eye movement until the eye reaches the restriction, and then will stop abruptly. A restriction also causes eyeball retraction and lid fissure narrowing, since the agonist muscle pulls the eye posteriorly against the restrictive leash. A tight medial rectus muscle will cause lid fissure narrowing on attempted adduction. Increased intraocular pressure can also be a clinical sign of restriction. As the eye rotates against the restriction, such as into abduction for a restricted medial rectus muscle, intraocular pressure will increase.

Box 14-3 Common Causes of Paralytic and Restrictive Strabismus

PARALYTIC

Cranial nerve palsy (IV, VI, and III)
Neuromuscular (myasthenia gravis, CPEO)
Slipped or lost muscle

RESTRICTIVE

Congenital fibrosis
Periocular scarring
Orbital fracture with muscle entrapment
Thyroid disease

INNERVATIONAL MISDIRECTION

Duane's syndrome
Synergistic divergence

Paresis

The inability of a muscle to generate a saccadic eye movement is an important indication of paresis. Even patients with severe restrictive strabismus will be able to generate a small-amplitude saccade in the direction of the restriction. Patients with muscle palsy show a slow saccade as compared to the fellow eye, or the muscle antagonist. In contrast to restriction that causes lid fissure narrowing, paresis causes lid fissure widening and relative proptosis since the patient looks in the field of action of the paretic muscle. A patient with a sixth nerve palsy, for example, will show lid fissure widening on attempted abduction. This is because the medial rectus muscle relaxes on attempted abduction (Sherrington's Law), and with the lateral rectus paretic it is loose, so the posterior pressure of the orbital fat pushes the eye forward. The active force generation test shows relative weakness of the paretic muscle. The examiner can compare agonist and antagonist muscle strength, as well as comparing the muscle strength of fellow eyes, to assess muscle function.

CYCLOPLEGIC REFRACTION

Cycloplegic refraction should be performed on every new strabismus patient. The standard regimen is cyclopentolate 1% and Neo-Synephrine 2.5% drops in each eye, times two, 5 minutes apart then perform the refraction 20 to 30 minutes after the last drop. For patients with dark eyes, the drops maybe repeated three times. Patients with blue eyes, or patients with albinism, should receive one set of drops. Remember that mydriasis does not mean cycloplegia. The mydriatic effect comes on sooner and lasts longer than the cycloplegic effect. If the patient shows varying refractive error during retinos-

MAJOR POINTS

Cortical binocular fusion controls eye alignment to lock the two eyes on a visual target through a feedback mechanism called *motor fusion.*

The *near reflex* includes accommodation, convergence, and pupillary miosis.

If a phoria is present, the patient has motor fusion. A base-out prism induces an exodeviation and evokes fusional convergence, a base-in prism induces an esodeviation and causes fusional divergence, and a base-up or base-down prism will evoke vertical fusional vergence.

A *positive angle kappa* is associated with a temporal displacement of the fovea, and an out-turning or temporal orientation of the eye for fixation.

Patients with a phoria have straight eyes and no shift to cover-uncover testing, but show a shift to the alternate cover testing. Patients with a tropia show a shift to both on cover-uncover testing and alternate cover testing.

Simultaneous prism cover test is used to measure the tropia component in patients with a small tropia and a larger phoria (i.e., monofixation syndrome).

In accordance with Herring's law, the deviation is smaller when the normal eye fixates (primary deviation), and larger when the eye with limited ductions is fixing (secondary deviation).

Accommodative convergence to accommodation ratio (AC/A ratio) is the amount of change in convergence for a specific amount of change in accommodation.

The heterophoria method compares the distance and near deviations along with the interpupillary distance to determine the AC/A ratio.

The clinical distance-near relationship is a simple comparison of the deviation in the distance to the deviation at near.

The lens gradient method determines the AC/A ratio by measuring the change in ocular deviation associated with a specific change in lens-induced accommodation.

Limitation of ocular rotation is either caused by restriction of eye movement or caused by a weak muscle.

copy, then it is likely that the patient has only partial cycloplegia and requires more drops. See Chapter 1 for more information on cycloplegic refraction.

SUGGESTED READINGS

Guyton DL: Exaggerated traction test for the oblique muscles, *Ophthalmology* 88:1035, 1981.

Jampel RS: The fundamental principle of the action of the oblique ocular muscles, *Am J Ophthalmol* 69:623,1970.

Wurtz RH, Richmond BJ, Judge SJ: Vision during saccadic eye movements: III visual interactions in monkey superior colliculus, *J Neurophysiol* 43:1168-1181,1980.

CHAPTER 15

Amblyopia and Sensory Adaptations

The developing infant brain is very plastic and vulnerable to environmental stimulation. Early stimulation with a clear retinal image to each eye and proper eye alignment is required for the development of binocular motor fusion, high-grade stereopsis, and excellent visual acuity of each eye. Strabismus or a blurred retinal image (monocular or binocular) in early infancy will disrupt normal visual development and lead to anatomic and functional changes to visual centers in the brain. In this chapter visual development and sensory adaptations to abnormal visual stimuli are discussed.

NORMAL VISUAL DEVELOPMENT

Monocular Visual Development

At birth, visual acuity is quite poor, in the range of hand motions to count fingers. This poor vision is in most part a result of an immaturity of visual centers in the brain, including the lateral geniculate nucleus and striate cortex. Rapidly, retinal stimulation with formed images stimulates specific dropout and growth of cortical connections and visual acuity improves. This early neural development gives rise to the organization of small, high-resolution, receptive fields in the central visual field. During the first few weeks, saccadic (fast or jerk) eye movements are responsible for refixation eye movements. By 6 to 8 weeks, central foveal fixation is established, along with accurate smooth pursuit. In humans, the first 2 months are associated with rapid visual improvement and this period is termed the *critical period of visual development*. The development of high resolution foveal vision is dependent on a clearly focused retinal image during early development. Abnormal visual stimulation (e.g., blurred retinal image from a congenital cataract) during this period can result in permanent damage to visual centers in the brain (see amblyopia in the following discussion). Visual acuity improves more slowly after the critical period and reaches 20/30 potential by approximately 3 years of age (Fig. 15-1).

Central fixation and accurate smooth pursuit are important clinical milestones of normal visual development. Most children will show central fixation and accurate smooth pursuit eye movements by 2 to 3 months of age, but some infants may show delayed visual maturation. Poor fixation at 5 to 6 months of age, however, is usually pathologic, and should prompt a full evaluation

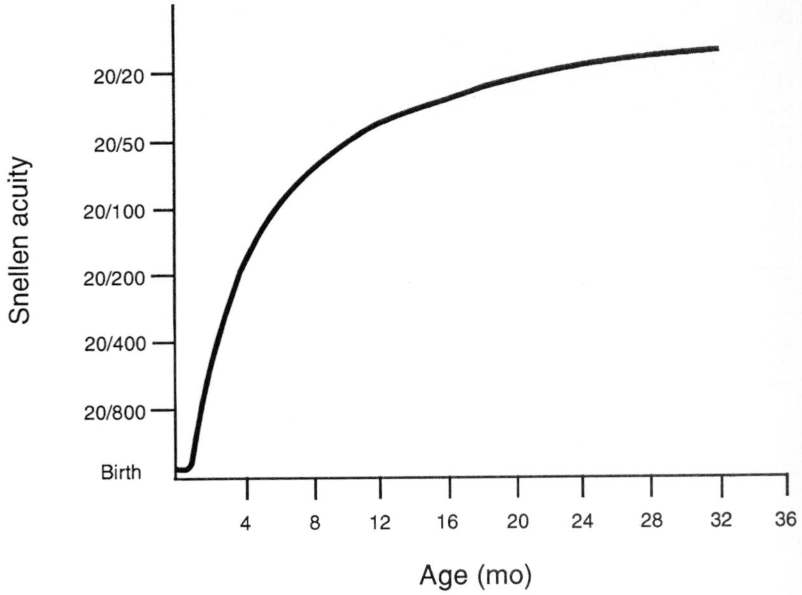

Fig. 15-1   Plot of Snellen visual acuity versus age in months. Note that visual acuity improves exponentially during the first few months of life, and that the improvement in visual acuity slows after 8 months to 1 year of age. Curve was drawn from a combination of preferential looking and visual evoked potential data.

for ocular motor or afferent visual pathway disease, including electrophysiology and neuroimaging studies.

Binocular Visual Development

Binocular visual development occurs in concert with improving monocular vision. Basic neuroanatomy tells us that the two eyes are linked to provide binocular vision. Optic nerve fibers from the nasal retina cross in the chiasm to join the temporal retinal nerve fibers from the fellow eye; together they project to the lateral geniculate nucleus and on to the striate cortex. This division of hemifields does not totally respect the midline, since in the foveal area there is significant overlap with some of the nasal foveal fibers projecting to the ipsilateral cortex and some of the temporal foveal fibers crossing to the contralateral cortex. In the striate cortex the afferent pathway connects to *binocular cortical cells* that respond to stimulation of either eye, and *monocular cortical cells* that respond to the stimulation of only one eye. In humans approximately 70% of the cells in the striate cortex are binocular cells, while the minority are monocular. Binocular cortical cells, along with neurons in visual association areas of the brain, produce single binocular vision with stereopsis. Animal studies demonstrate binocular cortical cells are present from birth. Refinement of neuroanatomic connections, and the development of normal binocular visual function, however, are dependent on appropriate binocular visual stimulation. Requirements for normal binocular visual development include *equal retinal stimulation* and *proper eye alignment*. Binocular vision and fusion has been found to be present between 1½ and 2 months of age, whereas stereopsis develops later, between 3 and 6 months of age.

Smooth Pursuit Asymmetry

In normal infants, monocular horizontal smooth pursuit in the temporal to nasal direction develops before pursuit movements in a nasal to temporal direction. During this time nasal to temporal smooth pursuit lags behind the visual target and frequent saccadic eye movements occur to keep up with the target. This is smooth pursuit asymmetry, and it is only seen under monocular conditions. Smooth pursuit asymmetry can be detected clinically by testing monocular optokinetic nystagmus (OKN). If smooth pursuit asymmetry is present, there will be a diminished OKN response with the drum rotating nasally to temporally as compared to temporally to nasally. Normally, smooth pursuit becomes symmetric between 3 to 6 months of age. If binocular visual development is disrupted during the first few months of life (e.g., congenital esotropia and a unilateral cataract) smooth pursuit asymmetry and OKN asymmetry will persist throughout life. Smooth pursuit asymmetry does not interfere with normal visual function or the ability to read, since it is not present under binocular viewing. It is, however, an important phenomenon that shows a physiologic link between ocular motor development and the development of binocular vision. Smooth pursuit asymmetry is a marker for disrupted binocular visual development and may be a helpful sign in older patients.

Single Binocular Vision and Stereopsis

Normal binocular vision is a process of integrating retinal images from two eyes into a single three-dimensional visual percept. Requisite to single binocular vision is appropriate eye alignment, so that similar images from each

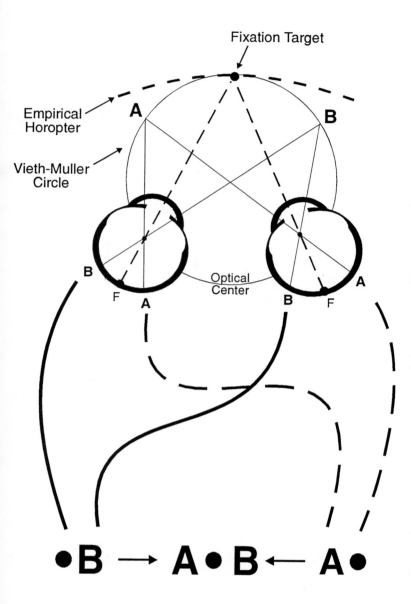

Fixation Target

Empirical Horopter

Vieth-Müller Circle

Optical Center

●B → A ● B ← A ●

Fig. 15-2 Vieth-Müller circle and the empirical horopter. By mathematical theorem, points on Vieth-Müller circle should project to corresponding retinal points. Point A stimulates nasal retina of left eye and temporal retina of right eye, and these retinal areas should mathematically correspond. Psychophysical experiments, however, show that the retinal architecture does not follow the mathematical circle of Vieth-Müller, and that points on the empirical horopter stimulate corresponding retinal points. The bottom of the figure shows the fusion of the images from each eye into a binocular perception.

eye fall on retinal points that project to the same cortical binocular cells.

Retinal areas from each eye that are physiologically linked to the same cortical binocular cells are called *corresponding retinal points.* When a subject with normal ocular alignment fixes on a target, the image falls on both foveae. Objects to the side of the fixation point (points A and B in Fig. 15-2) will project to corresponding retinal points if the peripheral objects lie on a circle that crosses through the optical centers of each eye. This mathematically determined circle of points is called the *Vieth-Muller circle.* As is often the case for mathematical explanations of biologic phenomenon, physiologic experiments have shown that the Vieth-Muller mathematical model only partially applies for visual perception. Psychophysical experiments indicate that the loci of points that stimulate corresponding retinal points are not a circle, but an ellipse. This elliptic line of points that

stimulate corresponding retinal points is called the *empirical horopter* (Fig. 15-2). Remember, the location of the horopter is determined by the point of fixation. Objects peripheral to the fixation point, which are oriented on the empirical horopter, will be seen singly as these objects fall on corresponding retinal points.

But what about objects located off the fine line of the empirical horopter? Objects in front of or behind the horopter will stimulate noncorresponding retinal points. Note that points behind the empirical horopter stimulate binasal retina (Fig. 15-3, *A*), and points in front of the horopter stimulate bitemporal retina (Fig. 15-3, *B*). In fact, the empirical horopter is infinitely thin and no three-dimensional object falls directly on this horopter line. Therefore virtually all objects stimulate noncorresponding retinal points. The brain, however, can combine or fuse images from slightly noncorresponding retinal points. There is a finite area in front of and behind

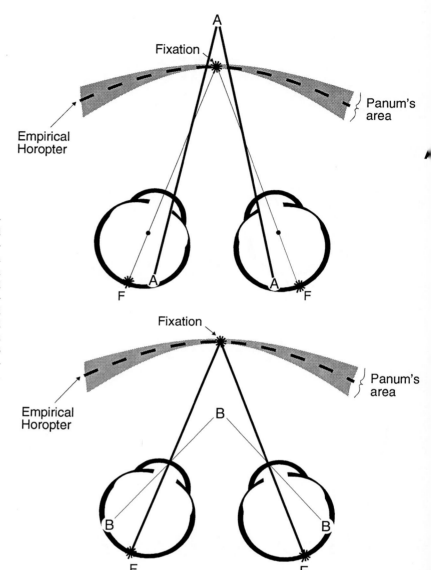

Fig. 15-3 Empirical horopter and Panum's fusional area. Objects that lie in front of or behind Panum's fusional area will stimulate noncorresponding retinal points. **A,** Patient fixating on the star in the center of the empirical horopter. Point A, which is distal to the horopter, stimulates binasal retinal points, which are noncorresponding. **B,** Patient fixating on the same spot; however, point B is proximal to Panum's fusion and point B stimulates bitemporal retinal points that are noncorresponding. Point A in **A** would cause uncrossed diplopia, whereas point B in **B** would cause crossed diplopia. This type of diplopia is termed *physiologic diplopia* (see Fig. 15-5).

the horopter line where objects stimulate noncorresponding retinal points, yet are still fusible into a single binocular image. This area is called *Panum's fusional area*. Objects within Panum's fusional area produce single binocular vision with stereoscopic or three-dimensional vision. The brain's ability to determine that images fall on slightly noncorresponding retinal points (within Panum's fusional area) produces *stereoscopic vision*. Note that bitemporal retinal disparity *within* Panum's fusional area produces stereoscopic vision with the image coming up towards the observer and binasal retinal disparity *within* Panum's area results in a stereoscopic image going away from the observer (Fig. 15-3). Fig. 15-4 shows how a three-dimensional cube produces slightly different images to each eye, which stimulates noncorresponding retinal points. The fovea has high spatial resolution, so even small displacements off the ho-

ropter line in the central visual field are detected, allowing for high-grade stereopsis. In contrast, as one moves to the peripheral fields, the receptive field size enlarges and the spatial resolution decreases so slight object displacements off the horopter are not detected. Therefore there is progressively poorer stereo acuity from peripheral visual fields. Central fusion (bifoveal fusion) refers to the normal state of cortically merged images from each macula producing high-grade stereo acuity of 40 to 50 seconds of arc and normal motor fusion.

The minimum stereoscopic resolution is approximately 30 seconds of arc disparity. Stereoscopic resolution depends on visual acuity, and the interpupillary distance. The farther apart the two eyes, the greater the stereoscopic potential. Additionally, the closer an object is to the eyes, the greater the relative separation of the eyes, and therefore the better the stereopsis. As objects

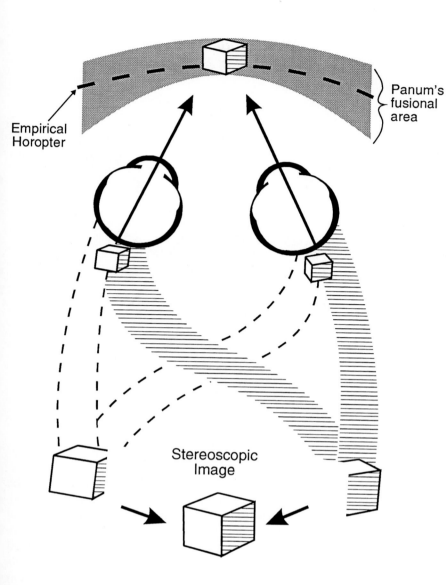

Fig. 15-4   Diagrammatic representation of stereoscopic vision. Note that any three-dimensional object will straddle the empirical horopter and parts of that object will be in front of or behind the empirical horopter. This stimulates noncorresponding retinal points that provide stereoscopic vision as long as the three-dimensional object falls within Panum's fusional area.

move away from the observer the relative interpupillary distance diminishes and the view of the target from each eye become similar, and stereopsis diminishes.

The perception of depth is not solely dependent on binocular stereo acuity. *Monocular cues* can provide information regarding depth and the distance of objects. Motion parallax, shadows, object overlap, and the relative size of objects give us monocular cues of depth. Monocular cues are so powerful that one-eyed patients or patients with large-angle strabismus (monocular vision) can successfully perform a variety of tasks that require keen depth perception. Professional athletes, microsurgeons, and others have been successful using monocular cues.

Physiologic Diplopia

Objects that are too far off the horopter line, and outside of Panum's fusional area, cannot be fused and double vision results (diplopia) (Fig. 15-5). This type of double vision caused by objects outside of Panum's fusional area is called *physiologic diplopia*. Note that in Fig. 15-5 the pencil is in front of Panum's fusional area and is stimulating the temporal retinas of each eye (bitemporal). Since the temporal retina projects to the nasal visual field, the observer perceives two pencils, with the left image coming from the right eye and the right image coming from the left eye, thus causing crossed diplopia. Physiologic diplopia would occur in everyday life; however, it is normally ignored or suppressed. You can experience physiologic diplopia simply by fixating on a distant object (several feet away) and then placing your finger or a pencil a few inches from your nose. Note that while looking at the distant object, the pencil will appear double. This is crossed diplopia, since when you close your right eye the left image disappears, and when you close the left eye the right image disappears. Objects located beyond Panum's fusional area cause binasal retinal stimulation and uncrossed diplopia. Panum's fusional area is narrow in the center and widens in the

Physiologic Diplopia

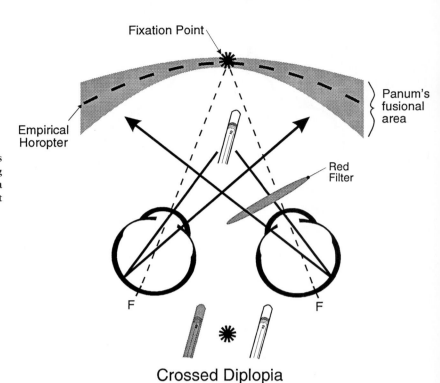

Fig. 15-5 Pencil is seen in front of Panum's fusional area. This stimulates noncorresponding bitemporal retinal points. Since temporal retina projects to the opposite field (*arrows*), the patient perceives crossed physiologic diplopia.

periphery. Relatively little object displacement off the horopter line in the central visual field elicits physiologic diplopia, whereas even large disparities in the peripheral visual field will be fused. This is because the receptive fields in the central foveal area are small with high spatial resolution, whereas in the peripheral retina receptive fields are large, with tolerance for larger image disparities.

ABNORMAL VISUAL DEVELOPMENT

Cortical Suppression

As discussed previously, visual system in the brain develops in response to early visual stimulation. Abnormal stimulation produced by strabismus, or a blurred retinal image during infancy or early childhood, disrupts normal visual development. The extent of the damage to visual development depends on the severity of the abnormal visual stimulus, the length of exposure to abnormal visual stimulation, and the level of visual maturity when the sensory insult began. The earlier the onset and the longer the duration, the more severe the impact on the neurologic development of the visual system.

Small image disparity is "good" since it provides stereoscopic vision (see previous discussion and Fig. 15-4). However, if the eyes are significantly misaligned, or one retinal image is blurred, the retinal images cannot be fused. The developing visual system adapts to the confusion of dissimilar retinal images by inhibiting cortical activity from one eye. This cortical inhibition usually involves the central portion of the visual field and is termed *cortical suppression*. Note that when the fixing eye is occluded, the fellow eye fixates and the suppression disappears.

AMBLYOPIA

Amblyopia occurs in approximately 2% of the general population and is the most common cause of decreased vision in childhood. The term *amblyopia* is derived from Greek, meaning dull vision (*amblys* = dull, *ops* = eye). The general term *amblyopia* can refer to poor vision from any cause, but in this text, and most ophthalmic literature, the term refers to poor vision caused by abnormal visual development secondary to abnormal visual stimulation. Other terms for *amblyopia* include *functional amblyopia* and *amblyopia ex anopsia*. For practical purposes amblyopia is defined as at least 2 Snellen lines difference in visual acuity; but amblyopia is truly a spectrum of visual loss, ranging from missing a few letters on the 20/20 line to hand motion vision.

Children are susceptible to amblyopia between birth

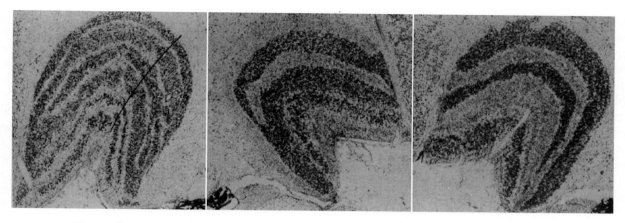

Fig. 15-6   Lateral geniculate nucleus of a normal monkey is on the left, with six nuclear layers. The two micrographs on the right are from an animal that had monocular lid suturing and monocular pattern deprivation. This monkey developed only three nuclear layers that correspond to the eye with normal visual experience. The layers from the eye with pattern deprivation have atrophied.

and 7 to 8 years of age. The earlier the onset of the abnormal stimulation, the greater the visual deficit. The critical period for visual development is somewhat controversial but is probably between 1 week to 3 months of age. A dense cataract or corneal opacity during this time is devastating and can result in severe amblyopia. Over time the visual plasticity decreases and by approximately 9 years of age the visual system is mature enough to be resistant to the effects of abnormal visual stimuli.

Functional amblyopia or "amblyopia" should be distinguished from *organic amblyopia,* which is poor vision caused by structural abnormalities of the eye or brain, such as optic atrophy, a macular scar, or anoxic occipital brain damage that are independent of sensory input. Functional amblyopia tends to be reversible when treated during early childhood, whereas organic amblyopia does not improve.

Pathophysiology

Amblyopia should not be viewed as an eye problem, but as brain damage caused by abnormal visual stimulation during the sensitive period of visual development. Basic research on animals has shown that retinal pattern distortion (image blur), and strabismus, which occurs during early visual development, can cause structural and functional damage to the lateral geniculate nucleus and striate cortex (Fig. 15-6).

Types

Amblyopia is best classified by its cause. Amblyopia is caused by disruption of visual development secondary to retinal image blur (pattern distortion), suppression or both. Suppression occurs in association with strabismus or unilateral image blur, and retinal image blur is caused

---

Box 15-1   Classification of Amblyopia

A. STRABISMIC AMBLYOPIA (STRONG FIXATION PREFERENCE—NOT ALTERNATING)

1. Congenital esotropia
2. Congenital exotropia
3. Accommodative esotropia

B. UNILATERAL RETINAL IMAGE BLUR (MONOCULAR PATTERN DISTORTION)

1. Anisometropia
2. Unilateral cataract
3. Unilateral corneal opacity (Peter's)
4. Unilateral vitreous hemorrhage or vitreous opacity

C. BILATERAL IMAGE BLUR (BILATERAL PATTERN DISTORTION)

1. Ametropic
   a. Bilateral high hypermetropia
   b. Meridional (astigmatic)
2. Media opacity
   a. Bilateral congenital cataracts
   b. Bilateral corneal opacities (Peters' anomaly)
   c. Bilateral vitreous hemorrhages.

---

by refractive error or a media opacity. If a patient with strabismus alternates fixation between eyes visual acuity will develop equally albeit separately without normal binocular function. Strong fixation preference for one eye, however, results is constant suppression of the fellow eye, resulting in poor vision of the suppressed eye (strabismic amblyopia), and poor binocularity. Box 15-1 provides a clinical classification of amblyopia.

Strabismic amblyopia Strabismus associated with strong fixation preference results in constant unilateral suppression of cortical activity related to the nonpreferred eye (deviated eye). Constant suppression in the visually immature patient results in poor vision of the nonpreferred eye (deviated eye), and loss of binocular vision. It occurs despite the fact that both eyes have clearly focused retinal images.

Strabismic amblyopia occurs in approximately 50% of patients with congenital esotropia (a constant tropia), but is very uncommon in patients with intermittent strabismus (e.g., intermittent exotropia) or those with incomitant strabismus (e.g., Duane's syndrome and Brown's syndrome) since they have central fusion. Strabismic amblyopia can be moderate to severe, and in some cases even result in eccentric fixation and visual acuity of 20/200 or worse.

Unilateral blurred retinal image Unilateral or asymmetric retinal image blur can produce amblyopia and loss of binocularity depending on the severity of the condition. The ophthalmic literature often refers to amblyopia associated with monocular image blur as pattern deprivation amblyopia. This usage is misleading since unilateral image blur results in pattern distortion and cortical suppression, and both contribute to the amblyopia.

Clinically, mild image blur such as that which is associated with mild anisometropia causes mild anisometropic amblyopia, and allows for the development of peripheral fusion and stereopsis (i.e., monofixation syndrome). However, a severely blurred image during infancy (e.g., unilateral congenital cataract or corneal opacity) can result in severe amblyopia with loss of binocular function and the development of secondary strabismus (esotropia, exotropia, or hypertropia).

Anisometropic amblyopia is caused by a difference in refractive errors that results in an unilateral or asymmetric image blur, and is one of the most common types of amblyopia. Most patients with anisometropic amblyopia have straight eyes and appear "normal," so the only way to identify these patients is through vision screening. Stereo acuity testing has had limited value in screening for anisometropic amblyopia because most patients have relatively good stereopsis (between 70 and 3000 second arc). Myopic anisometropia usually does not cause significant amblyopia unless the difference in refractive error is greater than 5.00 diopters. Hypermetropic anisometropia on the other hand is frequently associated with severe amblyopia. As little as +1.50 hypermetropic anisometropia can be associated with significant amblyopia, although moderate hypermetropic anisometropia (+3.00) can cause severe amblyopia with visual acuity of 20/200. Myopic anisometropic amblyopia is usually mild and amenable to treatment even in late childhood, whereas hypermetropic amblyopia is often difficult to treat past 4 or 5 years of age. This is probably because

high myopia is usually acquired after the critical period of visual development, and the more myopic eye is in focus for near objects. In contrast, patients with hypermetropic anisometropia always use the less hypermetropic eye because it requires less accommodative effort, and constantly suppress the more hypermetropic eye.

Bilateral blurred retinal image Pattern distortion in its pure form without suppression, occurs when there is bilateral, symmetric image blur, and no strabismus. Clinically the effects of pure image blur are seen in cases of bilateral high hypermetropia, bilateral symmetric astigmatism, or with bilateral ocular opacities such as bilateral congenital cataracts and bilateral Peters' anomaly. Bilateral pattern distortion causes bilateral poor vision but it does not preclude the development of at least some binocular fusion usually with gross stereopsis. If severe image blur occurs during the neonatal period so that essentially no pattern stimulation is provided, extremely poor vision and sensory nystagmus develops. In cases of dense bilateral congenital opacities, bilateral amblyopia and nystagmus will occur unless the image is cleared by 2 months of age. This type of nystagmus is called *sensory nystagmus*. It is associated with bilateral severe amblyopia, or other causes of congenital blindness such as macular or optic nerve pathology. Sensory nystagmus does not occur with cortical blindness because extra striate visual pathways supply the fixation reflex. Acquired opacities after 6 months of age usually do not cause sensory nystagmus since the motor component of fixation has already been established. The presence of sensory nystagmus indicates severe amblyopia, usually 20/200 visual acuity or worse.

Ametropic amblyopia (bilateral hypermetropic amblyopia) usually occurs with hypermetropia of +6.00 or more without significant anisometropia. In these cases, visual acuity is decreased in each eye, the eyes are usually straight, and the patients usually have gross stereopsis. When patients are first given their optical correction, visual acuity does not significantly improve. The lack of improvement with prescription of spectacle correction often leads the examiner to seek out an organic cause for the decreased vision. The treatment of bilateral high hypermetropic amblyopia is to prescribe full hypermetropic correction. In most cases, visual acuity will slowly improve if the glasses are worn full time, with final visual acuities usually in the range of 20/30 to 20/25.

Bilateral meridional amblyopia is similar to bilateral hypermetropic amblyopia in that it is a bilateral condition and is secondary to pattern distortion. Significant meridional amblyopia occurs with astigmatism of +3.00 or more. To avoid meridional amblyopia, it is suggested that astigmatisms of +2.50 or more should be treated in preschool children; astigmatisms over +3.00 to +4.00 should be treated even in infants.

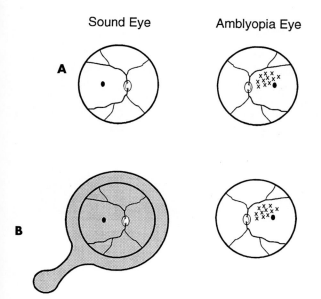

Sound Eye   Amblyopia Eye

A

B

Fig. 15-7   Diagram shows eccentric fixation. **A,** Sound eye fixes with the fovea and the amblyopic eye eccentrically fixates in area of fixation. **B,** Right eye is covered, and eccentric fixation persists with patient viewing in an eccentric area. Note that this is different from suppression and abnormal retinal correspondence, which is present only during binocular viewing, and disappears when the fixing eye is occluded.

Amblyopic Vision

The visual deficit associated with amblyopia has certain unique characteristics, including the "crowding phenomenon", the neutral density filter effect, and eccentric fixation. The *crowding phenomenon* relates to the fact that patients with amblyopia have better visual acuity reading single optotype than reading multiple optotypes in a row (linear optotypes). Often, patients with amblyopia will perform one or two Snellen lines better when presented with single optotypes versus linear optotypes. This crowding phenomenon may have something to do with the relatively large receptive field associated with amblyopia. A *neutral density filter* reduces overall luminance. The intraocular differences in visual acuity between the amblyopic eye and the sound eye diminish when the room lights are dimmed or when the patient views through a neutral density filter. For example, an amblyopic patient may have 20/20 vision in the right eye and 20/60 in the left eye under photopic conditions (four lines difference), but might have 20/50 right eye and 20/60 left eye under scotopic conditions (one line difference).

Patients with dense amblyopia develop *eccentric fixation,* and do not fixate with their fovea, but use a relatively large parafoveal area for viewing (Fig. 15-7). The area of eccentric fixation is not a pinpoint location as is the fovea, but a general area of viewing. The presence of

eccentric fixation is a clinical sign of severe amblyopia and has a poor visual prognosis. Remember that anomalous retinal correspondence is quite different than eccentric fixation. Anomalous retinal correspondence (ARC), as described previously, is a binocular sensory adaptation, which allows acceptance of images on noncorresponding retinal points (see the following discussion). ARC is only active during binocular viewing and when one eye is covered, fixation reverts back to the true fovea. Eccentric fixation, on the other hand, is dense amblyopia without foveation, and is present under monocular or binocular conditions.

Diagnosing Amblyopia

Testing vision   Linear acuity is desirable because single-optotype presentation under estimates the degree of amblyopia because of the crowding phenomenon. There are many ways to test visual acuity in preschool children, including Allen picture cards, HOTV, and illiterate E game. A visual acuity can often be obtained in children as young as 2 to 3 years old.

Fixation testing for amblyopia   Preverbal children can be tested for amblyopia by examining the quality of monocular fixation, or binocular fixation preference.

Monocular fixation testing   Normal children over 2 to 3 months of age should show central fixation with accurate smooth pursuit and saccadic refixation eye movements. Test for central fixation by covering one of the patient's eyes, then moving a target slowly back and forth in front of the child to observe the accuracy of fixation. A child with central fixation looks directly at the target, visually locks on the target, and accurately follows the moving target. Infants often find the human face a much more compelling target than toys or pictures, so try moving your head side to side to evaluate the quality of fixation. Central fixation indicates foveal vision usually in the range of 20/100 or better. *Eccentric fixation* on the other hand, means the fovea is not fixating and the patient is viewing from an extra-foveal part of the retina. Patients with eccentric fixation appear to be looking to the side, not directly at the fixation target, and they have poor smooth pursuit, so they do not accurately follow a moving target. Eccentric fixation is a sign of very poor vision and dense amblyopia, usually 20/200 or worse.

Visuscope   One way to identify the eccentric fixation point in older cooperative children is to use a *Visuscope,* which is a type of direct ophthalmoscope that projects a focused image onto the retina so the examiner can see the image on the retina. First the image is projected onto the parafoveal retina, then the patient is asked to look at the image. If the patient has central fixation the patient refixates to place the image precisely on the fovea. However, if the patient has eccentric fixation, the patient will view with the parafoveal retinal area and show wander-

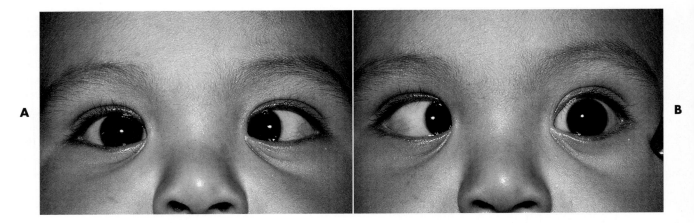

Fig. 15-8 Congenital esotropia with alternating fixation. **A,** Patient is fixing right eye. **B,** Patient spontaneously alternates to left eye. This is indicative of equal visual acuity.

ing unsteady fixation (see Fig. 15-7). The more peripheral the eccentric fixation, the denser the amblyopia.

Fixation preference testing This test is useful in preverbal strabismic children for identifying amblyopia that might be missed by monocular fixation testing. It is based on the premise that strong fixation preference indicates amblyopia. If a patient with strabismus spontaneously *alternates fixation,* using one eye then the other, this indicates equal fixation preference and no amblyopia (Fig. 15-8). In contrast, *strong fixation preference* for one eye indicates amblyopia. The stronger the fixation preference the worse the amblyopia.

In patients with a fixation preference, the degree of fixation preference can be estimated by briefly covering the preferred eye to force fixation to the nonpreferred eye. Remove the cover from the preferred eye, then observe how well and how long the patient will maintain fixation with the nonpreferred eye before refixating back to the preferred eye. If fixation immediately goes back to the preferred eye after the cover is removed, then this indicates strong fixation preference for the preferred eye and amblyopia of the deviated eye (Fig. 15-9). If the patient maintains fixation with the nonpreferred eye through smooth pursuit, through a blink or for at least 5 seconds, there is mild fixation preference and no significant amblyopia (vision within 2 Snellen lines difference). The ability to maintain fixation with the nonpreferred eye while following a moving target is a very reliable indicator of equal vision and no significant amblyopia.

The *reliability of fixation preference testing* has been shown to be quite good in patients with large-angle strabismus over 10 to 15 PD, accurately diagnosing amblyopia of two lines or more in over 90% of cases. Patients with small-angle strabismus, however, will show strong fixation preference in 50% to 70% of cases, even if the vision is equal to within two Snellen lines difference. This high over diagnosis rate in children with small-angle

strabismus is because they have the monofixation syndrome (see the following section). These patients have peripheral fusion but suppress one fovea so they show strong fixation preference even if vision is equal. The over diagnosis of amblyopia in patients with small-angle strabismus can be rectified by using the vertical prism test, which dissociates peripheral fusion and temporarily breaks down the monofixation syndrome.

Vertical prism test (induced tropia test) The vertical prism test is used in preverbal children with straight eyes or small-angle strabismus to accurately diagnose amblyopia. It is performed by placing a 15 PD prism base up or base down in front of one eye, thereby inducing a vertical tropia. With the induced vertical strabismus, fixation preference can be determined (Fig. 15-10). If the patient can hold fixation with either eye through a blink or through smooth pursuit eye movements, no significant amblyopia is present. Strong fixation preference indicates amblyopia.

Cross fixation Patients with a large-angle esotropia and tight medial rectus muscles will have difficulty bringing the eyes to primary position so the eyes stay adducted. These patients will "cross fixate." The right adducted eye fixes on objects in left gaze, and the left adducted eye fixates on objects in right gaze. Cross fixation has been said to be a sign of equal vision, but cross fixation does not guarantee equal vision. The ability to hold fixation past midline or hold fixation through smooth pursuit with either eye is a better criterion for equal vision.

Latent nystagmus Patients with strabismus often have latent nystagmus, which is a horizontal jerk nystagmus that occurs or gets worse with monocular occlusion. Thus covering one eye in a patient with latent nystagmus will increase nystagmus and diminish visual acuity. To evaluate monocular visual function blur one eye with a plus lens rather than occluding one eye. Blur-

Strong Fixation Preference OS
Will Not Hold Fixation OD
Amblyopia OD

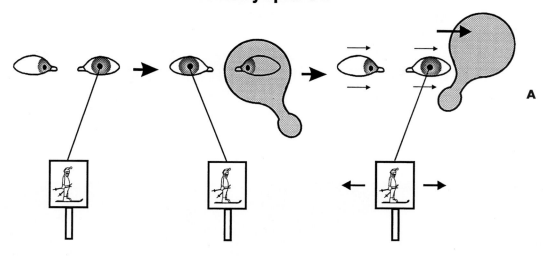

Mild fixation Preference OS
Holds Fixation OD
No Amblyopia

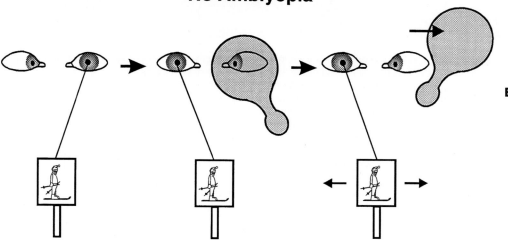

Fig. 15-9   **A,** Patient has strong fixation preference for the left eye (*left*) and amblyopia of the right eye. Temporarily covering the left eye (*center*) forces fixation to the right eye, but when the cover is removed the patient refixates to the left eye (*right*). **B,** Patient prefers to fix with the left eye (*left*). Occluding the left eye forces fixation to the right eye (*center*), and when occluder is removed (*right*) the patient maintains fixation with the nonpreferred eye, indicating no amblyopia.

ring one eye induces less nystagmus than occlusion. Use the minimum amount of plus necessary to force fixation to the fellow eye. The vertical prism test can identify which eye is fixing. Usually a +5.00 lens is sufficient to blur distance vision enough to force fixation to the fellow eye. Linear presentation of optotypes is difficult for pa-

tients with nystagmus because the optotypes tend to run together, so try a single-optotype presentation. Also take a binocular visual acuity measurement in addition to a monocular acuity in patients with nystagmus because binocular vision is usually better that monocular vision. To assess the best functional visual acuity potential in a

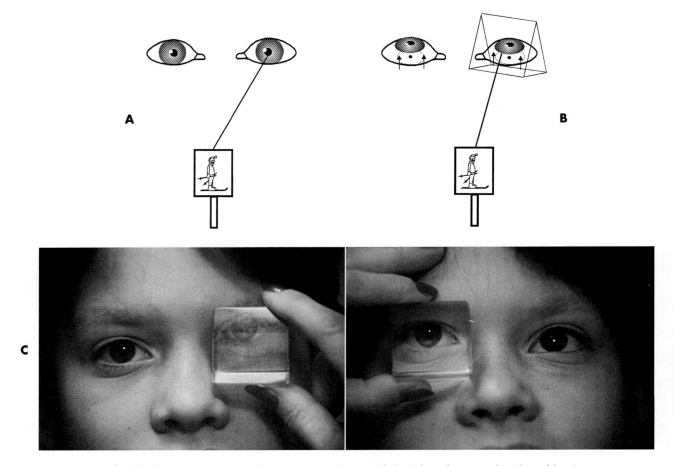

Fig. 15-10   A, Vertical prism test on a patient fixing with the left eye because of a right amblyopia. **B,** A vertical prism is placed in front of the left eye and since the left eye is fixing, the left eye elevates to pick up fixation. As per Hering's law, both eyes will elevate if the left eye is fixing. **C,** A vertical prism placed in front of one eye can identify which eye is fixing, and therefore can determine fixation preference. *Left,* One can identify that the right eye is fixing because the right eye is in primary position and the patient is ignoring the vertically displaced image in the left eye. *Right,* Patient is now fixing with the left eye and this can be identified since both eyes shift upward as the left eye, behind the prism, fixates on the vertically deviated image. This is a base-down prism, so the eyes move up to allow the left eye to fixate through the prism.

patient with nystagmus, test binocular vision while allowing the patient to adopt their preferred face turn or head tilt.

Treatment

Early treatment of amblyopia is critical for best visual acuity results. The basic strategy for treating amblyopia is to first provide a *clear retinal image,* and then *correct ocular dominance* if dominance is present, as early as possible during the period of visual plasticity (birth to 8 years). Correction of ocular dominance is accomplished by forcing fixation to the amblyopic eye by either patching or blurring the vision of the sound eye.

Clear retinal image   Patients with bilateral high hypermetropia (>5.00 D) should receive the full hypermetropic correction since amblyopic eyes do not fully accommodate. Patients given partial correction for high

hypermetropia often show very slow or no improvement in their amblyopia. Patients with bilateral large astigmatism (>2.50 D) will also have amblyopia secondary to the astigmatism or meridional amblyopia. Prescribe the full astigmatic correction to provide a clear retinal image. It is important to consider correcting astigmatisms of +2.50 to +3.00 or more in small children, even if the astigmatism is bilateral. Unilateral or asymmetric hypermetropia greater than +1.50 can cause anisometropic amblyopia. Treat anisometropic amblyopia by prescribing the hyperopic correction, then occlusion therapy if necessary.

Correct ocular dominance
Occlusion   Patching or occlusion therapy is based on covering the sound eye to stimulate the amblyopic eye. Strabismic patients without binocular fusion, can be treated with full-time occlusion; however, full-time occlusion may result in reverse amblyopia in children under

4 to 5 years of age. To prevent reverse amblyopia, do not use full-time occlusion for more than 1 week per the child's age in years without reexamining the vision of the good eye. For example, a 2-year-old child receiving full-time occlusion should be examined every 2 weeks. In children under 1 year of age, part-time occlusion may be preferable to avoid reverse amblyopia.

Amblyopic patients with essentially straight eyes (tropias <8 PD) and peripheral fusion (e.g., anisometropic amblyopia and microtropia monofixators) are best treated with part-time occlusion (4 to 6 hours a day). For anisometropic amblyopia initially prescribe spectacle correction and follow the patient each month for visual acuity improvement. If vision does not improve on monthly follow-ups, then part-time patching is started. Part-time occlusion or penalization therapy is preferred because these methods help to preserve fusion.

Penalization Penalization is a method for blurring the sound eye to force fixation to the amblyopic eye. Penalization actually switches ocular suppression and this can be demonstrated by Polaroid vectographic chart or by Worth 4-dot. Penalization only works if fixation is switched from the sound eye to the amblyopic eye. Blurring of the sound eye can be achieved by various methods. *Optical penalization* is based on over-plussing (prescribing more plus sphere than needed) to the sound eye to force fixation to the amblyopic eye for distance targets, yet the patient will usually use the sound eye for near targets. Optical penalization works well for mild amblyopia; however, some children will look over the glasses to use their sound eye. Atropine penalization is a stronger form of penalization and is useful even in dense amblyopia as long as the patient has significant hypermetropia of the good eye. Atropine 0.5% or 1% is placed in the sound eye each day, optical correction is removed from the sound eye, and the amblyopic eye is given full optical correction. If, under these conditions of penalization, the patient switches fixation to the amblyopic eye, then penalization will improve vision. Cyclopentolate can be used as an in-office test to predict if penalization will work. The in-office test consists of providing the amblyopic eye with full optical correction while cyclopleging the sound eye with cyclopentolate, and removing optical correction from the sound eye. If under these conditions fixation switches to the amblyopic eye, then the patient will improve with atropine penalization. Atropine penalization usually requires +3.00D or more hypermetropia of the sound eye to achieve significant blur to switch fixation. It is important to note that blurring the sound eye to a visual acuity lower than the amblyopic eye does not guarantee a switch in fixation to the amblyopic eye. Penalization in young children may result in reverse amblyopia, so patients 4 years or younger should be followed closely when undergoing atropine penalization therapy.

Box 15-2 **Clinically Encountered Sensory Adaptations**

Visually Mature
    Diplopia
    Confusion
    Rivalry
Visually Immature
    Monofixation
    Anomalous
        retinal
            correspondance
    Regional suppression

Pleoptics is a method of treating eccentric fixation associated with dense amblyopia. A bright ring of light is flashed around the fovea to temporarily "blind" or saturate the photoreceptors surrounding the fovea. This eliminates vision from the eccentric fixation point and forces fixation to the fovea. Pleoptic treatments are given several times a week to enhance occlusion therapy. Most practitioners have found pleoptics to be no better than standard occlusion therapy.

Active stimulation Some investigators have suggested active stimulation of the amblyopic eye as a way to improve vision of the amblyopic eye. A high-contrast spinning disc with square wave grading (CAM) was one method that has been tried. The CAM treatment has been found to be no better than standard occlusion therapy.

Prognosis

The prognosis for amblyopia depends on the age of the patient, severity of amblyopia, and type of amblyopia. The earlier the amblyopia occurs, and the longer it remains untreated, the worse the prognosis. Bilateral amblyopia responds better than unilateral amblyopia, and myopic anisometropic amblyopia responds better than hypermetropic amblyopia. Each case must be evaluated individually as to whether or not the child is too old to undergo amblyopia therapy. The general rule of thumb is every child under 9 years of age should undergo a trial of amblyopia therapy. Visual acuity improvement has been documented when children are treated in late childhood after 8 years of age.

SENSORY ADAPTATIONS

In addition to amblyopia, there are a variety of sensory adaptations that occur in response to clinical situations that disrupt binocular vision. The specific type of sensory adaptation depends on when the sensory anomaly

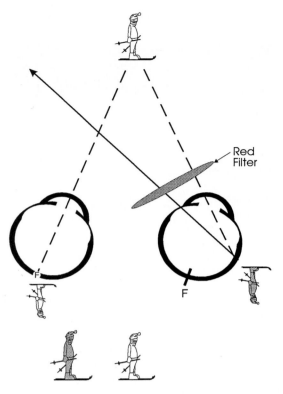

Crossed Diplopia

Fig. 15-11 Exotropia with image falling on the fovea of the left eye and on the temporal retina of the right eye causing crossed diplopia. A red filter over the deviated right eye produces a red image that is seen on the contralateral side (crossed diplopia).

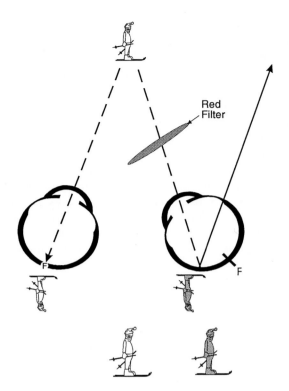

Uncrossed Diplopia

Fig. 15-12 Esotropia with uncrossed diplopia. Image falls on the fovea of the left eye and on the nasal retina in the deviated right eye. A red filter over the right eye causes the diplopic image on the right to be red.

occurred, and the severity and type of binocular disruption. Listed in Box 15-2 are sensory adaptations that are encountered clinically. They are divided into two sections based on the onset of the sensory insult.

Visually Mature

The following sensory adaptations occur after the development of bifoveal fusion, when the visual system is mature. These adaptations are associated with normal retinal correspondence. Visual-neural development is said to mature by around 9 or 10 years of age, and at this point there is not enough cortical plasticity for adaptations such as cortical suppression and abnormal retinal correspondence. There are some exceptions to this rule, however, and cases documenting prolonged visual plasticity have been reported (see the following discussion).

Diplopia Acquired strabismus in patients older than 8 to 9 years of age usually causes diplopia. The patient with diplopia will fixate with one fovea, and suppress the fovea of the deviated eye. The diplopic image comes from perifoveal retina of the deviated eye (Figs. 15-11 and 15-12). The foveal image from the fixing eye will be perceived as being located directly in front of the patient while the perifoveal retinal image from the deviated eye will project to its corresponding visual field. Exotropia

causes the image to fall temporal to the fovea, which projects to the nasal field producing *crossed diplopia* (Fig. 15-11). If a red cover is placed over the right eye of a patient with acquired exotropia, the red image will be seen to the left of the white image (i.e., crossed diplopia). Esotropia causes the image to fall on nasal retina, which projects temporally and causes *uncrossed diplopia* (Fig. 15-12). Remember e**X**otropia produces crossed diplopia because of the **X**, and the **S** in esotropia means **S**ame side diplopia (uncrossed). In cases of vertical strabismus, the hypertropic eye sees the lower image.

Aniseikonia Diplopia can also be caused by differences in retinal image size (*aniseikonia*) between fellow eyes. An acquired retinal image size disparity greater up to 7% is usually tolerated but aniseikonia over 10% may result in diplopia.

Confusion Confusion is a condition rarely seen clinically. Instead of diplopia, strabismic patients with confusion perceive two different images superimposed on each other. Confusion is caused by the simultaneous perception of two different images from the two foveae that are pointing to different objects of regard. Most patients with acquired strabismus do not experience confusion because they suppress the deviated fovea to regard the perifoveal image that matches the foveal image from the

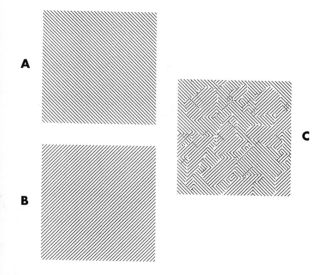

Fig. 15-13   Diagonal lines are presented to each eye with the lines oriented 90 degrees to each other (**A** and **B**). The combined binocular perception is a patchy pattern, with lines from each eye being seen; however, because of rivalry, crossing lines are not seen (**C**).

fixing eye (see diplopia previously discussed). However, patients with acquired strabismus and restricted visual fields (e.g., tunnel vision of unilateral glaucoma with acquired strabismus) often experience confusion. Because the peripheral field is eliminated in these patients, the patient is forced to use both foveae. It is likely that the foveal suppression associated with diplopia requires peripheral retinal stimulation and therefore foveal suppression is not possible when the peripheral field is eliminated.

Rivalry   Rivalry or, as it is sometimes termed, *retinal rivalry,* is produced when different images are presented to the central visual field of each eye in a visually mature subject with normal binocular vision. Instead of seeing two different images superimposed on each other (confusion), the subject perceives patchy drop-out of images where they overlap. Rivalry can be demonstrated by presenting parallel lines to each eye with the lines rotated 90 degrees in one eye (Fig. 15-13). The observer will perceive that some of the lines disappear in a spotty fashion since they cross over each other. You can experience rivalry by placing a pencil horizontally 2 inches in front of one eye and your index finger vertically 2 inches in front of the other eye. Note that there is patchy drop-out of either the pencil or the index finger where they overlap. The rivalry phenomenon is often described as retinal rivalry; however, it is a complex interaction involving cortical inhibition.

Prolonged visual plasticity   The dogma regarding the relatively short span of visual central nervous system plasticity has come into question. Veteran strabismologists know that some adult patients with acquired stra-

bismus can eventually learn to ignore or suppress their double vision. Do these patients actually develop suppression or do they consciously ignore their diplopia? In a study of acquired strabismus in adults, this author used the pattern VEP to document suppression of visual cortical activity in adult patients with acquired strabismus. Another example of prolonged plasticity is that adults with amblyopia can show significant visual acuity improvement after losing vision in their good eye.

Visually Immature

The following sensory adaptations occur when the binocularity is disrupted during the first few years of life, usually before 8 to 10 years of age. The specific type of sensory adaptation that occurs depends on the size of the strabismus, whether it is intermittent or constant, the age of onset of the strabismus, and the age the strabismus is corrected. Once childhood sensory adaptations are acquired they are usually present throughout the patient's life.

Throughout most of the discussion of sensory abnormalities we have presumed that motor strabismus is the primary event and that the brain develops sensory adaptations in response to the abnormal visual stimulation. This is probably true for the majority of strabismus cases, but strabismus can occur as a response to abnormal fusion. Patients with unilateral congenital cataracts routinely develop esotropia or exotropia, and patients with head trauma can lose central fusion and develop vertical or horizontal strabismus. It should be pointed out that some would argue for an abnormality of binocular fusion since the primary event in most types of infantile strabismus, and that strabismus is a consequence of congenitally abnormal fusion centers within the brain. The answer to this controversy—*which came first, the strabismus or the sensory fusion abnormality*—has not been resolved.

Monofixation syndrome   Small-angle strabismus (<10 PD), or mild to moderate unilateral retinal image blur, in young children and infants causes a suppression of the central visual field of the deviated or blurred eye, but binocular fusion in the peripheral fields (peripheral fusion) is maintained (Fig. 15-14). This sensory adaptation, first described by Marshall Parks, is termed *the monofixation syndrome.* Central suppression occurs because the central retina has small receptive fields and high spatial resolution potential, so relatively small differences in image clarity or retinal image position are recognized. In the peripheral fields, however, slight interocular image differences are not detected since the peripheral retina has large receptive fields and relatively low spatial resolution. Small retinal image discrepancies between fellow eyes are therefore not disruptive in the peripheral fields and peripheral fusion occurs. The size

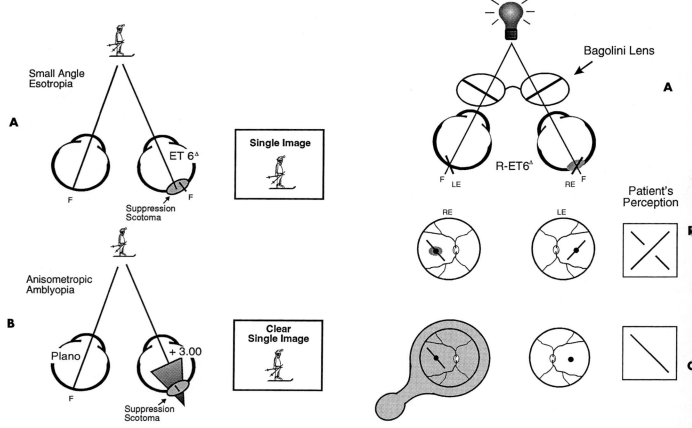

Fig. 15-14   Monofixation syndrome secondary to a small-angle esotropia (**A**) and hypermetropic anisometropia with amblyopia (**B**). In both cases, patient perceives a clear single image since the suppression scotoma eliminates the discrepancy from the esotropia and blurred image respectively.

Fig. 15-15   Monofixation with microtropia and the visual perception with Bagolini lenses. **A,** Right small-angle esotropia and suppression scotoma in the right eye. **B,** Note the patient's perception is one continuous line and one line with an interruption in the center. **C,** Effect of covering the fixing eye, which eliminated the suppression scotoma, and the patient sees a single continuous line from the left eye.

of the suppression scotoma is directly proportional to the amount of image disparity. If the intraocular image disparity is too great even peripheral fusion will be disrupted. Strabismus greater than 10 PD or severe unilateral image blur (e.g., unilateral dense cataract) will disrupt peripheral fusion, and these patients will lack the binocular fusion of the monofixation syndrome. Because patients with the monofixation syndrome have motor fusion, they often have a relatively large underlying phoria in addition to a small tropia, thus the term *phoria-tropia syndrome.*

Patients with monofixation syndrome usually have stereo acuity in the range of 3000 seconds to 70 seconds arc and the central suppression scotoma measures between 2 degrees and 5 degrees. *Bagolini striated lenses* is a sensory test that presents a linear streak of light to each eye oriented 90 degrees apart with each streak of light transecting the fixation light (Fig. 15-15, *A*). Patients with normal binocular vision describe a cross

through the center of a fixation light. In contrast, patients with the monofixation syndrome will describe a cross with a gap in the center of the line presented to the deviated eye (Fig. 15-15, *B*). The gap represents a central suppression scotoma of the nonfixing eye. It is important to note that as soon as the dominant fixing eye is occluded, the suppression scotoma vanishes and the patient fixes with their fovea (Fig. 15-15, *C*). The suppression scotoma is often referred to as a *facultative scotoma*, because its presence is dependent on fixation with the dominant eye. Worth 4-dot testing is another good way to document the monofixation syndrome (see the following discussion on Worth 4-dot testing).

Patients with monofixation syndrome usually have some degree of amblyopia. The amblyopia can be mild (one or two Snellen line difference) or quite severe (20/200). Even patients with 20/200 amblyopia can still maintain the monofixation syndrome with some peripheral fusion and gross stereopsis. Clinically, the monofixation

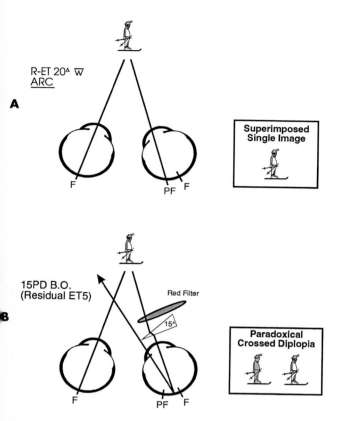

R-ET 20ᐟ W̄
ARC

A

Superimposed
Single Image

15PD B.O.
(Residual ET5)

Red Filter

15ᐟ

B

Paradoxical
Crossed Diplopia

F   PF   F

Fig. 15-16 Anomalous retinal correspondence with right eso-tropia. **A,** Left eye fixes with the fovea (F) and the right eye fixes with the pseudo-fovea (PF). The PF aligns with the esotropia and is located on nasal retina. Patient perceives a single image since the PF of the right eye corresponds with the true fovea of the left eye. **B,** Effect of placing a base-out prism to partially neutralize the esotropia. The patient fixes left eye and sees double since the image now falls temporal to the pseudo-fovea. Images temporal to the pseudo-fovea will project to the opposite visual field and will cause diplopia.

syndrome is frequently encountered in patients with an-isometropic amblyopia, unilateral astigmatism, unilateral partial cataract, and small-angle strabismus.

Anomalous retinal correspondence (ARC) With normal retinal correspondence *(NRC)* the anatomic cor-responding retinal points of each eye are functionally linked together in the occipital cortex to produce bin-ocular vision. Anomalous retinal correspondence *(ARC)* is associated with infantile strabismus where the angle of deviation is too large to allow peripheral fusion. The angle of deviation associated with ARC is usually be-tween 15 and 30 prism diopters. Like monofixation, ARC is a sensory adaptation, which acts to eliminate the con-fusion of images falling on noncorresponding retinal points. The brain adapts to the image misalignment by accepting the eccentric image location as the center of the eye. Thus ARC is a cortical change in the central reference point of the deviated eye from the anatomic fovea to a perifoveal location that corresponds to the

angle of deviation (Fig. 15-16, *A*). This new central point of reference in the deviated eye is called the *pseudo-fovea,* and it corresponds to the true fovea of the dom-inant fellow eye. The functional reorganization of the deviated eye is presumably done at the cortical level of visual processing. Thus ARC is a sensory adaptation where the brain reorganizes its retinal orientation to compensate for ocular misalignment. ARC allows retinal images to be cortically superimposed, even though the images are on anatomically noncorresponding retinal points. ARC is only present during binocular viewing and changes to foveal fixation during monocular fixation. In contrast to monofixation, which is associated with fu-sional vergence amplitudes and stereo acuity, patients with ARC do not have fusion vergence amplitudes and do not have stereopsis. They only have superimposition of retinal images without true fusion.

If a patient with ARC has their strabismus partially or fully corrected by surgery or a prism, this displaces the image off the pseudo-fovea onto retina that is cortically perceived as being off center (Fig. 15-16, *B*). The patient then sees double even if the image falls on the true an-atomic fovea. This type of diplopia is called *paradoxical diplopia* because even though the eyes are placed in alignment the patient sees double. Remember that under binocular viewing, the pseudo-fovea is the central orien-tation of the eye and images displaced off the pseudo-fovea will be perceived as off-center. Fig. 15-16 shows the retinal adaptation of a patient with 20 PD esotropia and ARC. Note that after partial correction of the eso-tropia with a 15 PD base-out prism, the image is now temporal to the pseudo-fovea (Fig. 15-16, *B*). This pa-tient will have crossed diplopia because the image falls on retina that is temporal to the pseudo-fovea, and the temporal retina projects to the opposite hemi-field. The patient will have crossed diplopia as long as the image is temporal to the pseudo-fovea, even if the eyes are per-fectly aligned so the image falls directly on the true fovea. Adult patients with ARC often experience diplopia after correction of their strabismus. An easy way to predict if a strabismic patient has ARC and will have postoperative paradoxical diplopia is to neutralize the angle of devia-tion with a prism. If the patient has diplopia with prism neutralization of the deviation, then the patient has ARC and the patient should be informed that postoperative diplopia will occur after the eyes are straightened. For-tunately, paradoxical diplopia is usually not as bother-some as true diplopia associated with normal retinal cor-respondence, and in most cases paradoxical diplopia will vanish within a few weeks after surgery. Only in rare circumstances is postoperative paradoxical diplopia so bothersome that it interferes with every day activities. Even so, in rare instances, persistent postoperative par-adoxical diplopia has required a reoperation to recreate the initial strabismus to eliminate paradoxical diplopia.

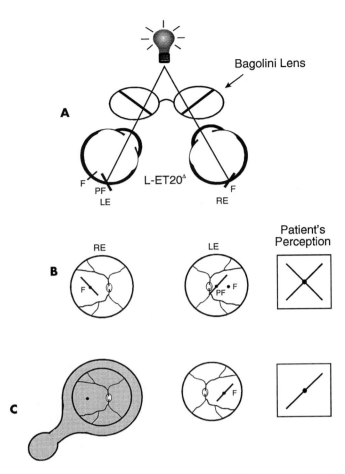

Fig. 15-17 Anomalous retinal correspondence as tested with Bagolini lenses. **A,** Bagolini lenses stimulating right fovea and left pseudo-fovea (PF). Note that the pseudo fovea is nasal to the true fovea (F). **B,** Retinal location of the Bagolini striation with the fovea of the right eye being stimulated and the pseudo-fovea of the left eye being stimulated. Patient's perception, however, is a cross since the pseudo-fovea corresponds to the true fovea. **C,** Right eye occluded. The patient now fixates with the true fovea of the left eye. Note that the pseudo-fovea has disappeared. Patient perceives a single line, which stimulated the visual center.

In cases where preoperative prism neutralization shows paradoxical diplopia that bothers the patient, the physician can prescribe press on prisms (prism adaptation) to see if the diplopia subsides over several weeks.

Bagolini striated lenses on a patient with a 20 PD esotropia and ARC is depicted in Fig. 15-17. The patient perceives a cross by superimposing the line from each eye even though the line in the deviated eye falls nasal to the true fovea through the pseudo-fovea. This cortical reorganization of ARC is only present during binocular viewing. Note that when the dominant eye is covered, the patient quickly reorients to the true anatomic fovea (Fig. 15-17, *C*). ARC should not be confused with eccentric fixation. Remember ARC is only present during binocular viewing where as eccentric fixation represents

a monocular loss of vision (amblyopia) and is present during both monocular and binocular viewing.

ARC provides crude binocular vision with superimposition of retinal images; however, there is not true fusion. Patients with ARC do not have fusional vergence amplitudes and they do not have stereo acuity. ARC can occur in association with intermittent strabismus. Some patients with intermittent exotropia, for example, have binocular vision with stereopsis when they are aligned but switch to ARC when they are tropic. In general, ARC is associated with good vision or only mild amblyopia.

Harmonious ARC is the term used for the situation as described previously, where the position of the pseudo-fovea completely compensates for the angle of strabismus (see Figs. 15-16 and 15-17). Put another way, the strabismic deviation equals the pseudo-foveal displacement from the true fovea. The amount of pseudo-foveal off set is termed the *angle of anomaly*. In patients with harmonious ARC, the angle of anomaly is equal to the strabismic deviation *(objective angle)*. Clinically, however, there are many cases where the angle of strabismus does not exactly match the location of the pseudo-fovea so the target image does not fall on the pseudo-fovea and this is called *unharmonious ARC* (Fig. 15-18). In these cases, it is likely that the angle of strabismus has changed (usually increased) after the formation of the pseudo-fovea and therefore the angle of the deviation measures greater than the eccentricity of the pseudo-fovea. Most patients with unharmonious ARC suppress the target image, so they do not experience diplopia. Others, perhaps those who had a change in the deviation off the pseudo-fovea in late childhood or adulthood, do experience diplopia. In Fig. 15-18, *A*, the angle of the strabismus measures 20 PD (objective angle) but the pseudo-fovea is only 15 PD from the true fovea (angle of anomaly = 15 PD). Thus the image is falling 5 PD nasal to the pseudo-fovea. A 5 PD base-out prism over the right eye places the image on the pseudo-fovea and eliminates the diplopia. The discrepancy between the location of the pseudo-fovea and the location of the target image is called the *subjective angle,* and in Fig. 15-18, *B,* the subjective angle is 5 PD. Note that neutralizing the subjective angle eliminates diplopia associated with unharmonious ARC, but neutralizing more than the subjective angle results in paradoxical diplopia (Fig. 15-18, *C*). See Chapter 4 under amblyoscope for further discussion.

Practically speaking, the differentiation between harmonious versus unharmonious ARC is not of great clinical importance; however, paradoxical diplopia after strabismus surgery is of clinical concern. Adult patients with long-standing strabismus should be examined for ARC by neutralizing the deviation with a prism.

Large regional suppression Children who have large-angle strabismus or severe unilateral retinal image blur, develop a large suppression scotoma to eliminate

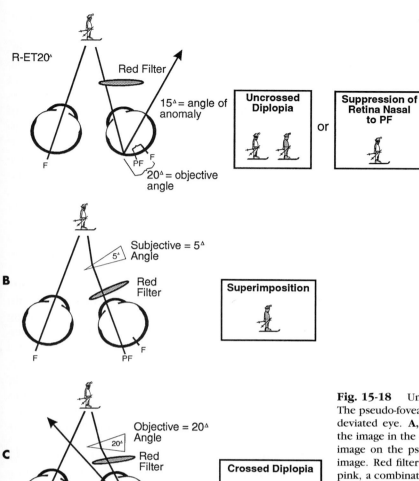

Fig. 15-18 Unharmonious ARC is shown in patient with esotropia. The pseudo-fovea (PF) is not in alignment with the retinal image in the deviated eye. **A,** Patient perceives uncrossed diplopia or suppresses the image in the deviated eye. **B,** A base-out prism is used to place the image on the pseudo-fovea. Patient perceives a superimposed single image. Red filter in front of the right eye causes the image to appear pink, a combination of the clear image left eye and the red image right eye. **C,** A 20 PD prism is placed base-out in front of the deviated eye to place the image on the true fovea. Patient has paradoxical diplopia and sees the red image on the contralateral side, giving crossed diplopia. (Remember that the pseudo-fovea is the center of reference.)

the image disparity. Patients with large-angle constant strabismus (e.g., congenital esotropia) will have essentially no binocularity, not even peripheral fusion or ARC. However, large regional suppression is not always constant and can be intermittent. Patients with large-angle strabismus and large fusional vergence amplitudes (e.g., intermittent exotropia) have intermittent strabismus and intermittent regional suppression. These patients switch from a state of binocular fusion, to a state of monocular vision and suppression. Another example of intermittent large regional suppression occurs in patients with congenital incomitant strabismus where the eyes are straight in one field of gaze (Duane's syndrome or congenital superior oblique palsy). These patients have binocular fusion when their eyes are aligned with a compensatory face turn but they suppress when they look into the field of gaze where they have strabismus. Patients with intermittent exotropia and Duane's syndrome who have de-

veloped suppression usually do not have diplopia when they are tropic.

SENSORY EXAMINATION

Stereo Acuity Tests

Contour stereo tests (Titmus test) Titmus stereo testing is a contour test and is one of the most widely used clinical tests for stereopsis. Contour stereo images are made up of two horizontally displaced identical figures one seen by each eye individually (Fig. 15-19). Stereo figures are nasally displaced to produce bitemporal retinal disparity resulting in stereo images that come up off the page toward the observer, whereas temporal figure displacements cause binasal retinal disparity with the stereo image appearing as a depression (going back away from the observer). Contour tests are the easiest to

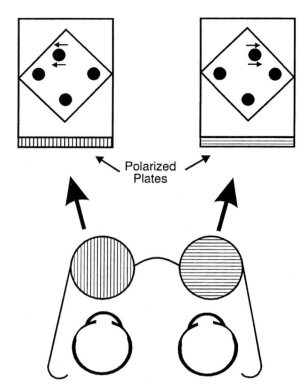

Fig. 15-19 Diagrammatic representation of a contour stereogram. Polarized glasses donned by the patient match the orientation of two polarized plastic plates, so one eye sees one plate and the fellow eye sees the other plate. The polarization is oriented vertically over the left eye and horizontally over the right eye, so the left eye views the left figure with the upper circle shifted to the left, and the right eye views the right figure with the upper circle shifted to the right. This temporal displacement of the circles stimulates binasal disparate retinal points, and produces the stereoscopic perception that the upper circle is recessed and goes back away from the observer. Titmus testing uses nasally displaced figures to produce stereoscopic images that come up off the page, toward the observer.

perceive, but they have the disadvantage of having monocular cues that allow even some stereo-blind patients to identify stereoscopic figures with large disparities (Fig. 15-20). Image displacement cues work well for large image disparities because the monocular displacement is obvious, but they are difficult to use on disparities less than 200 seconds arc (Fig. 15-21). The disparity range of the Titmus test is from 3,000 seconds arc (the fly), to 40 seconds arc (ninth circle); smaller disparities correspond to better stereo acuity. The presence of good stereo acuity is indicative of good visual acuity. Table 15-1 correlates stereo acuity to visual acuity.

One way to help verify that the patient does in fact have true stereo acuity is to retest with the Titmus test book turned 90 degrees and see if the patient still sees the stereoscopic target. With the test book turned 90 degrees, the displacements are vertical and targets are not stereoscopic, but the monocular cues are still present. If the patient identifies the stereoscopic target with the Titmus book turned 90 degrees; the patient is using monocular cues, and not true stereopsis. For further verification, turn the book 180 degrees (upside-down) and see if the patient notes that the stereo targets have returned, but are now projecting in an opposite direction, away from the patient. Rotating the book 180 degrees changes the stereo test from nasal to temporal displacement, resulting in binasal retinal disparity and stereoscopic images that move away from the observer.

The Titmus "fly" is useful in preverbal patients as young as 1 to 2 years. If a child startles to the fly coming out of the page, then this is suggestive of gross stereopsis. Also, if a child clearly picks up the wings of the Titmus stereo "fly" well off the page, this is good evidence for at least some peripheral fusion.

Randot stereo test Randot stereograms consist of

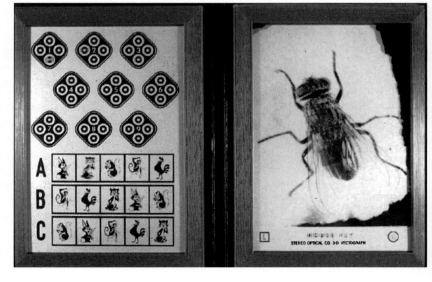

Fig. 15-20 Photograph of Titmus test showing stereoscopic fly, circles, and animals. This represents two polarized transparent plastic overlays with the stereoscopic images horizontally displacement. Note that there are two sets of fly wings, and the dot in circle group 1 and the cat in row A appear blurred. This is because there are two images horizontally displaced for each stereoscopic picture.

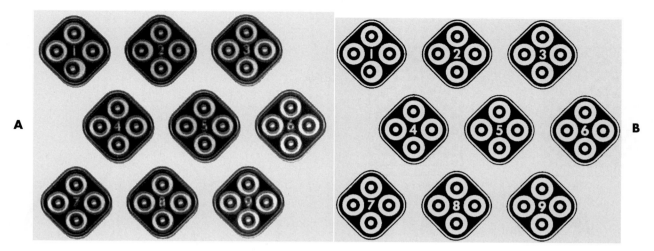

Fig. 15-21   Close-up photograph of the Titmus stereo circles. Note in figure A circle group 1 the bottom circle is shifted to the right, and that in figure B dot group 1 the bottom circle is shifted to the left. This causes a nasal shift of the circles and stimulates bitemporal disparate retinal points producing the perception that the circle comes up out of the page. The horizontal displacement can be seen monocularly and provides a monocular cue as to which circle is the stereo circle. Less horizontal displacement tests higher grades of stereo acuity (i.e., decreasing seconds of arc disparity corresponds to better stereo acuity). After dot group 4, the horizontal displacement is so small, it is difficult or impossible to detect the stereoscopic figure with monocular cues.

Table 15-1	Visual acuity needed for Titmus stereo acuity

Circles	(Seconds of Arc = V.A.)
9	40 sec = 20/25
8	50 sec = 20/30
7	60 sec = 20/40
6	80 sec = 20/50
5	100 sec = 20/60
4	140 sec = 20/70
3	200 sec = 20/80
2	400 sec = 20/100
1	800 sec = 20/200

two plates of randomly displayed dots, which are identical except that the dots that make up the stereoscopic figure are displaced horizontally in one plate relative to the other plate (Fig. 15-22). When viewed with polarized glasses, the dots from one plate are projected to one eye and the dots from the other plate are projected to the fellow eye. Retinal disparity from the displaced dots produces stereoscopic percept. If the dots are nasally displaced the stereoscopic figure will appear to come up out of the page, whereas temporally displaced dots produce figures that are recessed and go back away from the observer. The Randot test has almost no monocular cues, and a positive response indicates true stereopsis, with few false positive responses. The problem with Randot

stereo acuity testing is that some normal children have trouble seeing the Randot figures and falsely fail the test.

Diplopia Tests

Diplopia tests use one fixation target that is seen by both eyes. In patients with straight eyes, the target image will fall on both foveae (Fig. 15-23), but in strabismic patients the target image falls on the fovea of the fixing eye and an extrafoveal point in the nonfixing eye (Fig. 15-24). A color filter is placed over one eye (usually red) or both eyes (usually red right eye, green left eye) to tint the image of each eye. By distinctly tinting the retinal images of each eye, the examiner can tell which image corresponds to which eye. Lenses that place a streak of light on the retina (Maddox rod and Bagolini lenses) are also used.

Many diplopia tests disrupt fusion either by obscuring or eliminating peripheral fusion cues or by providing different images to each eye, which invokes retinal rivalry. Tests that disrupt fusion are referred to as dissociating tests. Box 15-3 lists diplopia tests, with the most dissociating test on top and least dissociating on the bottom. Note that with room lights out (scotopic conditions) tests that use color filters, such as the Worth 4-dot test and red filter test, become extremely dissociating since the only images seen by the patient are the test lights, and peripheral fusion cues are lost.

Red filter test   One of the simplest diplopia tests is the red filter test. Put a red glass over one eye and the patient is directed to fixate on a single light source, or an

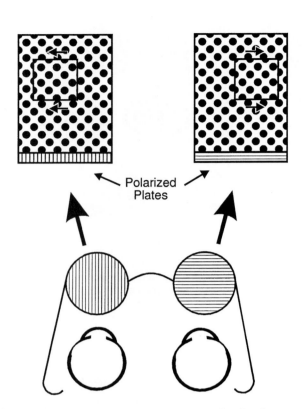

Fig. 15-22   Diagrammatic representation of a Randot stereogram. The left eye sees one set of dots and the right eye sees a second set of dots. The dots are identical, except for the dots within square area that have been horizontally displaced (temporally in the figure). Temporal displacement stimulates binasal disparate retinal points and produces the stereoscopic perception that the upper circle goes back away from the observer. The clinical test for Randot stereo acuity consists of nasal displacement and the stereo images appear to come up off the page.

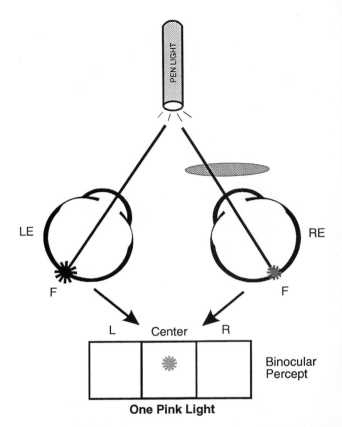

Fig. 15-23   Red filter test in a normal patient with straight eyes and normal retinal correspondence. Note that the image from the penlight falls on both foveae and the patient receives a single binocular image.

accommodative fixation target. Patients with straight eyes and normal retinal correspondence will see one pinkish red light (see Fig. 15-23). If a phoria is present, the red filter may dissociate the eyes, causing a manifest deviation and diplopia. The denser the red filter color, the more dissociating the test. Another way to make the standard red filter test more dissociating is to turn down the room lights. The red filter test is useful for identifying NRC, ARC, and suppression. *Esotropia NRC* causes uncrossed diplopia with the red light seen on the same side as the red filter (see Fig. 15-24, *A*) and *exotropia NRC* is associated with crossed diplopia since the red light is opposite to the red filter (see Fig. 15-24, *B*).

Strabismus associated with *suppression* results in the perception of a single light, either red or white, depending on which eye is fixing. In Fig. 15-25, *A*, the left eye is fixing so the patient sees one white light, and suppresses the red light falling on the right retina. If a dark red filter is placed over the fixing left eye, then fixation

switches to the right eye and the left eye is suppressed (Fig. 15-25, *B*). Patients who alternate fixation may report seeing two lights, a red alternating with a white. When a child with a manifest strabismus claims to see two lights, be sure to distinguish between diplopia where the red and the white lights are seen simultaneously, and alternating suppression where one light seen at a time.

During binocular viewing, patients with strabismus and *ARC* use a pseudo-fovea in the deviated eye that functionally corresponds to the true fovea of the fixing eye so they typically do not see double but see one pink light with red cover testing (Fig. 15-26). If a patient with strabismus sees one light on red cover testing (or in free view for that matter), this indicates suppression or ARC. Neutralizing the angle of strabismus with a prism can identify ARC. If partially or completely neutralizing the deviation results in diplopia, then the patient has ARC. For example, partial or full neutralization of the deviation in a patient with esotropia ARC moves the image temporal to the pseudo-fovea resulting in crossed diplopia (Fig. 15-27). Remember that during binocular viewing the pseudo-fovea corresponds to the true fovea of the fixing

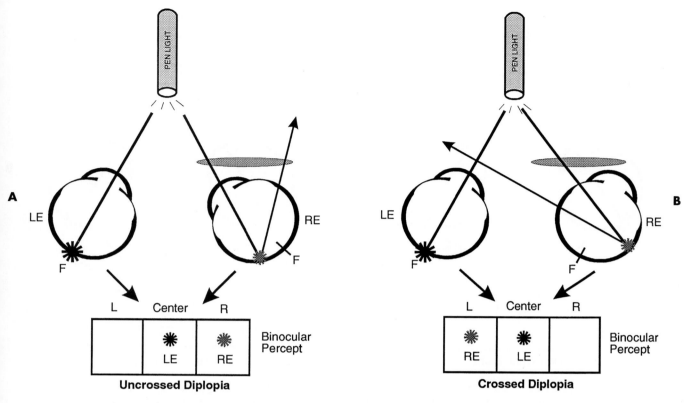

Fig. 15-24 **A,** A red filter test in a patient with normal retinal correspondence and an esotropia. The image from the penlight falls nasal to the fovea of right eye and the retinal image is projected temporally, thus producing uncrossed diplopia. **B,** Red filter test in a patient with right exotropia and normal retinal correspondence. The image from the penlight falls on temporal retinal and is projected nasally, thus giving crossed diplopia.

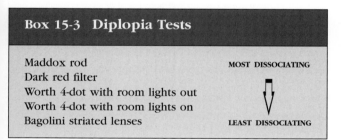

Box 15-3 Diplopia Tests

Maddox rod	MOST DISSOCIATING
Dark red filter	
Worth 4-dot with room lights out	
Worth 4-dot with room lights on	
Bagolini striated lenses	LEAST DISSOCIATING

eye, so the retina temporal to the pseudo-fovea projects to the nasal hemifield, therefore causing uncrossed diplopia, even if the image is falling on the true fovea. This diplopia is termed *paradoxical diplopia.*

It is important to perform prism neutralization on visually mature adults before strabismus surgery to rule out ARC and the possibility of postoperative diplopia. It is performed by simply neutralizing the deviation with a prism, and then having the patient view at the distance and near to see if the patient sees double. If neutralizing the deviation causes paradoxical diplopia, then ARC is present. Patients with diplopia on prism neutralization should be told they will probably experience diplopia

immediately after surgery, much like the diplopia they experience during prism neutralization. Patients who report bothersome diplopia in the office with prism neutralization can be fitted with press-on prisms, before surgery is undertaken, to determine their ability to eventually suppress the diplopia. If diplopia persists after several weeks of prism neutralization, then the surgeon may consider intentionally undercorrecting the deviation, or deferring surgery. In general, diplopia associated with ARC is well tolerated especially if the patient is appropriately informed preoperatively. Personally we have never had to undo a good surgical result because of paradoxical diplopia associated with ARC; however, some patients have declined surgery after experiencing diplopia with prism neutralization.

Another way ARC can be distinguished from NRC in patients with suppression is by placing a vertical prism (usually 15 PD base down) over the deviated eye (Fig. 15-28). A vertical prism causes patients with ARC to see two vertically displaced images with the red light directly over the white light. The lights are vertically aligned because the light in the deviated eye is over the pseudofovea, which directly corresponds to the true fovea (see Fig. 15-28, *A*). When a vertical prism is introduced to the

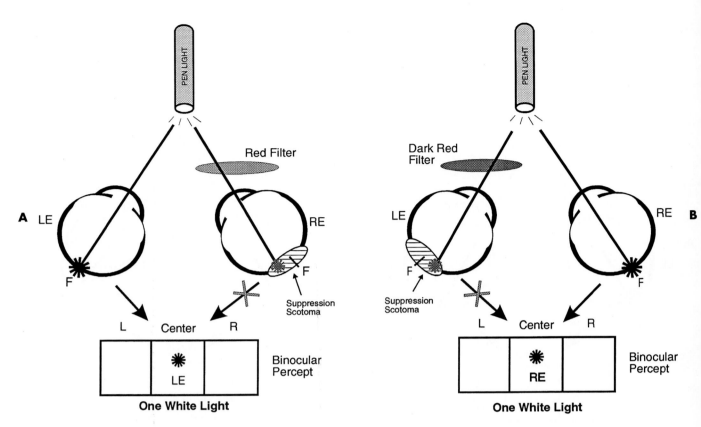

Fig. 15-25   Red filter test in a patient with childhood esotropia who developed suppression and a fixation preference for the left eye. **A,** Patient fixing left eye with a suppression scotoma of right eye. Note that the retinal image of the penlight falls within the suppression scotoma, and the patient only perceives one white light from the left eye. **B,** A dark red filter is placed over the left eye to shift fixation to the right eye. With right eye fixing, patient suppresses the image in the left eye and patient perceives one white light from the right eye.

Fig. 15-26   Red filter test in a patient with a right esotropia and ARC. Red filter is placed in front of the right eye and the image falls on the pseudo-fovea (P). Since the pseudo-fovea and fovea represent corresponding retinal points in a patient with ARC, the patient has a single binocular perception and sees one pink light.

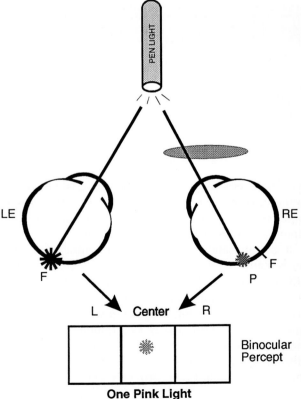

Paradoxical Diplopia

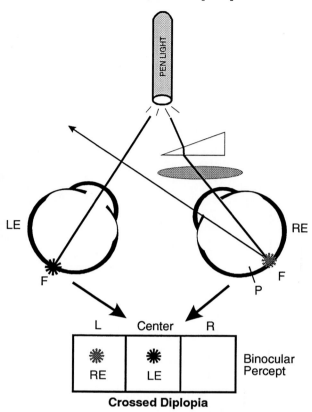

Crossed Diplopia

Fig. 15-27 *Paradoxical Diplopia.* Diagram of a patient with esotropia and ARC with the deviation being neutralized with a base-out prism. A red filter and base-out prism are placed over the right eye. The prism neutralizes the deviation by moving the retinal image of the penlight temporally, off the pseudo-fovea to the true fovea. Since the pseudo-fovea is the center of orientation, the image is perceived to fall on temporal retinal and is projected to the opposite field, thus resulting in crossed diplopia.

deviated eye of a patient with central suppression and NRC, the patient reports seeing two lights that are horizontally and vertically displaced because there is no pseudo-fovea, and the center of reference is the true fovea of each eye (see Fig. 15-28, *B*).

Worth 4-dot test The Worth 4-dot test consists of two green lights, one red light, and one white light as seen in Fig. 15-29. The patient wears red/green glasses, usually with the red lens over the right eye, and views a Worth 4 dot flashlight at one third of a meter, or a Worth 4-dot light box at 6 meters (20 feet). The near Worth 4-dots are separated by 6° at near (flashlight at one third meter) and by 1.25° for the distance (light box at 6 meters). The two green lights are seen by the eye with the green filter, the red light is seen with the eye with the red filter, and the white light is seen by both eyes. When the test is performed with the room lights out it is very dissociating since the white dot is the only binocular

fusion target. If the room lights are turned on, however, the patient can see the room environment with both eyes, thus providing strong fusion cues. This is why Worth 4-dot testing in the dark is much more dissociating than testing with the room lights on.

The normal fusion response is seeing four lights, two red and two green (see Fig. 15-29). Another normal response is one red light, two green lights and one light that flickers between red and green. The light that flickers is the white light that is seen by both eyes, and the flicker is caused by color rivalry. Patients with acquired strabismus and diplopia will see five lights, three green and two red (exotropia = crossed diplopia, esotropia = uncrossed diplopia). Patients with suppression report either three green lights or two red lights, depending on which eye is fixing. In Fig. 15-30 the left eye is fixing and the right eye is suppressed, so the patient sees three green lights. If the right eye was the preferred eye and the left eye was suppressed, then the patient would see two red lights. Patients who alternate fixation usually describe seeing two red lights, alternating with three green lights, but a few patients will report the sum total of the alternating lights, that is, five lights. Thus alternating suppression can be confused with diplopia, because patients with diplopia also report seeing five lights. Patients with large scotomas (scotomas greater than 6°) will suppress both the distance and near Worth 4-dot.

Patients with the monofixational syndrome have a small central suppression scotoma (<5°) and peripheral fusion. They will, therefore, fuse the near Worth 4-dot, which subtends 6°, because the dots fall outside the scotoma (Fig. 15-31), but suppress the distance Worth 4-dot, which subtends only 1.25° and projects within the scotoma (Fig. 15-32). One of the best uses of the Worth 4-dot test is identifying central suppression and peripheral fusion associated with the monofixation syndrome; however, remember to leave the room lights on to promote fusion.

The Worth 4-dot flashlight can be used to plot the size of suppression scotomas. By moving the flashlight closer to the patient the lights subtend a larger angle (i.e., stimulate more peripheral retina) and by moving the flashlight farther away the lights subtend a smaller angle (i.e., stimulate more central retina). Table 15-2 shows the stimulus angle for the Worth 4-dot flashlight at various distances from the patient.

Bagolini lenses Bagolini striated lenses are clear powerless lenses with a linear scratch through the center that provides a streak of light on the retina when a point light source is viewed. One lens is placed over each eye, and the lenses are oriented obliquely at 45° and 135°. Since the lenses are otherwise clear, they are not dissociating. Bagolini lenses, therefore, have the advantage of providing a free binocular view without dissociation. Normal patients with straight eyes and NRC, and those

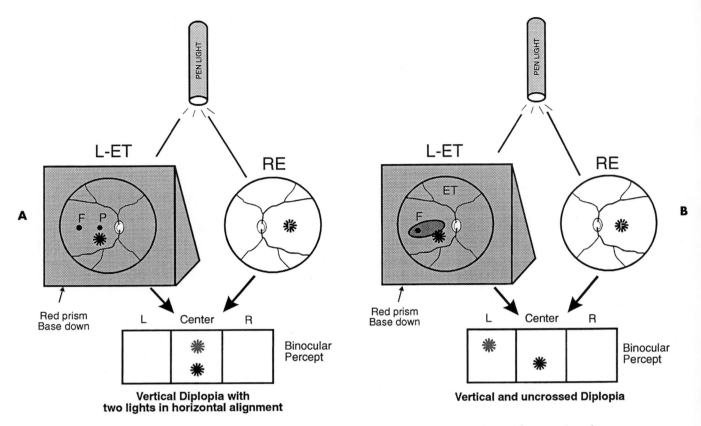

Fig. 15-28   Vertical prism red filter test for suppression versus ARC. **A,** Patient with esotropia and ARC is presented with a base-down vertical prism and a red filter over left eye. The prism deflects the retinal image below the pseudo-fovea and the patient perceived two images, vertically one on top of the other. Remember the pseudo-fovea is the center of vision during binocular viewing. **B,** Patient with esotropia and suppression of left eye. A base-down prism is placed in front of the left eye, which displaces the retinal image inferiorly, out of the central scotoma. The patient perceives two images, vertically and horizontally displaced. Note that there is no pseudo-fovea and the true foveae are at the center of vision.

with strabismus and ARC will report seeing a cross with Bagolini lenses (Fig. 15-33, *A*). Patients with strabismus and ARC see a cross because one line goes through the true fovea and one line goes through the pseudo-fovea during binocular viewing. Patients who have large regional suppression will report seeing only one line (Fig. 15-33, *B*). The monofixation syndrome, on the other hand, is associated with a cross, but one line will have a gap centrally (Fig. 15-33, *C*). Patients with NRC, heterophoria, and diplopia will show the response of either an A or a V. Since esotropia is associated with uncrossed diplopia, esotropia will cause the right line to move to the right, thus creating a "V" (Fig. 15-33, *D*). Exotropia produces an "A" because exotropia is associated with crossed diplopia and the right line moves to the left (Fig. 15-33, *E*).

Maddox rod test   The Maddox rod is described in Chapter 14 as a means for measuring subjective torsion, but it also can be used for measuring phorias. The single Maddox rod test is performed by placing the Maddox rod over one eye and having the patient view a pen light. Align the streak vertically to detect horizontal deviations and horizontally for vertical deviations. If the streak of light is seen to pass through the pen light, the patient is orthophoric or has ARC. This is one of the most dissociating tests since there are essentially no binocular fusion cues because the image forming the Maddox rod is totally distorted. Virtually any phoria will break down with the Maddox rod test; therefore the test does not distinguish between phorias and tropias. To make the diagnosis of phoria versus tropia, the physician must assess the eye alignment objectively before moving on to the dissociating diplopia test.

Haploscopic Tests

In contrast to diplopia tests where there is one stationary fixation target that is viewed by both eyes, haploscopic tests have two fixation targets, one for each eye, and the targets can be moved separately to align them

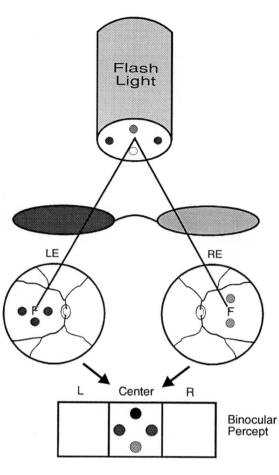

Fig. 15-29 Worth 4-dot flash light. The top light is red, the two horizontal lights are green, and the bottom light is white. The filter over the right eye is red and left eye is green. In a normal patient with straight eyes, three lights are projected to the left eye and two lights to the right eye. Patient fuses the white light seen by both eyes and perceives four lights.

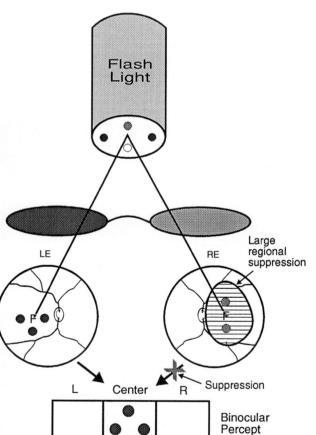

Fig. 15-30 Worth 4-dot in a patient with large regional suppression of right eye. The two dots fall within the suppression scotoma, so the patient perceives three dots from the left eye.

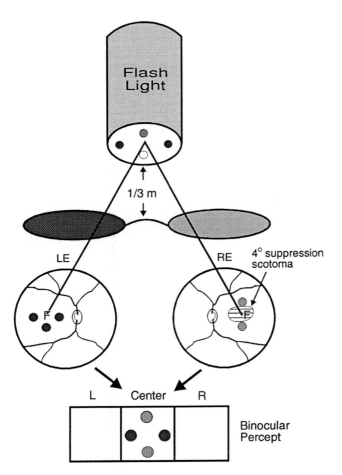

Fig. 15-31   Near Worth 4-dot test in a patient with monofixation syndrome and 8 PD (4°) esotropia. The near Worth 4-dot subtends 6° and the dots fall outside the scotoma. Patient perceives four dots.

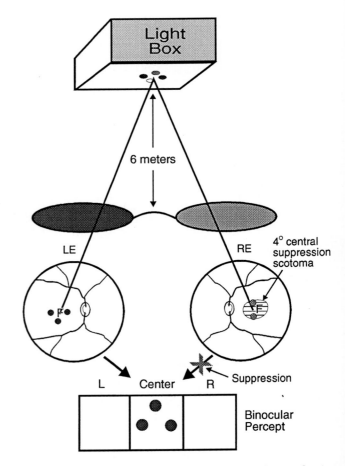

Fig. 15-32   Distance Worth 4-dot in a patient with monofixation syndrome, esotropia of 8 PD (or 4°). The distance Worth 4-dot subtends 1.25 degrees and two dots fall within the central suppression scotoma. Patient therefore perceives three dots from the left eye and no dots from the right eye.

with each fovea. There are various ways to separately stimulate each eye. One way to create haploscopic vision is to place a mirror in front of each eye, with the mirrors angled so the right eye sees the right temporal field and the left eye sees the left temporal field. Mirror separation of vision is the principle of the amblyoscope. Another commonly used method is to have the patient wear color-tinted glasses, a red filter for one eye and a green filter for the other eye. Two moveable targets are presented to the patient, one red and one green. The eye with the red filter sees only the red target and the eye with the green filter sees only the green target; thus separate visual stimuli are presented to each eye. This is the principle of the Lancaster red/green test (see Chapter 14). If strabismus is present, either the mirrors can be angled or the red/green targets moved so the fixation target is aligned with each fovea. Haploscopic tests include the Lancaster red/green test, the amblyoscope, and the afterimage test.

Amblyoscope   The amblyoscope provides a haplo-

Table 15-2	Stimulus angle for the Worth 4-dot flashlight

Worth 4-dot distance from patient*	Worth 4-dot angle
1/6 meter	12 degrees
1/3 meter (14 inches)	6 degrees*
1/2 meter	4 degrees
1 meter	2 degrees

*Standard near Worth 4-dot flashlight.

scopic view, allowing presentation of images to each eye independently. There are mirrors at the elbow of the amblyoscope arms that reflect images from transparent picture slides into each eye (Fig. 15-34). The arms of the amblyoscope can be moved to measure either subjective or objective angle. The *subjective angle* is the angle in

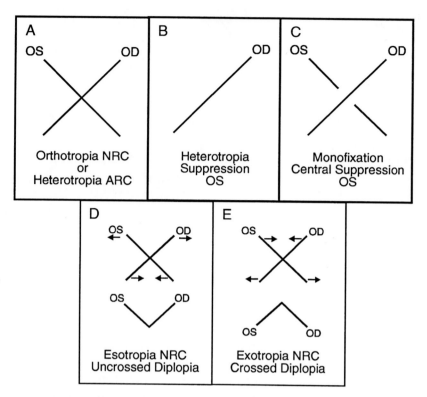

Fig. 15-33   Diagram of the patient's perception of Bagolini testing. **A,** A cross is perceived in orthotropia with normal retinal correspondence or strabismus with ARC. **B,** Patient with strabismus and large suppression scotoma sees one line. **C,** Patient with monofixation syndrome and small central scotoma will see one continuous line and one line broken in the center, which corresponds with the eye with the suppression scotoma. **D,** Patient with esotropia and uncrossed diplopia reports a V. **E,** Patient with exotropia and crossed diplopia reports an A-type configuration.

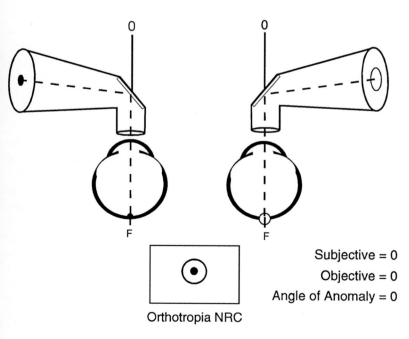

Fig. 15-34   Diagram of amblyoscope, testing a patient with normal retinal correspondence and orthotropia. A black dot is a target to the left eye and a ring is the target to the right eye. Patient sees the black dot inside the ring without moving the arms of the amblyoscope.

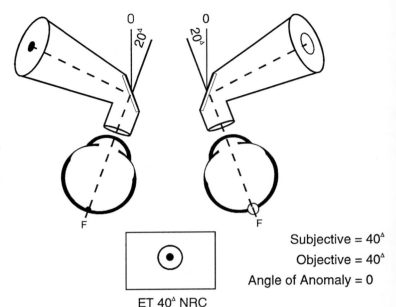

Fig. 15-35   Patient with NRC and esotropia. The arms of the amblyoscope are angled so the image falls on each fovea and the patient perceives the dot inside the circle. Each arm is moved 20^Δ (10 degrees) for a total of 40 PD.

Subjective = 40^Δ

Objective = 40^Δ

Angle of Anomaly = 0

ET 40^Δ NRC

degrees the examiner must move the amblyoscope arms to allow the patient to see the two pictures as being superimposed. The *objective angle* is measured by alternating target presentation from right eye to left eye and moving the arms of the amblyoscope until there is no refixation eye movement. The objective angle equals the deviation as measured by the alternate prism cover test. Note that the subjective angle is determined under binocular viewing, whereas the objective angle is measured during monocular viewing.

Normal retinal correspondence   In a strabismic patient with NRC and diplopia, the subjective and objective angle are the same (Fig. 15-35). This is because patients with NRC always use the fovea as the center of reference. Patients with NRC and *dense large regional suppression* will not have a measurable subjective angle, since they suppress one eye, making subjective superimposition of the images impossible. The subjective angle can be measured in patients with the *monofixation syndrome* and a small central suppression scotoma, by using targets that stimulate peripheral retina.

Anomalous retinal correspondence (harmonious)   Patients with strabismus and harmonious ARC have the pseudo-fovea positioned to compensate for the angle of deviation so there is no subjective misalignment (Fig. 15-36). These patients have a significant objective angle but the subjective angle is zero. The subjective angle is zero because the subjective angle is measured under binocular conditions and reflects the alignment of the true fovea of the fixing eye to the pseudo-fovea of the deviated eye. Patients with harmonious ARC will see the targets from each eye as superimposed with the amblyoscope arms set to zero (parallel), even though there is a large objective angle (see Fig. 15-36). The objective angle is

measured by alternate cover (monocular viewing) so the objective angle reflects the misalignment based on the true fovea of each eye.

The displacement of the pseudo-fovea off the true fovea is called the *angle of anomaly* (see Fig. 15-36). Since in harmonious ARC, the location of the pseudo-fovea completely compensates for the objective deviation, the subjective angle is 0, and the objective angle equals the angle of anomaly. For example, in Fig. 15-36, the objective angle is ET 20 PD and the subjective angle is zero, then the angle of anomaly (i.e., distance of the pseudo-fovea from the true fovea) is 20 PD (20–0 = 20).

Unharmonious ARC   In patients with unharmonious ARC, the pseudo-fovea is located in a position that does not fully compensate for the objective deviation. These patients will either see double or will suppress the image that does not fall on the pseudo-fovea (Fig. 15-37). The subjective angle is measured by moving the arms of the amblyoscope until the two images are superimposed. When the images are superimposed, the image of the fixing eye is on the true fovea, and the image in the nonfixing eye is on the pseudo-fovea. The subjective angle is the number of degrees from the zero position the amblyoscope arm needs to move to place the image on the pseudo-fovea. For example, in Fig. 15-37 the subjective angle (I-P) is 10 PD, and the objective angle (I-F) is 30 PD. Since the angle of anomaly is equal to the objective angle minus the subjective angle, the angle of anomaly is 20 PD (30 minus 10).

The amblyoscope is a useful tool since it can measure fusional vergence amplitudes, angle of deviation, area of suppression, retinal correspondence, and even torsion. Some degree of instrument convergence, however, is usually present when using the amblyoscope.

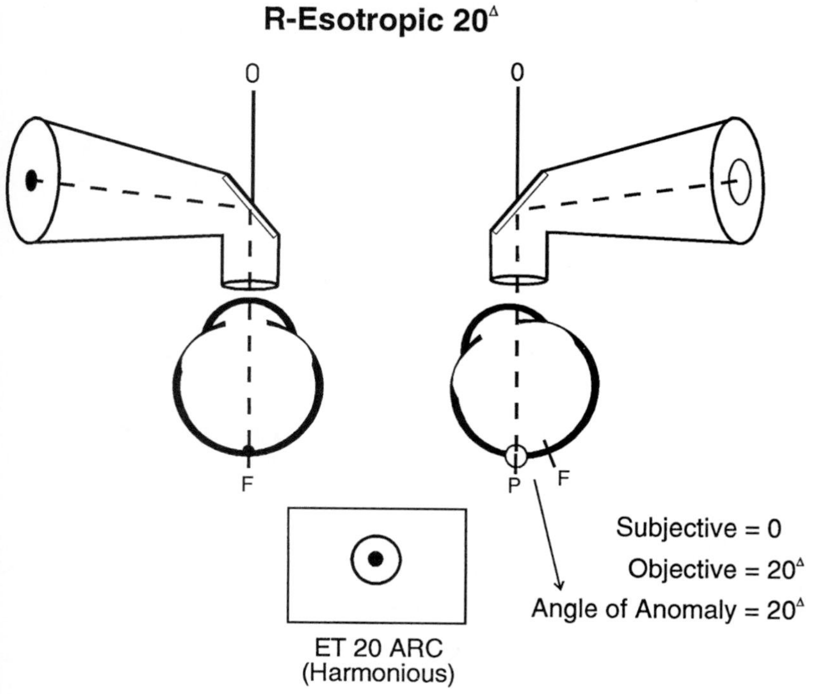

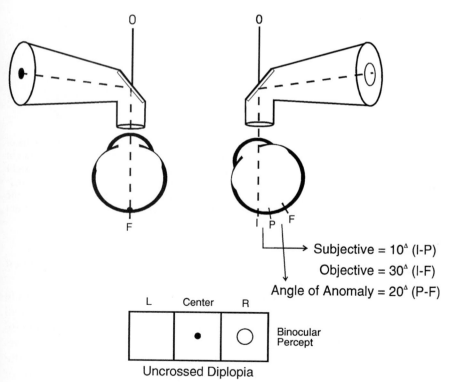

R-Esotropic 20$^\Delta$

Subjective = 0

Objective = 20$^\Delta$

Angle of Anomaly = 20$^\Delta$

ET 20 ARC
(Harmonious)

Fig. 15-36   Patient with harmonious ARC and right esotropia. The arms of the amblyoscope do not have to be angled for the patient to see the dot inside the ring, since the pseudo-fovea is directly in alignment with the ring target. The patient perceives the black dot in the center of the circle with the arms of the amblyoscope aligned to 0. The alternate cover test shows the objective angle to be 20 PD.

Subjective = 10$^\Delta$ (I-P)

Objective = 30$^\Delta$ (I-F)

Angle of Anomaly = 20$^\Delta$ (P-F)

L   Center   R

Binocular
Percept

Uncrossed Diplopia

Fig. 15-37   Patient with unharmonious ARC and 30 PD of esotropia. In this diagram the arms of the amblyoscope are set at 0 and are not angled. Since the image (I) is falling nasal to the pseudo-fovea, the patient perceives uncrossed diplopia as diagrammed in the rectangle at the bottom of the figure. If the arm of the amblyoscope in front of the right eye was moved 10° in to place the image on the pseudo-fovea, the patient would perceive the ring around the dot.

Other Tests for Suppression and Fusion

Afterimage test   The afterimage test is a fovea to fovea sensory test that does not use a haploscopic apparatus, but in which each eye is stimulated separately. Each fovea is marked individually during monocular viewing with a linear strobe light that bleaches the retina and causes a linear afterimage shadow through the true fovea that lasts approximately 10 seconds. The center of the linear strobe light is masked to spare the fovea; thus the afterimage line has a break in the middle. Testing is performed by having the patient occlude one eye while the other eye fixates on the central masked part of a strobe light held in front of the patient (Fig. 15-38). One eye is stimulated to produce a vertical afterimage; next the fellow eye is stimulated with a horizontal strobe light. After both eyes have been independently stimulated the patient is asked where they see the afterimage lines while they are binocularly viewing. Since the stimulus is presented under monocular conditions, the stimulus always marks the true fovea of each eye unless there is eccentric fixation with dense amblyopia.

Patients with NRC will, therefore, always see a cross, whether they are orthophoric, esotropic, exotropic, or hypertropic, because their center of reference is the fovea under monocular or binocular conditions (Figs. 15-39, *A* and *B*). Patients with ARC, however, use their true fovea during monocular viewing but during binocular viewing the deviated eye switches to the pseudo-fovea. Consequently even patients with ARC have each fovea marked by the monocular afterimage stimulation. When binocular vision is reestablished, the pseudo-fovea takes over since the center of reference for the deviated eye and the tagged "true fovea" is regarded as a peripheral point. With esotropia the true fovea of the deviated eye is temporal to the pseudo-fovea and projects to the nasal hemifield, causing crossed diplopia, since the right afterimage is seen on the left (Fig. 15-39, *C*). Exotropia is just the opposite, with the fovea nasal to the pseudo-fovea and nasal retina projects to the ipsilateral hemifield, so the right afterimage is seen on the right (Fig. 15-39, *D*).

Vectograph test   The vectographic test is an excellent test for suppression. The test consists of two superimposed polarized slides of letters that are projected onto an aluminized screen that reflects the images while preserving polarization. Polarized glasses are worn by the patient, who is asked to read the letters on the screen. The polarization of the glasses and the projected slides are oriented so some of the letters are only seen by the right eye, some are only seen by the left eye, and some are seen by both eyes. Patients with normal bifoveal fusion will see all the letters. If suppression is present, the letters projected only to the suppressed eye will not be seen. Some patients with suppression will

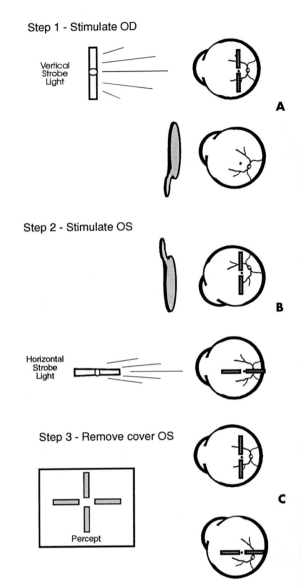

Fig. 15-38   Afterimage test of a patient with NRC. The results of the afterimage test are the same whether the patient has straight eyes, ET, XT, or a hyperdeviation if the patient has NRC. **A,** Right eye is stimulated with a vertical strobe while the left eye is covered. **B,** Left eye is stimulated with a horizontal strobe light while the right eye is covered. **C,** The cover is removed and the patient reports seeing a cross.

alternate fixation and will see all the letters, albeit separately.

Four base-out test   This test is performed by placing a 4 PD base-out prism over one eye to induce fusional convergence. Normals show biphasic fusional convergence eye movements. First is a conjugate version movement of both eyes in the direction of the apex of the prism, and second, a fusion convergence movement of the eye without the prism (it moves "in" towards the nose) (see Chapter 14). With the four base-out test, the examiner must look carefully for the second convergence

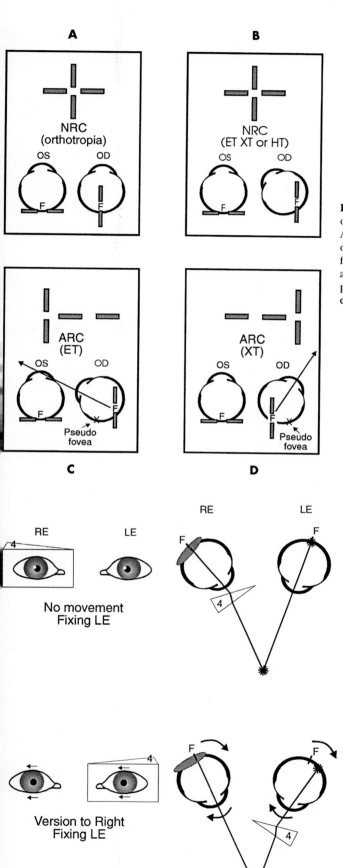

Fig. 15-39   Perception of afterimage test in patients with NRC orthotropia (**A**), NRC and strabismus (**B**), ARC esotropia (**C**), and ARC exotropia (**D**). Note that the stimulation for the afterimage test occurs under monocular conditions and that the light always tags the fovea, even in patients with ARC. After the stimulation the patient is again given binocular vision, so the patient switches back to the pseudo-fovea and the image tagged on the fovea appears to be in an eccentric location (**C** and **D**).

Fig. 15-40   Four base-out prism test performed on a patient with a large suppression scotoma right eye and no motor fusion. **A,** Placing a 4 PD base-out prism in front of the right eye has virtually no effect on the eye movements since the image moves within the suppression scotoma. **B,** Placing the 4 PD base-out prism in front of the fixing eye results in a version movement with both eyes moving in the direction of the apex of the prism, but since there is not fusion there is no convergence movement.

▶ MAJOR POINTS ◀

During the first few weeks of life, saccadic (fast or jerk) eye movements are responsible for refixation, and by 6 weeks of age, smooth pursuit movements develop.

The first 2 to 3 months of life are associated with rapid visual improvement and this period is termed the *critical period of visual development.*

Objects that are outside Panum's fusional area cannot be fused and produce physiologic diplopia.

The brain's ability to determine which images fall on disparate retinal points within Panum's fusional area produces the perception of stereoscopic vision.

Amblyopia should not viewed as an eye problem, but as brain damage caused by abnormal visual stimulation during the sensitive period of visual development (birth to 9 years).

Patients with bilateral hypermetropic amblyopia do not fully accommodate, and therefore it is important to give them their full hypermetropic correction, even in the absence of strabismus.

Myopic anisometropia usually does not cause significant amblyopia unless the difference in refractive error is greater than 5.00 diopters. Hypermetropic anisometropia of as little as +1.50 D is frequently associated with amblyopia.

The crowding phenomenon relates to the fact that patients with amblyopia have better visual acuity reading single optotypes than reading multiple optotypes in a row (linear optotypes).

In patients with latent nystagmus, it is preferable to blur one eye with a plus lens rather than occlude one eye to assess monocular visual acuity, because blurring of one eye causes less nystagmus than occlusion.

The basic strategy for treating amblyopia is to first provide a *clear retinal image,* and then *correct ocular dominance* if dominance is present, as early as possible.

Full-time occlusion may result in reverse amblyopia in children under 4 years of age, so do not use full-time occlusion for more than 1 week per the child's age in years without reexamining the vision in the good eye.

Acquired strabismus in patients older than 8 to 9 years of age usually causes diplopia (crossed = XT, uncrossed = ET).

Monofixation syndrome: Small-angle strabismus (<10 PD), or mild to moderate unilateral retinal image blur, causes suppression of the central visual field of the deviated or blurred eye, but peripheral fusion and gross stereopsis is maintained.

Eccentric fixation occurs in dense amblyopia, usually 20/200 or worse, with nonfoveal fixation during monocular or binocular viewing.

ARC is a sensory adaptation in which the brain reorganizes its retinal orientation to compensate for ocular misalignment, by cortically establishing a pseudofovea in the deviated eye that lines up with the fovea of the fixing eye. ARC is only present during binocular viewing and changes to foveal fixation during monocular fixation.

Patients with the monofixation syndrome have peripheral fusion, so they fuse the near Worth 4-dot, which subtends 6°, but suppress the distance Worth 4-dot, which subtends only 1.25° because the dots fall within the scotoma.

---

movement for it is the sign of fusion. Patients with large regional suppression show no movement of either eye when the prism is placed over the deviated eye (Fig. 15-40, *A*). When the prism is placed over the fixing eye a version (not vergence) movement in the direction of the apex of the prism occurs, but there is no subsequent correctional fusion convergence movement (Fig. 15-40, *B*).

Patients with the monofixation syndrome and a small central scotoma usually show no movement when the 4PD prism is placed over the nondominate eye. Because these patients have peripheral fusion, monofixators occasionally show a normal fusional convergence movement. A prism over the fixing eye always results in a version movement in monofixators and some will also show fusional convergence movement as well. Normal patients with bifoveal fusion often show atypical responses to the four base-out test. Some normals fail to

fuse the 4 PD base-out prism, showing an initial version movement but there is no secondary fusional convergence movement. These patients often alternate fixation and report alternating diplopia. Other normals seem to ignore the induced phoria and show no movement when the 4PD prism is placed over one eye. Thus a secondary fusional convergence movement on four base-out testing indicates fusion (central fusion or even peripheral fusion), but because of frequent atypical responses in normals, absence of a convergence movement does not necessarily mean an absence of fusion.

SUGGESTED READINGS

Hubel KH, Weisel TN: Receptive field, binocular interaction and functional architecture in the cat's visual cortex, *J Physiol* 160:106-154, 1962.

Oliver M, et al: Compliance and results of treatment for amblyopia in children more than 8 years old, *Am J Ophthalmol* 102:340-345, 1986.

Parks MM: The monofixational syndrome, *Trans Am Ophthalmol Soc* 67:609-657, 1969.

Raab E: Refractive amblyopia, *Intl Ophthalmol Clin* II:155, 1971.

Repka MX, Ray JM: The efficacy of optical and pharmacological penalization, *Ophthalmology* 100:769-775, 1993.

Sondhi N, Archer SM, Helveston EM: Development of normal ocular alignment, *J Pediatr Ophthalmol Strabismus* 25:210-211, 1988.

Tychen L. Lisberger SG: Maldevelopment of visual motion procession in humans who had strabismus with onset in infancy, *J Neurosci* 6:2495-2508, 1986.

Vereecken EP, Brabant P: Prognosis for vision in amblyopia after the loss of the good eye, *Archives Ophthalmol* 102:220, 1984.

von Noorden GK: Amblyopia caused by unilateral atropinization, *Ophthalmology* 88:131-133, 1981.

Wright KW, Guyton DL: A test for predicting the effectiveness of penalization on amblyopia. In Henkind P, editor: *Acta: XXIV International Congress of Ophthalmology,* Philadelphia, 1983, JB Lippincott.

Wright KW, Edelman PM, Walonker F, et al: Reliability of fixation preference testing in diagnosing amblyopia, *Arch Ophthalmol* 104:549, 1986.

Wright KW, Walonker F, Edelman P: 10-diopter fixation test for amblyopia, *Arch Ophthalmol* 99:1242-1246, 1981.

Zipf RF: Binocular fixation pattern, *Arch Ophthalmol* 94:401-405, 1976.

Esotropia

Esotropia is an inward turning of the eyes. In contrast to our innate strong fusional convergence (amplitudes >30 prism diopters [PD]), our normal fusional divergence is weak, measuring only 4 to 6 PD. A tendency for the eyes to cross (esotropia) is therefore not easily controlled, since our fusional divergence mechanism is weak. Exphoria, a tendency for the eyes to drift out on the other hand, usually can be controlled by fusional convergence. Patients with an exodeviation tend to have intermittent strabismus and good stereo acuity, whereas patients with an esodeviation tend to have a constant tropia and poor stereo acuity. Esotropia can be divided into the categories listed in the chapter outline, with congenital esotropia and accommodative esotropia being the most common.

CONGENITAL ESOTROPIA (INFANTILE ESOTROPIA)

Congenital esotropia is characterized by a large-angle esotropia that is constantly manifest and occurs during the first few months of life (Fig. 16-1). By definition, the esotropia must be present before 6 months of age. In some cases the esotropia can develop several weeks after birth and, because of this, the more inclusive term *infantile esotropia* has also been used.

In most cases congenital esotropia occurs as an isolated problem in an otherwise healthy child; however, it can be associated with systemic diseases such as Down syndrome, albinism, and cerebral palsy. The differential diagnosis of esotropia occurring in infancy includes Moebius syndrome, congenital fibrosis syndrome, Duane's syndrome, infantile myasthenia gravis, and congenital sixth nerve palsy. Congenital sixth nerve palsy is rare and usually spontaneously resolves over a few weeks. Neurologic processes such as hydrocephalus and intracranial tumors can present with infantile esotropia. Most clinical studies on congenital esotropia exclude patients with neurologic or systemic disease. Thus congenital esotropia is usually defined as a primary esotropia not associated with a sixth nerve palsy, a neurologic condition or a significant restriction. One type of esotropia easily confused with congenital esotropia is in-

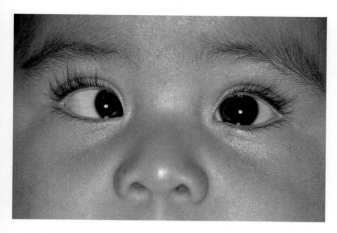

Fig. 16-1   Sixth month old with congenital esotropia. This is a large-angle constant esotropia.

fantile accommodative esotropia (see the following section). These two entities can be difficult to separate since many infants with classic congenital esotropia are significantly hypermetropic (average +2.50) and accommodative esotropia can occur under 6 months of age.

Differential Diagnosis

Box 16-1 lists the differential diagnosis of infantile esotropia.

Normal Neonatal Alignment

It is well known that newborns usually do not have straight eyes. A large population study (Sondhi, et al 1988) documented that approximately 30% of normal neonates have straight eyes, approximately 70% have a small variable exotropia, and less than 1% have esotropia. In that study only 2 out of 2271 neonates had an esotropia at birth and, in both cases, the esotropia resolved by 2 months of age.

Etiology

Suffice it to say, the etiology of congenital esotropia remains unknown. There are probably many types and causes of congenital esotropia. Costenbader suggested that hypermetropia with over convergence plays an important role. He found that of 500 children with congenital esotropia over half had moderate to severe hypermetropia ranging from +2.25 to over +5.00. It is likely that many of the high hypermetropes in Costenbader's study were infantile accommodative esotropias and the patients acquired the esotropia in the first few months after birth.

Another theory on the cause of congenital esotropia is a congenital absence of fusion potential at the cortical level (*Worth theory*). This theory places the blame on a primary cortical fusion deficit that causes a secondary esotropia. Primary cortical fusion loss, however, usually results in a variable small-angle strabismus, either exotropia, esotropia, or hypertropia, not the large-angle constant deviation consistently seen in congenital esotropia. In addition, patients with monocular congenital cataracts lose fusion on a central sensory basis and develop exotropia as often as esotropia. A stronger argument against a primary fusion deficit is that fusion can be achieved in patients with congenital esotropia when surgery is performed in early childhood and infancy.

Others believe that congenital esotropia represents a primary motor dysfunction in infants and these infants do have cortical potential for fusion (*Chavasse theory*). They speculate that the lack of high-grade stereopsis and poor fusion so often associated with congenital esotropia is due to disruption of binocular visual development caused by the esotropia.

The authors' hypothesis is that there are many factors that play a role in causing congenital esotropia. Factors such as early weakness of the lateral rectus muscle, hypermetropia causing accommodative convergence, and a lack of strong cortical fusion, will all predispose an infant to the development of esotropia. Our guess is that most infants with esotropia have the cortical potential for high-grade stereopsis, although some may not. Since there is no way to distinguish between these groups, we should give children with congenital esotropia the benefit of the doubt and treat them all as if they have fusion potential.

Clinical Features

Congenital esotropia is usually a large-angle constant esotropia that measures between 30 and 70 PD and occurs either at or soon after birth. There is a small subset

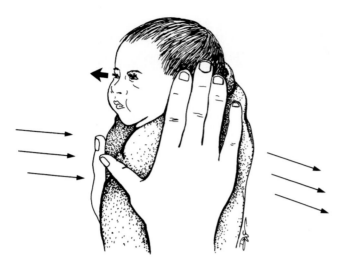

Fig. 16-2 Diagram of an infant in examiner's hands. Infant is moved to the right, which stimulates eye movement to the left. If the right eye fully abducts, then lateral rectus function is normal and there is no significant restriction of the medial rectus muscle. This is an excellent way to examine ductions in an otherwise uncooperative infant.

of infants who develop a relatively small variable esotropia with minimal hypermetropia. These are difficult to manage because of the variable angle of deviation and the poor compliance with low-power hypermetropic spectacles in this young age group. Some of these patients with small-angle esotropia may spontaneously resolve. In general, congenital esotropia rarely resolves spontaneously after 2 months of age, especially if the deviation is constant and larger than 30 PD.

Patients may alternate fixation or show a fixation preference for one eye. Strong fixation preference for one eye indicates significant amblyopia and should be treated by patching the preferred eye before strabismus surgery. Amblyopia occurs in approximately 40% to 50% of children with congenital esotropia.

Patients with congenital esotropia often show some limitation of abduction. In these cases, it is important to verify the abduction deficit by vestibular stimulation with the doll's head maneuver or spinning the infant. Vestibular stimulation is best performed in infants by gently spinning the child. Spinning the child to the examiner's right will cause the eyes to move to the left, thus testing abduction of the patient's right eye (Fig. 16-2). Many children who show an abduction deficit to voluntary abduction will have full abduction by vestibular stimulation. If an abduction deficit persists, assess lateral rectus function by examining the abduction saccade. If there is a brisk abduction saccade, then the lateral rectus is functioning and the limited abduction is restrictive, probably secondary to tight medial rectus muscles. A slow or absent abduction saccade indicates a weak lateral rectus, possibly caused by a sixth nerve palsy or Duane's syn-

drome. Optokinetic stimulation (drum or tape) is a good way to stimulate saccadic eye movements.

Cross-Fixation

Patients with limited abduction and tight medial rectus muscles adopt a face-turn to fixate with eye in adduction. This is similar to patients described by Ciancia (see Ciancia syndrome). These patients may *cross-fixate,* fixing with the right eye for objects in the left visual field and with the left eye for objects in the right visual field. Cross-fixation was once seen as a sign of equal vision but Dickey et al (1991) have reported that cross-fixators can have amblyopia. Patients truly have equal vision if they can hold fixation with either eye through smooth pursuit, without refixating to the fellow eye.

Associated Motor Abnormalities

Box 16-2 lists the motor abnormalities associated with congenital esotropia. These three associated findings may occur individually or in any combination, and usually become manifest sometime after 1 year of age.

Inferior oblique overaction is covered in Chapter 18.

Dissociated vertical deviation (DVD) is elevation, abduction, and extortion of an eye when the binocularity is suspended by monocular occlusion. This tendency for the eye to drift up and out may spontaneously manifest when the patient is fatigued or day dreaming. This is not a true hypertropia since there is no contralateral hypotropia. Note that with a true hypertropia there is a corresponding hypotropia of the nonfixing eye. DVD is a monocular vertical deviation that is almost always bilateral, albeit often very asymmetric. Cover-uncover testing of both eyes shows a bilateral hyperphoria. DVD therefore violates Hering's law of yoke muscles because one eye moves without a similar movement in the same direction from the fellow eye. DVD is most often associated with congenital esotropia, but may occur in virtually any condition that disrupts binocular vision (i.e., monocular congenital cataract, unilateral optic nerve hypoplasia). On version testing, DVD can look like inferior oblique overaction because one side gaze vision of the adducting eye is blocked by the bridge of the nose. This dissociates the eyes causing the DVD of the adducting eye to be manifest. The two can be distinguished since DVD has no corresponding hypotropia of the opposite eye, and the hyperdeviation is the same in abduction and adduction. In inferior oblique overaction there is a hypotropia of the opposite eye and the deviation increases in lateral gaze. DVD and inferior oblique overaction often coexist with congenital esotropia. The cause of dissociated vertical deviation is unknown, but it is associated with abnormal binocular visual development.

The treatment of DVD is surgical if it manifests greater than approximately 50% of the time and or is a cosmetic problem. DVD is almost always bilateral and surgery is usually performed bilaterally. Large recessions of the superior rectus muscles are most commonly performed to correct DVD. Strabismus surgery rarely, if ever, cures DVD, but can improve the condition. Unilateral surgery of the amblyopic eye is indicated if there is amblyopia of three lines or more. If DVD and inferior oblique overaction coexist, then an anterior transposition of the inferior oblique is indicated, since this will address both problems with one procedure.

Dissociated horizontal deviation (DHD), which may be unilateral or bilateral, is a horizontal form of DVD often seen after surgery for congenital esotropia. This is a monocular dissociated condition like DVD, but the abduction component of DVD is exaggerated, with little or no vertical component. Cover-uncover testing may show no shift or even a small esotropia one eye, and an exotropia of the fellow eye. Prolonged occlusion produces an increasing exodeviation. Look for DHD in congenital esotropia patients who have a postoperative intermittent exodeviation especially if the deviation is different depending on which eye is fixing. The treatment of DHD is recession of the ipsilateral lateral rectus muscle.

Latent nystagmus manifests when one eye is occluded, the eyes are dissociated by blurring the vision of one eye, or by suppression of one eye associated with manifest strabismus. This is a jerk-type nystagmus with the fast phase towards the fixing eye. Velocity recordings show that the velocity of the slow phase decreases towards the end of the slow phase eye movement (decreasing velocity slow phase). Latent nystagmus is associated with conditions that disrupt early binocular visual development, such as congenital esotropia and congenital monocular cataracts.

Smooth pursuit asymmetry is a monocular phenomenon in which temporally directed smooth pursuit eye movements are slow and lag behind the fixation target compared to nasally directed smooth pursuit eye movements. Smooth pursuit asymmetry is a normal finding in infants less than 3 months of age, but smooth pursuit should become symmetric by 6 months of age. Patients who have disruption of binocular visual development, as in congenital esotropia or dense unilateral amblyopia, retain smooth pursuit asymmetry throughout life. Virtually all patients with congenital esotropia will have persistent smooth pursuit asymmetry. Smooth pursuit asymmetry is seen by comparing monocular OKN responses from both temporally and nasally directed stimuli.

Inheritance

The inheritance of congenital esotropia remains undefined; however, it is well known that it runs in families. Affected family members may have congenital esotropia, but often other types of strabismus are found including accommodative esotropia and congenital superior oblique palsy. Inheritance patterns for congenital esotropia are variable, which probably speaks to the heterogeneity of this syndrome.

Other Types

Pseudo-esotropia Pseudo-esotropia is a condition where the eyes are orthotropic, but appear to be crossed. This usually occurs in infants who have a wide nasal bridge with prominent epicanthal folds (Fig. 16-3). Pseudo-esotropia usually resolves by 2 or 3 years of age because the epicanthal folds diminish as the bridge of the nose enlarges. Patients with a small interpupillary distance may also appear to be esotropic, especially when the eyes are in side-gaze or are focusing at near. Often parents bring photographs that show the child's eye "turned in." Close examination of these photographs often reveal that the photograph was taken with the child's head turned and the eyes in side-gaze, with the eye that is turned nasally buried under the epicanthal fold. Children with pseudo-strabismus should also have a full ocular examination since some patients will have a true tropia. It is important to follow these children, since a small percentage will end up having a true esodeviation.

Infantile accommodative esotropia Accommodative esotropia can occur in babies as young as 2 months of age and is often classified under the diagnosis congenital esotropia. These infants should be immediately treated with their full hypermetropic correction (see infantile accommodative esotropia in the following section).

Ciancia syndrome Ciancia syndrome is a large-angle congenital esotropia with cross-fixation and both eyes appear to be "stuck" in towards the nose. It consists of the characteristics given in Box 16-3. In Ciancia syndrome the abduction deficit is secondary to tight medial rectus muscles. Clinical examination shows good lateral rectus function evidenced by normal brisk abduction saccades. Forced ductions at the time of surgery shows

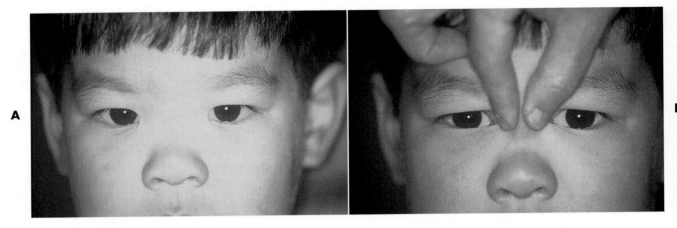

Fig. 16-3   Pseudo-strabismus. **A,** Note the large epicanthal folds giving the appearance of esotropia. **B,** Pinching the epicanthal skin folds demonstrates the eyes are well aligned.

Box 16-3   Characteristics of Ciancia Syndrome

Large-angle deviation (>60 PD)
  Limited abduction bilaterally (with good abduction saccades)
  Fixing eye in adduction
  Nystagmus on attempted abduction with minimal or no nystagmus in adduction
  Face-turn to the side of the fixing eye (Fig. 16-4)

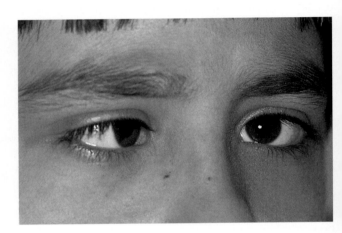

Fig. 16-4   Ciancia syndrome. Patient has a large-angle esotropia, bilateral tight medial rectus muscles, and limited abduction. On attempted abduction there is exaggerated end-point nystagmus with the fast phase to the fixing eye. Vision is most comfortable with the eye in adduction so the patient fixes in adduction and has a face-turn towards the fixing eye.

moderately tight medial rectus muscles. The abduction nystagmus is a jerk-end-point nystagmus with the fast phase in the direction of the fixing eye and only occurs when the fixing eye abducts. This nystagmus is often minimal and may represent an exaggerated end-point nystagmus since the lateral rectus muscle pulls against the tight medial rectus muscles. Ciancia found that approximately one third of his patients with congenital esotropia had this syndrome. It is likely that many of the patients described by Ciancia would have been classified as large-angle congenital esotropia with cross-fixation in American publications. The reason for the face-turn in these patients with a large-angle esotropia and the fixing eye in adduction is probably not to dampen nystagmus, since the nystagmus is usually minimal if present at all. The face-turn is because the medial rectus is tight and will not allow abduction.

Surgically correcting the esotropia associated with Ciancia syndrome is difficult, since undercorrections are frequent. One of the problems is measuring the full deviation because both eyes are "stuck" in adduction, and it is difficult to get the fixing eye into primary position for a true measurement. The surgery of choice is large medial rectus recessions between 6 to 7 mm from the insertion site.

Congenital fibrosis syndrome   This is a congenital restrictive strabismus, often inherited as an autosomal dominant trait (Fig. 16-5). Congenital fibrosis syndrome may cause virtually any horizontal or vertical strabismus and is associated with extremely tight fibrotic rectus muscles on forced duction testing. It frequently presents as a large-angle congenital esotropia with severe limitation of abduction of one or both eyes. This has also been termed *strabismus fixus*. Even though abduction is severely restricted, OKN stimulus or the doll's head maneuver will show abduction saccadic eye movements of brisk, albeit small, amplitude indicating intact lateral rectus function.

Treatment

The treatment of congenital esotropia is usually surgical. Occasionally, infants with esotropia may be cor-

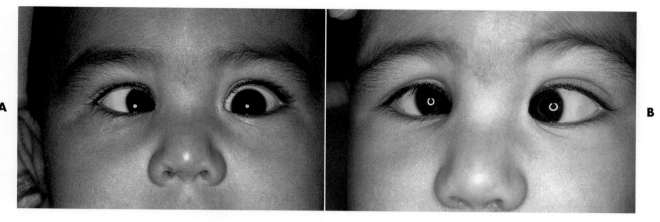

Fig. 16-5   **A,** Patient with congenital esotropia caused by congenital fibrosis syndrome (strabismus fixus) right eye. **B,** The right eye cannot abduct. At the time of strabismus surgery, forced ductions showed a very tight right medial rectus muscle. Surgical exposure of the right medial rectus was extremely difficult because of the total lack of abduction.

rected with hypermetropic spectacle correction. Spectacles should be tried in small-angle cases (ET <40) if hypermetropia is > +2.00, and in patients with large-angle esotropia (>40 PD or more) if the hypermetropic correction is > +3.00.

It is important to fully treat amblyopia before performing surgery with the end point of patching being "holds fixation well" with either eye by fixation preference testing. If the child is cosmetically straightened by the surgery, the parents may feel the problem is cured and they may not return for amblyopia treatment. The only situation when surgery is indicated in the face of residual amblyopia is a tight medial rectus muscle that causes one eye to be buried in the medial canthus even when the good eye is patched. This blocks the vision of the amblyopic eye and makes effective amblyopia therapy impossible. This unusual problem most frequently occurs in association with strabismus fixus of congenital fibrosis syndrome or, rarely, Ciancia syndrome.

The standard surgical approach is bilateral medial rectus recessions. The amount of recession is usually based on the near deviation, since it is difficult to obtain accurate distance measurements in infants. In older patients with irreversible significant amblyopia, limit surgery to the amblyopic eye by performing a recession of the medial rectus muscle and a resection of the lateral rectus muscle.

Timing of surgery and treatment goal   The best time to operate on congenital esotropia remains controversial, with most authorities advocating surgery around 6 months of age. The goal of surgery for congenital esotropia has been to establish peripheral fusion (the monofixation syndrome). To obtain fusion, the esotropia must be corrected to within 8 to 10 PD of orthotropia. Ing was one of the first pediatric ophthalmologists to demonstrate the importance of early surgery for establishing binocular fusion. Ing reported approximately

80% of congenital esotropic patients achieved peripheral fusion if aligned by 2 years of age. In contrast, patients aligned after 2 years of age had less than a 20% chance of obtaining peripheral fusion. Historically, the best sensory result obtainable with congenital esotropia has been peripheral fusion with monofixation syndrome, and bifoveal fixation and high-grade stereopsis were thought to be virtually impossible.

Basic science research by Crawford and von Noorden (1979, 1980, 1983, and 1984) suggests that our classic approach of waiting until 6 months to 2 years may preclude normal bifoveal fusion. These studies have shown that as little as 2 to 3 weeks of prism-induced esotropia will cause permanent loss of binocular cells in infant monkeys. Clinical studies suggest early surgery may result in better binocular fusion. Alignment by 1 year of age resulted in 35% of congenital esotropias developing random-dot stereo acuity (high-grade) versus 0% for those aligned after 1 year. High-grade stereo acuity, even stereopsis of 40 seconds arc, has been shown to be obtainable if the eyes are aligned very early, between 13 and 19 weeks of age (Fig. 16-6). Together with the basic science data, these clinical studies suggest that some patients with congenital esotropia do have the potential for high-grade stereopsis and that early surgery, even as young as 3 months of age, may be beneficial.

Postoperative care   All patients with congenital esotropia should be followed closely for amblyopia even if good motor alignment is achieved. The goal of surgery is to obtain alignment within 8 to 10 PD of orthotropia to allow for the establishment of peripheral fusion and the monofixation syndrome. Deviations larger than 10 PD preclude the development of even peripheral fusion. Postoperative tropias greater than 10 PD should be treated either with further surgery or spectacle correction.

Consecutive exotropia   An initial small-angle exotro-

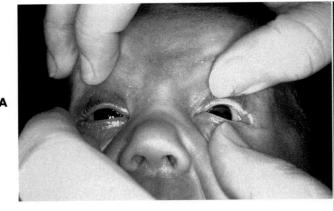
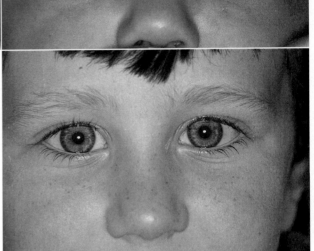
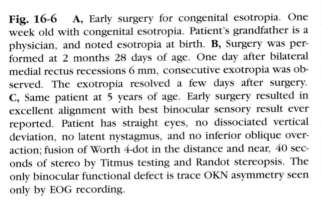

Fig. 16-6   **A,** Early surgery for congenital esotropia. One week old with congenital esotropia. Patient's grandfather is a physician, and noted esotropia at birth. **B,** Surgery was performed at 2 months 28 days of age. One day after bilateral medial rectus recessions 6 mm, consecutive exotropia was observed. The exotropia resolved a few days after surgery. **C,** Same patient at 5 years of age. Early surgery resulted in excellent alignment with best binocular sensory result ever reported. Patient has straight eyes, no dissociated vertical deviation, no latent nystagmus, and no inferior oblique overaction; fusion of Worth 4-dot in the distance and near, 40 seconds of stereo by Titmus testing and Randot stereopsis. The only binocular functional defect is trace OKN asymmetry seen only by EOG recording.

pia is probably desirable in infants young enough to have fusion potential; however, a persistent exotropia after 4 to 6 weeks may require additional surgery. If the consecutive exotropia is incomitant or associated with an adduction deficit, consider the possibility of a slipped muscle. The treatment of choice for a consecutive exotropia without a slipped muscle is bilateral lateral rectus recessions. If there is an adduction deficit, explore for the possibility of a slipped medial rectus.

Residual esotropia   A residual esotropia greater than 10 to 15 PD that persists longer than 6 to 8 after weeks after surgery should be treated. The first line of treatment is to give the full hypermetropic spectacle correction if the cycloplegic refraction is +1.50 or more. If there continues to be a significant esotropia after glasses are prescribed or there is not enough hypermetropia to warrant glasses, then surgery should be considered, especially if the child is under 2 years of age and there is fusion potential. If the initial recession was 5 mm or less, I prefer a re-recession of one or both of the medial rectus muscles. A bilateral 2 mm re-recession corrects roughly 20 to 25 PD of residual esotropia. Patients with residual esotropia and initial recessions greater than 5 mm should be managed with lateral rectus resections, doing slightly less than described on the standard charts. Remember that you are resecting against a previously recessed medial rectus muscle, so do a slightly smaller resection to avoid an overcorrection.

Prognosis   There are only a few long-term outcome studies on congenital esotropia. Studies that look at short-term outcomes of 6 months to 1 year claim a 70% to 80% success rate. With a 5-year follow up, however, the incidence of reoperation for a horizontal misalignment increases to 40%. Add to that the incidence of vertical strabismus surgery for DVD and inferior oblique muscle overaction, the chances that a child will need a reoperation is probably well over 50%.

The binocular sensory outcome is also relatively poor. Except for a handful of cases, the best result is monofixation with peripheral fusion and only gross stereopsis. Ing's report showed that 80% of congenital esotropic patients achieved peripheral fusion if aligned by age 2 years, but only cases with good postoperative alignment were included in the study. Monofixation and peripheral fusion does not guarantee long-term stability, since a high percentage of patients will lose binocular fusion over time. Very early surgery may improve binocular sensory results.

Investigational role of botulinum   In addition to surgery, some practitioners have advocated the use of botulinum for the treatment of congenital esotropia. The theoretic advantage would be to create an incomitant deviation so the patient could adopt a face-turn and obtain fusion. This is a good theoretic strategy; however, there are some problems involved with the use of botulinum including secondary ptosis and the temporary effect of the botulinum injection. Most studies have shown that multiple injections are needed to sustain the effect. The treatment of choice for patients with congenital esotropia remains surgical; however, investigations continue regarding the use of botulinum.

ACCOMMODATIVE ESOTROPIA

The term *accommodative esotropia* applies to esotropia caused by over-convergence in response to accommodation. In most cases, accommodative esotropia is associated with significant hypermetropia of +2.00 or more and is termed *hypermetropic accommodative esotropia* or *refractive esotropia*. Prescribing the full hypermetropic spectacle correction will improve or, in many cases, totally correct the esotropia. Some patients with accommodative esotropia have a *high AC/A ratio esotropia*. These patients have a greater deviation at near versus distance. They are usually hypermetropic but may be emmetropic or even myopic.

Acquired esotropia deserves an urgent consultation. Delay of treatment will reduce the chances for reestablishing binocular fusion. In addition, acquired esotropia may represent a neurologic process, so urgent evaluation is important.

Hypermetropic Accommodative Esotropia

Etiology   Hypermetropic accommodative esotropia is caused by accommodative convergence associated with hypermetropia. These children have straight eyes as infants, but as they learn to accommodate to correct for their hypermetropia, they over converge and develop esotropia. For example, a child with hypermetropia of +3.00 would have to accommodate 3 diopters to create a clear retinal image for distance viewing. If the AC/A ratio is 6 (normal), the accommodative convergence will produce an esodeviation of 18 PD. Depending on the patient's interpupillary distance and divergence fusional amplitudes, this patient may develop an esodeviation.

Clinical features   Accommodative esotropia usually presents as an acquired intermittent esotropia. The onset is from infancy to late childhood, most commonly occurring around 2 years of age. The size of deviation is variable and is typically smaller than congenital esotropia, usually measuring between 20 and 40 PD. Cycloplegic refraction reveals hypermetropia between +1.50 and +6.50 diopters. Parents often give a history that the eyes are straight some of the time; however, when the child is tired or focusing at near objects the eyes cross. The esotropia is initially intermittent, but may quickly increase to become a constant deviation. Patients with constant esotropia may lose fusion potential and are prone to develop amblyopia.

Cycloplegic refraction   An accurate cycloplegic re-

fraction is required to determine the full hypermetropic correction. Young children are often difficult to refract and repeat cycloplegic refractions help ensure accuracy. Cyclopentolate is the standard cycloplegic agent. Consider using atropine in patients with a darkly pigmented iris who show variable retinoscopy readings. Cyclopentolate is given topically, one or two doses for a lightly pigmented iris, and two or three doses for a dark iris. The refraction is performed 30 minutes after the last dose. Atropine is given twice a day for 3 days and the refraction is done on the third day. The mydriatic effect of these drugs lasts much longer than the cycloplegic effect, so a dilated pupil does not mean complete cycloplegia.

Treatment of hypermetropic accommodative esotropia   The treatment of hypermetropic accommodative esotropia is to prescribe the full hypermetropic correction (see Example 1). In both juvenile onset and infantile onset accommodative esotropia, full hypermetropic correction should be prescribed as soon as the esotropia is identified, even giving glasses to children as young as 2 months of age.

Example 1
2 year old with esotropia for 2 months
Full ductions and versions
Cycloplegic refraction = +4.50 OU

Without correction (sc)	With correction (cc) + 4.50 OU
Dsc ET 30	Dcc E 4 (phoria-fusing)
Nsc ET 35	Ncc E 2 (phoria-fusing)

Treatment
Prescribe Spectacles + 4.50 sphere OU

It is important that the child wears the optical correction full time. Children who intermittently remove their glasses will not relax their accommodation and will have blurred vision with their appropriate hypermetropic correction. For children who have difficulty relaxing accommodation and thus do not accept their hypermetropic correction, it may be helpful to prescribe a short course of cycloplegics such as *atropine* or cyclopentolate. We also have found that extended-wear contact lenses are useful in selected children who will not wear their spectacles. Parents should be told that the glasses are prescribed to straighten the eyes by relaxing the overfocusing caused by the farsightedness. The glasses may not necessarily improve visual acuity.

If, after prescribing full hypermetropic correction, the eyes are straightened to within 10 PD distance and near, and the patient obtains binocular fusion, nothing more needs to be done. Continue with the full hypermetropic correction. Some ophthalmologists advocate reducing the plus lens until an esophoria is induced. This is done to try to build fusional divergence and wean the child out of glasses. I have not seen this practice eliminate the need for spectacles, but I have all too frequently seen it turn a well-controlled deviation into a manifest esotropia. By reducing the plus, you run the risk of producing a manifest esotropia and losing binocular fusion.

Remember, children with accommodative esotropia have tenuous fusion. To establish the best binocular function, the goal must be to align the eyes to orthotropia.

If, after wearing full hypermetropic spectacles for 4 to 8 weeks, a residual esotropia of greater than 10 PD to 15 PD is present for distance and near (the patient is not fusing), which is termed *partially accommodative esotropia,* then surgery is indicated (see the following section). In some cases the full hypermetropic correction will align the eyes for distance; however, a residual esotropia will persist at near. These patients have a high AC/A ratio and bifocals are indicated (see the following section).

High AC/A Ratio Esotropia

A subgroup of patients with accommodative esotropia will have a high AC/A ratio and have a significantly larger esotropia at near. High AC/A ratio esotropia usually occurs in patients with hypermetropia, but may occur in patients with myopia or no refractive error. If the eyes are straight in the distance (<10 PD), a bifocal add is given to correct the near deviation and promote near fusion.

Example 2
4 year old with esotropia for 2 months
Full ductions and versions
Cycloplegic refraction = +3.50 OU

Without correction (sc)	With correction (cc) + 3.50 OU
Dsc ET 25	Dcc E 4 (phoria-fusing)
Nsc ET 55	Ncc ET 25
	Ncc & +3.00 add E 3 (phoria-fusing)

Treatment
Prescribe bifocals (+ 3.50 sphere upper; +3.00 add, OU)

Prescribing bifocals A bifocal plus add is indicated for patients who are fusing in the distance but have an esotropia at near that is large enough to interfere with near fusion (>8 to 10 PD). The plus add will relax near accommodation, thus reducing convergence. If the AC/A ratio is 7 (high) then a +3.00 add will reduce the near esotropia by 21 PD. In Example 2 the +3.00 add reduced the residual near deviation with correction to an esophoria of 3 PD allowing binocular fusion. Usually start with a +3.00 add (that is the maximum). Over time, the bifocal add can be diminished slowly to promote divergence. Reduce the add to produce a small esophoria of no more than 4 to 6 PD. This will stimulate divergence, while maintaining comfortable binocular fusion. In many cases, the bifocal can be eliminated by 10 to 12 years of age. The best bifocal is a flat-top that bisects the pupil. A common mistake is to prescribe a low bifocal, which is easily overlooked by the child (no pun intended).

Remember that bifocals will not treat a manifest esotropia in the distance. If a patient has an esotropia in the distance greater than 10 PD with full hypermetropic correction and is not fusing, then surgery is indicated, not bifocals. Bifocals, however, may be needed postoperatively if a near esotropia persists.

Partially Accommodative Esotropia

If, after wearing full hypermetropic correction, a residual esotropia (> 10 PD) for distance and near exists, it is known as partially accommodative esotropia (Fig. 16-7). The treatment is surgery: bilateral medial rectus muscle recessions.

Example 3
3 year old esotropia for 2 months
Full ductions and versions
Cycloplegic refraction = +3.50 OU

Dsc ET 30	Dcc ET 20
Nsc ET 35	Ncc ET 25

Treatment
Strabismus surgery = bilateral medial rectus recessions

After wearing the +3.50 sphere for 6 weeks, the patient in Example 3 still has a significant esotropia in the distance (20 PD). This residual esotropia cannot be fused and should be addressed surgically. Bifocals are not indicated, since they will not correct the distance deviation. Preoperatively, it is important to re-refract these patients to make sure that the full latent hypermetropia is corrected.

Surgery for partially accommodative esotropia Bilateral medial rectus recession is the procedure of choice for partially accommodative esotropia. There is, however, controversy regarding how to determine the target angle. Historically, surgery has been performed for the residual deviation measured with correction in the distance (i.e., *standard surgery*). In Example 3 the standard surgery target angle is ET 20. Unfortunately, this standard surgery approach results in a high undercorrection rate of approximately 25%. Because of this unacceptably high undercorrection rate, many surgeons are augmenting their surgical numbers for partially accommodative esotropia. The idea of surgery is not to eliminate hypermetropic correction by overcorrection, but to get the eyes straight and fusing with full hypermetropic correction. Parents should be advised that spectacles will be required postoperatively.

Augmented surgery Various formulas are used to augment standard surgery. I have studied results using a target angle determined by averaging the near deviation with correction and the near deviation without correction. In Example 3 the augmented surgery target angle is 30 PD ([35+25]/2). Results comparing standard surgery to my augmented surgery formula showed a 26% undercorrection for standard surgery, whereas augmented surgery resulted in a 93% success rate with 7% overcorrected. Three out of the 40 augmented surgery patients

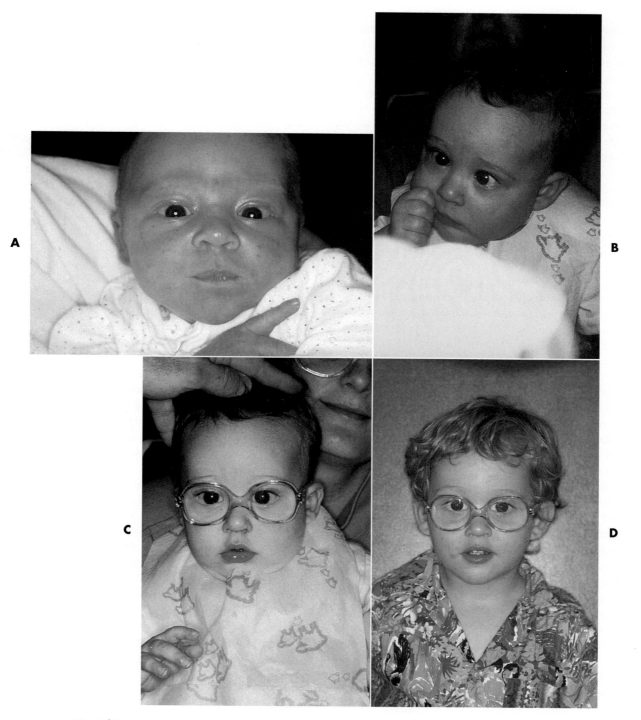

Fig. 16-7   Infantile accommodative esotropia. The patient is the author's youngest son. **A,** At 6 weeks of age, the patient's eyes were well aligned with normal motility. **B,** At 2½ months of age a variable esotropia occurred. Deviation measured between essentially straight eyes and an esotropia of 40 prism diopters. **C,** Cycloplegic refraction at 2½ months of age revealed a +5.00 refractive error OU. Patient was given full hypermetropic correction. However, a small residual esotropia persisted. Note that the left eye is deviated and the Bruckner reflex shows a brighter reflex left eye. Augmented surgery was performed at 5½ months of age by the author. **D,** Patient 3 years after surgery with straight eyes, excellent binocular function with stereoacuity measured by Randot testing. At the time of this writing he is 9½ years old and is still well aligned.

studied required a reduction in plus spectacle power to correct a small consecutive distance exotropia, and there was only one persistent overcorrection with a minimum follow-up of 1 year. The patients who were overcorrected all had a high AC/A ratio, were well aligned at near, and had an intermittent exotropia in the distance. The augmented surgery formula is based on the near measurement, so it is not surprising that patients with a high AC/A ratio have a tendency for overcorrection in the distance. To determine the target angle, I now recommend averaging the near deviation without correction (largest deviation) and the distance deviation with correction (smallest deviation), or using prism adaptation in these difficult to manage high AC/A ratio patients (see the following section).

Prism adaptation Another method for determining the amount of surgical correction in patients with partially accommodative esotropia is using prism adaptation. Prism adaptation consists of prescribing base-out prism for the residual esotropia after prescribing full hypermetropic correction. In Example 3 the initial press-on prism would be 20 PD base out. The patient returns in approximately 2 weeks after wearing the prisms. If the esotropia has increased, then the prisms are increased. This continues at 1- to 2-week intervals until the deviation has stabilized. The surgeon operates on the full prism-adapted angle as determined by the press-on prisms. Operating on the larger adapted-angle reduces the undercorrection rate. Results of a multi-center study on prism adaptation showed that standard surgery resulted in approximately 75% successful correction rate and operating on the prism-adapted angle resulted in an 85% success rate. The disadvantage of prism adaptation is the cost and time involved with prescribing press-on prisms and reexamining the patient until the deviation stabilizes.

Postoperative care Postoperative care would be similar to that described previously under congenital esotropia. The goal is to achieve binocular fusion since most patients with acquired strabismus have fusion potential. Patients who are aligned for distance but have an esotropia greater than 8 to 10 PD at near may be candidates for bifocals. If a small-angle esotropia persists, consider prescribing hypermetropic correction, even as little as 1.50 diopters. A small consecutive exotropia can be managed by reducing the plus of hypermetropic spectacles, but do not "cut the plus" more than 3.00 diopters.

Miotics In selected patients, miotic drops such as phospholine iodide (i.e., Echothiophate Iodide) may be indicated to treat accommodative esotropia. Miotics, such as phospholine iodide, are cholinesterase inhibitors and increase the effectiveness of locally released acetylcholine. Topical phospholine iodine has a parasympathomimetic affect on the iris sphincter and ciliary muscles causing miosis and pharmacologic accommodation. Acetylcholine released in the ciliary body will last longer and produce more accommodation for a given amount of innervational stimulation. Thus miotics reduce the accommodative effort necessary to provide a clear retinal image and likewise reduce the amount of associated reflex convergence. Miotics truly reduce the AC/A ratio and esotropia associated with hypermetropia.

Miotics can be tried if the patient has a high AC/A ratio and has minimal hypermetropia. In the vast majority of cases, however, bifocal spectacles are the treatment of choice. Another indication for the use of miotics is in children who cannot wear spectacles or contact lenses. This is most useful for short periods of time, perhaps during the summer months when children are swimming. Miotics are occasionally used as a diagnostic test to determine if an esotropia will respond to hypermetropic optical correction. If the miotics fail to correct the deviation, this would identify a nonaccommodative component. Unfortunately, the only way to know if spectacles will correct the deviation is to actually prescribe spectacles. When using miotics, it is preferable to start with a low dose of phospholine iodide, 0.03%, one drop every morning. If this dose is not sufficient to correct the esotropia, the dose may be increased to twice a day or use phospholine iodide 0.125%.

Adverse effects of miotics Phospholine iodide, even when given topically, is systemically absorbed and will lower cholinesterase activity in the blood for several weeks. This is of significance in patients who undergo general anesthesia with succinylcholine. Phospholine iodide prolongs the effect of the succinylcholine and may prolong respiratory paralysis after surgery. Succinylcholine should be avoided if phospholine iodide has been used within 6 weeks before surgery. Systemic side effects of miotics may include brow ache, headaches, nausea, and abdominal cramping. If the lower dose of phospholine iodide is used, these complications are infrequent.

Ocular side effects of phospholine iodide include iris cysts along the pupillary margin in 20% to 50% of cases, which can occur anywhere from several weeks to several months after treatment. Iris cysts tend to regress after discontinuing phospholine iodide; however, this author has seen persistent iris cysts several years after stopping phospholine iodide therapy. Phenylephrine used in combination with phospholine iodide may prevent iris cysts. Other rare and unusual complications include lens opacities, retinal detachment in adults, and angle-closure glaucoma.

Infantile Accommodative Esotropia

Infantile accommodative esotropia is frequently confused with congenital esotropia. The key to diagnosing infantile accommodative esotropia is the presence of straight eyes for the first 2 to 3 months, a variable angle esotropia at the onset, and hypermetropia (>2.00). Treatment is to immediately prescribe the full hypermetropic correction as determined by a good cycloplegic refraction and treat amblyopia if present. If spectacles do not align the eyes to within 10 PD, then strabismus surgery is indicated (see partially accommodative esotropia). Approximately half the patients will be corrected with spectacles alone and half will require surgery. This author is personally very familiar with this disorder since his youngest son developed accommodative esotropia at 2½ months of age and required surgery (see Fig. 16-7).

The prognosis for binocular fusion in patients with accommodative esotropia is quite good since most patients have had straight eyes for several years. The treatment goal for accommodative esotropia is establishing binocular fusion and stereopsis.

ACQUIRED NONACCOMMODATIVE ESOTROPIA

Primary esotropia may be acquired during childhood or adulthood not in association with hypermetropia. Initially, these deviations are variable and intermittent. However, over time (weeks, months, or even years), the esodeviation becomes constant. It is important in cases of acquired esotropia to rule out the possibility of an intracranial tumor, Arnold-Chiari malformation, or a neurologic process such as myasthenia gravis. A divergence paralysis pattern with a larger esotropia in the distance than at near is a red flag to the possibility of a mild sixth nerve paresis and a neurologic disorder.

The treatment for acquired nonaccommodative esotropia is usually surgery and the prognosis for reestablishing binocular fusion is relatively good. Undercorrections are frequent in this group and prism adaptation will help reduce the number of patients with a residual esotropia.

ESOPHORIA

Small esophorias (8 to 10 PD) can cause significant asthenopic symptoms. These patients usually complain of headaches and fatigue when reading for long periods of time. Small esophorias are best treated with hypermetropic correction for near, or base-out prisms. A reading add relaxes accommodation and convergence, thus correcting the esophoria. Base-out prisms will also correct the esophoria; however, patients tend to adapt to the prisms and require increasing prisms over time. If prisms are prescribed, prescribe slightly less than the full deviation to stimulate some divergence. In cases of a large esophoria, surgery may be required. In these cases it is helpful to use prism adaptation to disclose the full underlying esophoria. In any case of a symptomatic esophoria, a cycloplegic refraction is indicated, since latent hypermetropia is a common cause for an acquired esodeviation.

ESOTROPIA, NYSTAGMUS, AND FACE-TURN

Nystagmus may be associated with esotropia. These patients will often adopt a face-turn to dampen the nystagmus and improve visual acuity. Specific types of esotropia, nystagmus, and face-turn syndromes have been described including (1) manifest latent nystagmus, (2) congenital nystagmus with constant esotropia, (3) nystagmus compensation syndrome, and (4) Ciancia syndrome (see the previous section on congenital esotropia). The face-turn is used to position the fixing eye at the null point. In the case of manifest latent nystagmus, nystagmus compensation syndrome, and Ciancia syndrome, the null point is always in adduction. Consequently, the fixing eye in these cases is always adducted and the face-turn is towards the side of the fixing eye (Fig. 16-8).

Manifest Latent Nystagmus

Latent nystagmus that spontaneously becomes apparent or when manifest without monocular occlusion is called *manifest latent nystagmus*. The null point for latent nystagmus or manifest latent nystagmus is always in adduction. Patients with strabismus and manifest latent nystagmus will place the fixing eye in adduction to improve vision. This produces a face-turn to the side of the fixing eye. Patients with esotropia, nystagmus, and face-turn caused by manifest latent nystagmus have latent nystagmus and an intermittent esophoria, both of which are controlled by peripheral fusion. At times, the patient has straight eyes or a microtropia with peripheral fusion, the latent nystagmus is controlled and there is no face-turn. Other times (i.e., when the patient is fatigued) the esophoria breaks down to an esotropia and the manifest esotropia results in cortical suppression and loss of peripheral fusion. Loss of peripheral fusion changes the latent nystagmus to a manifest latent nystagmus causing the patient to adopt a face-turn to place the fixing eye at the null point, which is in adduction (Fig. 16-9).

The treatment of manifest latent nystagmus with face-turn is to enhance binocular fusion to avoid the tropia phase of the esotropia. Methods for enhancing binocular fusion in patients with esotropia include providing hypermetropic correction in patients with an accommodative component or operate for the residual esodeviation. In an article by Zubcov (1990), five patients with esotropia and manifest latent nystagmus underwent strabismus surgery resulting in straight eyes, which converted the

Fig. 16-8   A, Patient with esotropia, nystagmus, and face-turn. In this case, the null point of the nystagmus is in adduction. The patient adopts a face-turn to the right to place the fixing right eye in adduction. **B,** Companion drawing of the patient in *A*. Note that the right eye is fixing in adduction and that the face-turn is to the same side as the fixing eye.

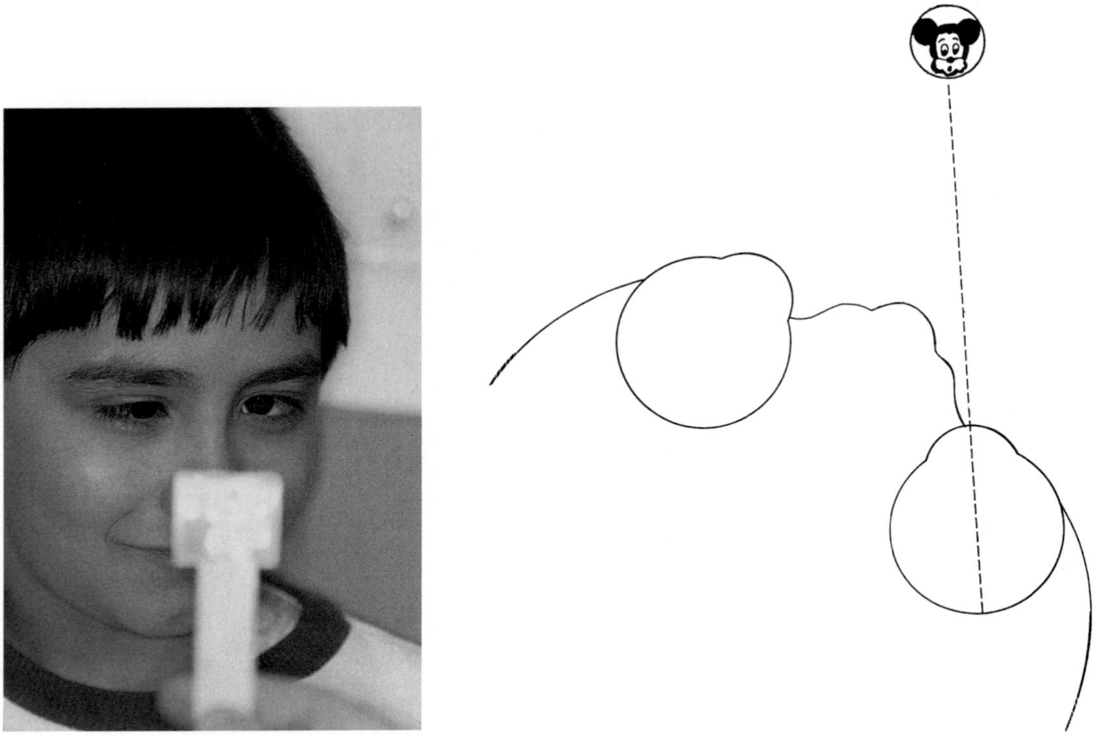

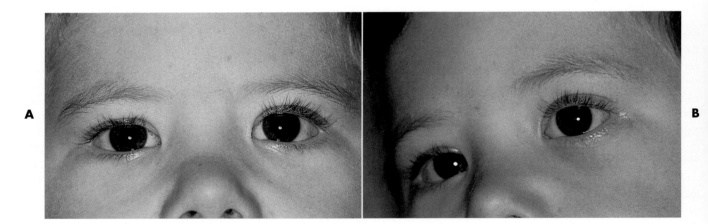

Fig. 16-9   Patient with Down syndrome and previous surgery for congenital esotropia. Patient now has an intermittent esotropia with peripheral fusion and the monofixation syndrome. **A,** Patient is fusing with an esophoria after surgery and has latent nystagmus, which is controlled as long as the patient is fusing. Note that there is no face-turn. **B,** Now the patient is focusing on an accommodative target and is manifesting an esotropia. The esotropia disrupts fusion and changes the latent nystagmus into a manifest latent nystagmus. The null point of manifest latent nystagmus is in adduction, so the fixing eye (the right eye) moves into adduction and the patient develops a face-turn to the right.

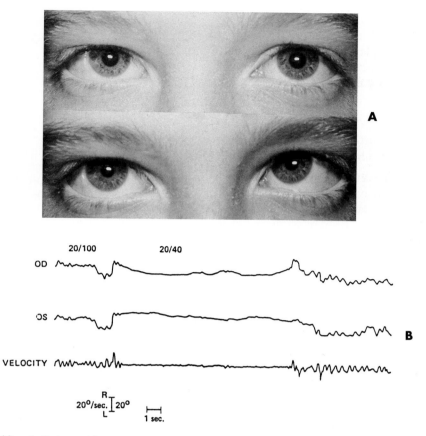

Fig. 16-10   A, Patient with nystagmus compensation syndrome. *Top,* Patient with congenital nystagmus, straight eyes, and mid-dilated pupils. When patient tries to read near target, the patient
invokes accommodative convergence to dampen the nystagmus and an esotropia occurs. Visual
acuity improves to 20/40 at near *(bottom)* **B,** Electrooculograph of a patient with congenital nystagmus and nystagmus compensation syndrome. At the beginning of the tracing, the congenital
nystagmus shows large amplitude and visual acuity is 20/100. The patient then uses accommodative
convergence to dampen the nystagmus, an esotropia occurs, and visual acuity improves to 20/40 at
near. The amplitude of the nystagmus increases as patient relaxes accommodative convergence and
the congenital nystagmus recurs. (**A,** Courtesy of G.K. von Noorden; From von Noorden GK, Munoz
M, Wong SY: *Am J Ophthalmol* 104:391,1987.)

manifest latent nystagmus back to latent nystagmus. Four
out of the five patients also showed improvement in binocular visual acuity because of the decreased nystagmus.

Congenital Nystagmus with Constant Esotropia

Patients with congenital nystagmus may have an associated esotropia. These patients commonly adopt a face-
turn to place the fixing eye at the null point. The null
point in congenital nystagmus may be in any gaze position. If the null point is in adduction, fixing right eye, the
face-turn will be to the right. Null point in abduction
causes the fixing eye to abduct, and the face-turn is to the
left. A vertical null point position causes a compensatory
chin depression or chin elevation. Obviously, there is no
face-turn if the null point is in primary position.

Congenital nystagmus is a jerk or pendular nystagmus.
The characteristics of congenital nystagmus are different
from manifest latent nystagmus. With congenital nystagmus, there is an increasing velocity of the slow phase and
no change in the nystagmus on unilateral occlusion or
binocular dissociation. The nystagmus switches direction on side gaze with the fast phase to the right in right
gaze and fast phase to the left in left gaze. Congenital
nystagmus and latent or manifest latent nystagmus can
occur concurrently.

The treatment for the face-turn with esotropia is to
perform strabismus surgery to *move the null point of the
fixing eye* to primary position. Then, if necessary, move
the nonfixing eye to match. For example, if there is a
right esotropia of 40 PD (20°), right eye fixing in adduction, with a face-turn to the right 20° (see Fig. 16-8), then
recess the right medial rectus and resect the right lateral

rectus for 40 PD. This will move the right eye to primary position and correct the face-turn and the esotropia at the same time. If the esotropia had measured more than 40 PD, then add a medial rectus recession left eye for the amount not corrected by the recessed and resected right eye.

Nystagmus Compensation Syndrome (Nystagmus Blockage Syndrome)

Some patients with congenital nystagmus and straight eyes may use accommodative convergence to dampen their nystagmus. In rare circumstances, this can produce an esotropia. In the past, this rare syndrome of an esotropia caused by accommodative convergence to dampen or "block" nystagmus has been termed *nystagmus blockage syndrome* or *nystagmus compensation syndrome*. These patients present with straight eyes and congenital nystagmus. On viewing near targets, they manifest a variable esodeviation since they use accommodative convergence to dampen the nystagmus to improve vision. Key observations include variable angle esotropia, intermittent esotropia only at near, and pupillary miosis, which occurs with the esotropia (Fig. 16-10). Many patients who have previously been reported in the literature as having nystagmus blockage syndrome or nystagmus compensation syndrome actually had manifest latent nystagmus. Some practitioners have doubted the existence of congenital nystagmus with accommodative convergence causing esotropia; however, von Noorden (1987) has documented this syndrome with EOG recordings. There is no good surgical treatment for this esotropia at near; however, von Noorden has suggested a small medial rectus recession with Faden (posterior fixation suture).

CYCLIC ESOTROPIA

Cyclic esotropia is a very rare type of esotropia with most pediatric ophthalmologists only seeing one or two cases in their entire career. This is an acquired esotropia that occurs at virtually any age, but most frequently occurs between 2 to 6 years of age. These patients cycle between straight eyes and esotropia every 48 or 24 hours. To help establish a pattern, ask the parents to plot on a calendar the days when the eyes are crossed versus the days when the eyes are straight. When the eyes are aligned, the patient has good binocular vision and stereoacuity. Cyclic esotropia is usually progressive and over several months to years, the esodeviation finally becomes constant in most cases. Some cases of cyclic esotropia are associated with hypermetropia and in these cases, the full cycloplegic correction should be given. In cases where there is no significant hypermetropia surgery for

MAJOR POINTS

- By definition, the congenital esotropia must be present before 6 months of age. It is a large-angle esotropia that can develop from birth to several weeks after birth. Because of this, the more inclusive term *infantile esotropia* has also been used.
- Strong fixation preference for one eye indicates significant amblyopia and should be treated by patching the preferred eye before strabismus surgery.
- Amblyopia occurs in approximately 40% to 50% of children with congenital esotropia.
- It is important to fully treat amblyopia before performing surgery with the end point of patching being "holds fixation well" with either eye by fixation preference testing.
- The triad of classical motor abnormalities associated with congenital esotropia includes *inferior oblique overaction* (70%), *dissociated vertical deviation (DVD)* (75%), and *latent nystagmus* (50%). Another associated finding that has more recently been described is *persistent smooth pursuit asymmetry*.
- The goal of surgery for congenital esotropia is alignment within 8 to 10 PD of orthotropia in infancy to allow for the establishment of peripheral fusion and the monofixation syndrome.
- Accommodative esotropia is treated by prescribing the full plus.
- A bifocal plus add is indicated for patients who are fusing in the distance but have an esotropia at near.
- If, after wearing full hypermetropic correction, a residual esotropia (> 10 PD) for distance and near exists, a partially accommodative esotropia is present. The treatment is surgical, bilateral medial rectus muscle recessions.
- Cyclic esotropia can be acquired at virtually any age, but most frequently occurs between 2 to 6 years of age. These patients have straight eyes except on a 48- or 24-hour cycle when they develop an esotropia.
- In cases of acquired esotropia with divergence paresis the practitioner must rule out intracranial tumors, Arnold-Chiari malformation, and neurologic process such as myasthenia gravis.

the full deviation should be performed to provide appropriate eye alignment and preserve binocularity and fusion. Sporadic cases associated with central nervous system disease have been reported (Pillai and Dhand, 1987).

DIVERGENCE PARESIS

Divergence paresis produces an esodeviation that is greater in the distance than near. It can occur idiopathically as a primary strabismus. An important cause for divergence paralysis is a mild sixth nerve palsy, causing an esodeviation in the distance. An acquired esodeviation with a divergence paresis pattern is a red flag for possible neurologic disease. Divergence paresis has been associated with pontine tumor, head trauma, myesthenia gravis, and Arnold-Chiari syndrome. Neuroimaging studies, as well as a neurologic consultation, are indicated to rule out possible neurologic disease.

SENSORY ESOTROPIA

Sensory esotropia is an esotropia occurring secondary to unilateral blindness. It has been the general teaching that, if the vision loss occurred before 2 years of age, the patient will develop esotropia and after 2 years will develop exotropia. This has not been borne out, though, since many infants with unilateral visual loss develop exotropia. Surgery for sensory esotropia is a recession medial rectus muscle and a resection lateral rectus muscle of the blind eye.

SUGGESTED READINGS

Aiello A, Borchert MS, Wright KW: Independence of optokinetic nystagmus asymmetry and binocularity in infantile esotropia, *Arch Ophthalmol* 112:1580-1583, 1994.

Archer SM, Sondhi N, Helveston EM: Strabismus in infancy, *Ophthalmology* 96:133-137, 1989.

Arthur BW, Smith JT, Scott WE: Long-term stability of alignment in the monofixation syndrome, *J Pediatr Ophthalmol Strabismus* 26:224-231, 1989.

Baker JD, Parks MM: Early onset accommodative esotropia, *Am J Ophthalmol* 90:11, 1980.

Birch EE, Stager DR, Everett ME: Random dot stereo acuity following surgical correction of infantile esotropia, *J Pediatr Ophthalmal Strabismus* 32:231-235, 1995.

Ciancia AO: La esotropia con limitacion bilateral de la abduccion en el lactante. Leido en la Sociedad Argentina de Oftalmolgia el dia 19 de septiembre de 1962. Beunos Aires.

Costenbader FD: Infantile esotropia, *Trans Am Ophthalmol Soc* 59:397, 1961.

Crawford MLJ, von Noorden GK: Optically induced concomitant strabismus in monkeys, *Invest Ophthalmol Vis Sci* 19: 1105, 1980.

Dell'Osso LF, Ellenberger Jr. C, Abel LA, et al: The nystagmus blockage syndrome, *Invest Ophthalmol Vis Sci* 24:1580, 1983.

Helveston EM: Cyclic strabismus, *Am Orthoptic J* 23:4851, 1971.

Ing, MR: Early surgical alignment for congenital esotropia, *Tr Am Ophth Sci* 79:625-663, 1981.

Magoon E: Chemodenervation of strabismic children, *Ophthalmology* 96:931-934, 1989.

Pollard ZF: Accommodative esotropia during the first year of life, *Arch Ophthalmol* 94:1912, 1976.

Pratt-Johnson JA, Tillson G: Acquired central disruption of fusional amplitude, *Ophthalmology* 86:2140, 1979.

Prism Adaptation Research Group: Efficacy of prism adaptation in the surgical management of acquired esotropia, *Arch Ophthalmol* 108:1248-1256, 1990.

Scott WE: Temporary surgical overcorrection of infantile esotropia, Trans New Orleans Acad Ophthal 1986.

Smith JT, Scott WE: Long-term stability of alignment in the monofixation syndrome, *J Pediatr Ophthalmol Strabismus* 27, 1990.

von Noorden GK, Munoz M, Wong SY: Compensatory mechanisms in congenital nystagmus, *Am J Ophthalmol* 104:387-397, 1987.

Wright KW, Edelman PM, Terry A, et al: High grade stereo acuity after early surgery for congenital esotropia, (abstract) *Invest Ophthalmol Vis Sci* 34:710, 1993.

Wright KW, Bruce-Lyle L: Augmented surgery for esotropia associated with high hypermetropia, *J Pediatr Ophthalmol Strabismus* 30:167-170, 1993.

Zubcov AA, Reinecke RD, Gottlob I, et al: Treatment of manifest latent nystagmus, *Am J Ophthalmol* 110:160-167, 1990.

Exotropia

Exodeviations are quite common and they are not necessarily pathologic. Small exophorias are found in high frequency in the normal population, and 70% of normal newborn infants have a transient exodeviation that resolves by 2 to 4 months of age. Normal fusional convergence amplitudes are strong, measuring between 30 to 40 prism diopters (PD), compared to divergence (8 PD) and vertical vergence (1 to 2 PD). Strong convergence facilitates control of exodeviations and is probably why most exodeviations and are intermittent associated with high-grade stereo acuity.

INTERMITTENT EXOTROPIA

Clinical Features

Intermittent exotropia is an acquired exodeviation intermittently controlled by fusional convergence. Unlike a pure phoria, intermittent exotropia spontaneously breaks down into a manifest exotropia (Fig. 17-1). Intermittent exotropia is the most common type of exodeviation and is usually first observed by the parents in early childhood. Patients with intermittent exotropia tend to manifest their deviation when they are tired, have a cold

or the flu, or when they are daydreaming. Adult patients may become exotropic after imbibing alcoholic beverages or taking sedatives. Symptoms of intermittent exotropia include blurred vision, asthenopia, visual fatigue, and rarely diplopia in older children and adults. Many patients will experience photophobia and squint to bright light. Squinting to bright sunlight is thought to be a way of eliminating diplopia or confusion when the exotropia is manifest.

The natural history of intermittent exotropia remains obscure since there are no longitudinal prospective studies and only a few retrospective studies of untreated intermittent exotropia. von Noorden found that 75% of 51 untreated patients showed progression over an average follow-up period of 3.5 years, while 9% did not change, and 16% improved. The most we can say about the natural history is that in the majority of cases intermittent exotropia does not get better; it either stays the same or progresses. If the tropic phase increases, patients may develop dense suppression and, over time, this may lead to a constant exotropia with loss of fusional potential. Only in rare cases does intermittent exotropia spontaneously resolve.

Sensory Adaptations

As a rule, during the phoric phase of intermittent exotropia, the eyes are perfectly aligned and the patient will have bifoveal fusion with excellent stereo acuity, ranging between 40 and 60 seconds arc. This excellent bifoveal fusion develops because the eyes are well-aligned in early infancy when the critical binocular cortical connections are being established and the deviation is intermittent, allowing reinforcement of fusion. During the tropia phase when the exotropia is manifest, most patients will show large regional suppression of the temporal retina. Anomalous retinal correspondence during the tropia phase and normal retinal correspondence during the

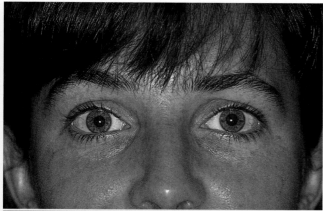

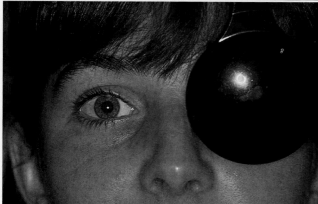

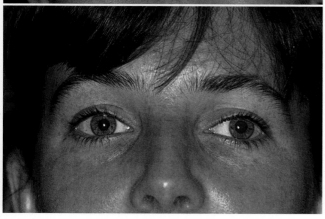

Fig. 17-1 **A,** Patient with intermittent exotropia and straight eyes in the phoric phase. Patient has 40 seconds arc stereo acuity. **B,** Occluder of the left eye disrupting fusion and manifesting the exotropia. Under the occluder, the left eye is deviated temporally. **C,** Occluder removed and the left eye is deviated temporally showing the exotropia. Patient is in the tropic phase and suppresses left eye.

phoria phase has also been demonstrated in some patients with intermittent exotropia. A minority of patients with intermittent exotropia have the monofixation syndrome and do not develop normal bifoveal fusion with high-grade stereopsis. A rare patient will even have significant amblyopia. In these cases it is likely that a constant tropia became manifest in infancy or anisometropia

---

Box 17-1 The Three Classic Categories of Intermittent Exotropia

Basic
Pseudo-divergence excess
True divergence excess

---

contributed to the amblyopia. Patients with late onset exotropia after 6 to 7 years of age may experience diplopia because the exotropia occurs after the loss of plasticity that allows suppression.

Classification

Intermittent exotropia has been classically categorized into three subtypes based on the difference between the distance and near deviation. The three classic categories are listed in Box 17-1.

It is important to note that the term *divergence excess* as previously used is only descriptive and is not meant to imply a mechanism for the distance-near disparity. The cause of distance-near disparities seen with intermittent exotropia is probably superimposed excess convergence on the basic exodeviation, not divergence excess. In addition to binocular fusional convergence, convergence mechanisms that reduce the near deviation include, *tonic fusional convergence* (near convergence that continues even when one eye covered), *accommodative convergence* (AC/A ratio), and *proximal convergence* (instrument convergence).

1. ***Basic intermittent exotropia*** is present when the deviation in the distance is within 10 PD of the near deviation. Patients with a basic deviation have normal tonic fusional convergence, accommodative convergence (normal AC/A ratio), and proximal convergence, so their deviation is essentially the same for distance and near.

2. ***Pseudo-divergence excess*** is present when the patient has a larger exotropia for the distance than near but the near deviation increases to within 10 PD of the distance deviation after 30 to 60 minutes of monocular occlusion. For example, an exotropia measures 30 PD in the distance and 10 PD at near to alternate cover testing. Following monocular patching for 30 minutes (see patch test in the following section) the patient measures XT 30 PD in the distance and XT 25 PD at near. This occurs because patients with pseudo-divergence excess have increased tonic fusional convergence, which acts more at near. The prolonged monocular occlusion dissipates tonic fusional convergence, thereby disclosing the full latent deviation, which in pseudo-divergence is the same for distance and near. The relatively brief period of monocular oc-

clusion that occurs with alternate cover testing is not enough to break up the tonic fusional convergence. Pseudo-divergence excess is quite common. Over 80% of patients with a divergence excess pattern actually have pseudo-divergence excess as disclosed with the patch test.

3. *True divergence excess* is present when the distance deviation is more than 10 PD greater than the near deviation, even after performing the patch test. In this case, the distance deviation would measure 30 PD, near deviation 10 PD and, after a 30-minute patch test, the distance deviation would be 30 PD and the near deviation 15 PD. The author (KWW) and Dr. Eugene De Juan studied the causes of true divergence excess at the Wilmer Clinic at Johns Hopkins Hospital in 1982. We found that most of the patients with true divergence excess had a high AC/A ratio as determined by the +3.00 add test (see the following discussion) after a 30-minute patch test. In a similar study, Kushner (1988) found approximately 60% of patients with a true divergence excess had a high AC/A ratio, and 40% had a normal AC/A ratio. The group with a high AC/A ratio was prone to postoperative overcorrection (75% overcorrection) if the distance measurement was used as the target angle.

Measuring the Angle

Obtaining reproducible measurements in a patient with intermittent exotropia can be difficult, since the angle of deviation is often variable when measured by routine alternate cover prism testing. If it is late in the day and the patient is tired, tonic fusional convergence (see Chapter 15) will be weak, and the deviation will be easily uncovered by alternate cover testing. On the other hand, if the patient is wide awake and alert, strong tonic fusional convergence will control the deviation and may make it difficult to elicit. Patients with intermittent exotropia should be measured using prolonged alternate cover testing to suspend tonic fusional convergence. If after prolonged alternate cover testing, there is significant angle variability or a significant distance/near discrepancy, then a patch test is indicated. In contrast, patients who show consistent measurements and no significant distance-near disparity do not need the patch test.

Patch test   The *patch test* is used to reduce tonic fusional convergence to differentiate pseudo-divergence excess from true divergence excess and to reduce angle variability. One eye is covered for 30 minutes to 1 hour, then the deviation is measured without allowing binocular fusion.

+3.00 near add test (lens gradient method)   Most patients who have a divergence excess pattern actually have pseudo-divergence excess but rare patients have true divergence excess caused by a high AC/A ratio. The

+3.00 near add test uses the lens gradient method to measure the AC/A ratio, thus identifying the high AC/A ratio patients. These patients are the ones that will continue to have a distance-near disparity postoperatively, and may require bifocal spectacles after surgery for a consecutive esotropia at near. Consider using the +3.00 near add test in patients who have a distance deviation greater than near deviation of 15 PD or more after the patch test (i.e., those with true divergence excess). After the patch test, while still dissociated, remeasure the deviation at near with a +3.00 add. If the +3.00 add increases the near XT by 20 PD or more the diagnosis is high AC/A ratio true divergence excess intermittent exotropia.

Far distance measurement   Measuring the deviation to far fixation reduces measurement variability and helps uncover the full deviation by reducing near convergence. Have the patient fixate on an object at a distance of 20 feet or more, and then perform alternate cover testing. If you don't have a 20-foot lane, have the patient look down a hallway or fixate through a window to a far distant target. Combining the patch test and far distance measurement can greatly reduce undercorrections and has improved our overall results.

Treatment

Nonsurgical treatment   In general, nonsurgical treatments for intermittent exotropia are not very effective. One method is to prescribe 2 to 3 diopters of myopic correction in excess of what is required by cycloplegic refraction. Over-minusing induces accommodative convergence thus reducing the exodeviation. Another method is part-time monocular occlusion therapy. By occluding the dominant eye, the patient is forced to use the nonpreferred eye, thus providing "anti-suppression" therapy. Use alternate-day occlusion in patients with equal fixation preference. Although others have found success with this procedure, in the author's experience, 30% to 40% patients have responded to occlusion therapy, but in virtually every case, the intermittent exotropia returned when the patching was stopped. Part-time occlusion therapy may be tried in younger patients as a method for delaying surgery, but it is only a temporary measure. Convergence exercises are useful for convergence insufficiency but not for most cases of intermittent exotropia.

Indications for surgery   As with any strabismus, the indications for surgery include preservation or restoration of binocular function and cosmesis. In intermittent exotropia one of the most important indications for therapeutic intervention is an increasing tropia phase, since this indicates deteriorating fusional control. If the frequency or duration of the tropia phase increases, this indicates diminished fusional control and the potential for losing binocular function. Progression should be monitored by documenting the size of the deviation, the frequency it is manifest, and the ease of regaining fusion after dissociation from the cover-uncover test. Deteriorating fusional control is an indication for treatment. Additionally, if the exotropia is manifest more than 50% of waking hours, surgery is probably indicated, since this indicates unacceptably poor fusional control.

There is controversy about the management of children under 4 years of age because, in contrast to infantile esotropia, these patients have intermittent fusion and excellent stereopsis. A study comparing surgery at various ages showed a significant increase in the incidence of amblyopia and loss of stereopsis when a consecutive esotropia occurred after surgery in children under 4 years of age. Since the desired result is an initial consecutive esotropia, younger children who have surgery for intermittent exotropia are at risk for developing amblyopia and losing binocularity. Thus it is probably better to wait in young children unless the exotropia is present more than 50% of waking hours or is increasing in size, frequency, or duration. Patients under 4 years of age can undergo surgery for intermittent exotropia, but they must be followed closely.

Surgical treatment For all three types of intermittent exotropia (i.e., basic, pseudo-divergence excess, and true divergence excess) bilateral lateral rectus recessions work well. Symmetric surgery is usually preferred over monocular resect-recess procedures, since a recession-resection procedure may produce lateral incomitance with a significant esotropia to the side of the operated eye. In adults, this incomitance can produce diplopia in side gaze, which may persist for months to even years. In contrast, in amblyopic patients with acuities of 20/50 or worse, a recession-resection procedure on the amblyopic eye is preferred to avoid surgical risk to the good eye.

Role of the patch test Historically, the patch test was important to distinguish between the three subgroups of intermittent exotropia because patients with basic or pseudo-divergence excess intermittent exotropia would receive a monocular recess-resect procedure, whereas patients with true divergence excess would undergo bilateral lateral rectus recessions. Parks has shown that bilateral lateral rectus recessions works well for all three types of intermittent exotropias, so the patch test is probably not very important for determining whether a recess-resect, or a bilateral recession should be performed. The patch test is, however, very useful in patients with a distance-near disparity to distinguish pseudo-divergence from true divergence excess to determine how much lateral rectus recession should be performed.

Amount of surgery

Basic deviation Surgery for patients with basic intermittent exotropia should be based on the full distance deviation as determined by alternate cover testing:

Ncc XT 25
Dcc XT 30

Target angle = XT 30

Pseudo-divergence excess Surgery based on distance deviation after patch test.

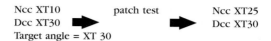

Ncc XT10   patch test   Ncc XT25
Dcc XT30   Dcc XT30
Target angle = XT 30

True divergence excess (high AC/A ratio) These patients are difficult to manage since totally correcting the distance deviation often leads to a persistent esotropia at near. Surgery for true divergence excess should be based on a deviation somewhere between the distance and near deviations after the patch test. Patients with true divergence excess and a high AC/A ratio should be told they have a significant risk for a persistent near overcorrection at near, and they may require a reoperation, a bifocal add, or miotic drops postoperatively.

Ncc XT10   patch test   Ncc XT15
Dcc XT30   Dcc XT35
Target angle = XT 10 to 25

Lateral incommitance Lateral incommitance is a difference in size of the deviation on lateral gaze. Intermittent exotropia is commonly associated with lateral incommitance, with a smaller exotropia in right and left gaze. Some have suggested reducing the amount of recession in patients with lateral incommitance, especially if the deviation in lateral gaze is 50% less than the deviation in primary position. It is the author's experience that small to moderate amounts of symmetric lateral incommitance is common, but its presence should not change the surgical plan.

A- and V-patterns: oblique overaction Intermittent exotropia may be associated with A- and V-patterns, and inferior and superior oblique overaction. For inferior oblique overaction with a V-pattern weaken the inferior obliques at the time of the horizontal surgery. Beware, however, of performing superior oblique tenotomies or tenectomies in patients with intermittent exotropia and bifoveal fusion, since this may result in a consecutive superior oblique paresis with intractable cyclo-vertical diplopia. If significant superior oblique overaction and an A-pattern is present, consider an infra placement of the lateral rectus muscles or the Wright superior oblique tendon expander procedure, rather than a tenotomy or tenectomy of the superior oblique muscle. It is generally not required to alter the amount of horizontal surgery when simultaneous oblique surgery is performed.

Small vertical deviations associated with intermittent exotropia should be ignored since these vertical phorias less than 8 PD usually disappear after surgery. Patients with large-angle intermittent exotropia may have an *X-pattern* with the exotropia increasing in up gaze and down gaze relative to the deviation in primary position. This pattern may be explained by tight lateral rectus muscles causing a leash effect similar to the up-shoot and down-shoot seen in Duane's syndrome (see Chapter 19). The X-pattern associated with intermittent exotropia is usually small, and it is best to ignore the pattern and simply perform bilateral lateral rectus recessions for the deviation in primary position.

Postoperative care Immediately after surgery, a small consecutive esotropia of 8 to 10 PD is desirable. Even a large consecutive esotropia up to 20 PD may resolve without further surgery. Be sure to warn the parents and or patients before surgery that postoperative diplopia may occur so they are not surprised. Postoperative diplopia associated with the initial over correction usually resolves in 1 to 2 weeks. In children under 4 years of age, part-time alternate patching of each eye helps prevent amblyopia and may facilitate straightening of the eyes. If a residual esotropia persists past 2 to 3 weeks, then the patient should be treated with prism glasses to neutralize the esotropia. Prescribe just enough prism to allow fusion, but leave a small residual esophoria to encourage divergence. If after 6 to 8 weeks the esotropia persists, then a reoperation should be considered. Advancement of lateral rectus muscle is indicated if there is limited adduction or lateral incommitance that is consistent with a slipped muscle. Otherwise, bimedial recessions are usually the procedure of choice for a consecutive esotropia, especially if the esotropia is greater at near. If the consecutive esotropia is present only at near, the practitioner may consider a bifocal add, miotics, or even a base-out prism to correct the near esotropia but create a small exodeviation in the distance. Failing this, small bimedial rectus recessions is the next option with or without Faden procedure.

Patients with a residual exotropia over 15 PD in the first postoperative week will probably not improve and many will require additional surgery. Most surgeons wait 8 to 12 weeks before reoperating on the residual exotropia. Re-recess both lateral rectus muscles if the primary surgery was bilateral recessions of 6 mm or less. If the primary recession were greater than 6 mm, then perform bilateral medial rectus resections, but be conservative because overcorrections are common after resecting against a large recession. I usually reduce the amount of surgery by 1 mm from the standard resection tables.

Prognosis

The success rate of intermittent exotropia is dependent on the length of follow-up. The longer the follow-up, the higher the incidence of undercorrection. Short-term studies with 6 months to 1 year follow-up report success rates of approximately 80%, whereas studies with 2 to 5 year follow-up have shown a 50% to 60% success rate with one surgery. The majority of undesirable results are a result of undercorrections. Hardesty (1990) reported an 80% success rate after no more than two surgeries with a 10-year follow-up. Hardesty attributes the long-term success to the aggressive use of postoperative prisms for both overcorrections and undercorrections to maintain constant fusion and to prevent suppression. The prognosis for the true divergence excess high AC/A ratio patients is not as good as for the pseudo-divergence excess or basic exotropic patients.

CONVERGENCE INSUFFICIENCY

Clinical Features

Convergence insufficiency is the inability to maintain convergence on objects as they approach from distance to near. Symptoms usually first appear during or after the teenage years and include asthenopia, reading difficulty, blurred near vision and diplopia. Alternate cover testing will disclose a near exophoria and essentially no distance deviation. The exophoria at near intermittently breaks down into a tropia especially after prolonged near work such as reading. When tropic, most patients will see double, while some do not since they have learned to suppress. Even patients with suppression can experience asthenopia and are often symptomatic.

Patients with convergence insufficiency will show a remote near point of convergence. The *near point of convergence (NPC)* is how close one can bring a fixation target to the nose and maintain fusion. The *break point* occurs when the target is so close that fusion breaks, and an exotropia becomes manifest. The normal NPC is between 5 to 6 cm from the bridge of the nose. Patients with convergence insufficiency will have a remote break point, ranging from 10 to 30 cm, or more. Convergence insufficiency may also be associated with reduced fusional convergence amplitudes. Normal fusional convergence amplitudes for near are between 30 to 35 PD but patients with convergence insufficiency usually break when tested with less than 20 PD base-out prism. Some patients with convergence insufficiency will initially show fairly good near point of convergence and convergence fusion amplitudes at near; however, on repeated testing, they fatigue. The diagnosis of convergence insufficiency should not be based solely on one test trial but on repeated testing.

Treatment

The best treatment for convergence insufficiency is orthoptic convergence exercises. The two most useful convergence exercises are near-point exercises (pencil push-ups), and prism convergence exercises. Near-point exercises consist of presenting a target at a remote distance, where it is easily fused, and then slowly bringing the target towards the patient until they reach their break point (Fig. 17-2). With prism convergence

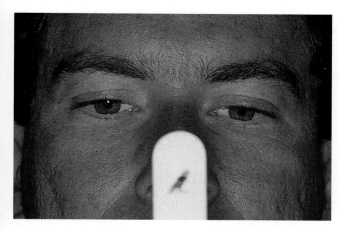

Fig. 17-2   Near-point convergence exercise showing accommodative target at near. Patient starts with the target at arm length and then brings the target towards the nose, converging on the accommodative target.

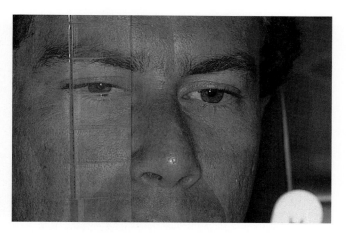

Fig. 17-3   Prism convergence exercise at near. A base-out prism is presented in front of one eye to induce convergence. The amount of prism is increased until the patient reaches the blur point, then the break point.

exercises a prism bar oriented base-out is presented to one eye to induce fusional convergence (Fig. 17-3). First use a small prism that can be easily fused while the patient fixates on a near target. Increase the base-out prism until the patient notes blurred vision (blur point), and then increase until fusion breaks (break point). Both convergence exercises should be repeated 15 to 20 times during each exercise session and sessions should be repeated two to three times per day. Convergence exercises stimulate fusional convergence only if the patient appreciates diplopia and the break point. Patients who do not appreciate diplopia can be treated with red-glass convergence exercises. A red filter is placed over the dominant eye, and a light is used as the fixation target. The red filter and light will help the patient recognize diplopia.

Convergence exercises have been found to be extremely helpful and curative in patients with convergence insufficiency as long as these exercises are followed. Improvement of symptoms usually occurs after a few weeks of exercises, but some cases may take several months before symptoms are relieved. In the author's experience, most patients with convergence insufficiency can be managed by exercises alone, and it is the rare case that requires surgery. Always try orthoptic exercises first, second, and third. Some advocate surgery if exercises fail to alleviate the symptoms; however, this author has never operated for convergence insufficiency unless there is a distance exotropia of 10 PD or greater. The surgery for convergence insufficiency without a distance exotropia is a small medial rectus resection of one or both medial rectus muscles. In the author's experience this surgery is not very effective and often results in a consecutive esotropia with diplopia in the distance.

ACCOMMODATIVE INSUFFICIENCY

Accommodative insufficiency is not a strabismus, but does cause asthenopia and blurred near vision and will occasionally occur in combination with convergence insufficiency. Presbyopia is the most common type of accommodative insufficiency usually occurring after 40 years of age. Latent hypermetropia can cause early-onset presbyopia and asthenopia, so be sure to perform a cycloplegic refraction on patients who complain of asthenopia.

Primary accommodative insufficiency can rarely occur in children and young adults. Accommodative insufficiency can be secondary to a systemic disorder such as Parkinson's disease, lithium, or local ciliary body dysfunction associated with Adie's pupil.

According to Duane's standard curve of accommodation, normal patients under 20 years of age should be able to accommodate at least 10 diopters or read the 20/40 line on the near card at 10 cm. Patients with accommodative insufficiency will have remote near point of accommodation. There are no good exercises for treating accommodative insufficiency; however, some have tried accommodative exercises. A near bifocal add is the treatment of choice, but prescribe the lowest power that relieves the symptoms to stimulate some accommodation. Prescribing a strong reading add only weakens the patient's remaining accommodation.

CONGENITAL EXOTROPIA

Congenital exotropia is extremely rare and most ophthalmologists will see only one or two cases during their

MAJOR POINTS

Small exophorias are commonly found in the normal population.

Unlike a pure phoria, intermittent exotropia spontaneously breaks down into a manifest exotropia.

During the phoric phase of intermittent exotropia, the eyes are perfectly aligned and the patient will have bifoveal fusion with excellent stereo acuity ranging between 40 and 60 seconds arc. During the tropia phase of intermittent exotropia most patients will show large regional suppression of the temporal retina.

For pseudo-divergence excess patients surgery is based on distance deviation after the patch test. Surgery for true divergence excess should be based on a deviation somewhere between the distance and near deviations after the patch test.

Beware of performing superior oblique tenotomies or tenectomies in patients with intermittent exotropia and bifoveal fusion, since this may result in a consecutive superior oblique paresis with intractable cyclovertical diplopia.

Patients under 4 years of age can be safely operated on for intermittent exotropia, but they must be followed closely, since a persistent consecutive esotropia can cause loss of stereopsis and amblyopia in this age group.

The best treatment for convergence insufficiency is orthoptic convergence exercises.

Congenital exotropia is rare but can occur in patients with craniofacial anomalies, ocular albinism, or cerebral palsy.

If a patient loses vision in one eye, the blind eye may drift out (sensory exotropia).

SENSORY EXOTROPIA

If a patient loses vision in one eye, the blind eye may drift out (sensory exotropia). Patients with dense amblyopia may also develop a sensory exodeviation. It is often said that if the visual loss occurs before 4 years of age, an esotropia develops, and vision loss after 4 years of age results in an exodeviation. This rule, however, is violated as often as it holds true. Patients with unilateral congenital cataracts show an even distribution between esodeviations and exodeviations. Treatment of sensory exotropia is a recession-resection procedure of the eye with the decreased vision.

SUGGESTED READINGS

Archer SM, Sondhi N, Helveston EM: Strabismus in infancy, *Ophthalmology* 96:133-137, 1989.

Chrousos GA, O'Neill JF, et al: Accommodative deficiency in healthy young adults, *J Pediatr Ophthalmol Strabismus* 25: 176-179, 1988.

Edelman PM, Murphree AL, Brown MH, et al: Consecutive esodeviation...then what? *Am Orthoptic J* 38:111-116, 1988.

Freeman RS, Isenberg SJ: The use of part-time occlusion for early onset unilateral exotropia, *J Pediatr Ophthalmol Strabismus* 26:94, 1989.

Hardesty H: Management of intermittent exotropia, *Binoc Vis Quart* 5:145, 1990.

Hardesty HH, Boynton JR, Keenan P: Treatment of intermittent exotropia, *Arch Ophthalmology* 96:268, 1978.

Kushner BJ: Exotropic deviations: a functional classification and approach to treatment, *Am Orthoptic J* 38:81-93, 1988.

Parks MM: Comitant exodeviations in children. In *Strabismus Symposium*, New Orleans Academy of Ophthalmology. St Louis, 1962, Mosby.

Raab EL, Parks MM: Recession of the lateral recti: early and late postoperative alignments, *Arch Ophthalmol* 82:203, 1969.

von Noorden GK: *Binocular vision and ocular motility: theory and management of strabismus,* St Louis, 1985, Mosby.

Wright KW, De Juan E: Patch test with and without +3.00 near add. Wilmer Institute, Johns Hopkins, 1981. In K. Wright (editor): *Pediatric ophthalmology and strabismus,* St Louis, 1995, Mosby.

Wright KW, Min BM, Park C: Comparison of superior oblique tendon expander to superior oblique tenotomy for the management of superior oblique overaction and Brown syndrome, *J Pediatr Ophthalmol Strabismus* 29(2):92-97, 1992.

entire career. Congenital exotropia can occur in patients with craniofacial anomalies, ocular albinism, or cerebral palsy. The treatment for congenital exotropia is to treat amblyopia if present, then bilateral lateral rectus recessions, which should be performed after 6 months of age. Congenital exotropia should not be confused with the variable small-angle exodeviation seen in 70% of normal newborns. Congenital exotropia is a large-angle constant exodeviation, has a relatively poor prognosis for fusion, and has a much higher incidence of amblyopia than intermittent exotropia.

CHAPTER 18

A- and V-Patterns and Oblique Muscle Overaction

A- and V-patterns of strabismus are changes in the horizontal deviation as the patient looks up and down. They are usually associated with oblique dysfunction, either overaction or paresis. Primary oblique muscle overaction is when an oblique muscle is too strong for its antagonist and there is no known cause. Secondary oblique overaction is caused by a paresis of the antagonist muscle. A superior oblique paresis results in inferior oblique overaction, and inferior oblique paresis results in superior oblique overaction. This chapter covers the management of A- and V-patterns and primary oblique muscle overaction.

A- AND V-PATTERNS

Clinical Features

A-patterns are defined as increasing divergence in down gaze (>10 prism diopters [PD]), whereas V-patterns are increased divergence (>15 prism diopters) in up gaze. The type of A- or V-pattern helps identify the cause. Superior oblique paresis produces a V-pattern, arrow subtype, with convergence in down gaze. The arrow pattern subtype indicates a lack of abduction in down gaze, the field of action of the superior oblique muscles. Inferior oblique overaction, on the other hand, has a V-pattern, Y subtype, with increased abduction in up gaze. The Y-pattern occurs because the field of action of the inferior oblique muscles is up gaze and they are abductors. Lambda subtype is typically associated with superior oblique overaction, with increased abduction in down gaze, because the field of action is in down gaze. These patterns usually require bilateral oblique dysfunction to become manifest.

Etiology

Oblique muscle overaction or paresis usually causes A- and V-patterns, but primary patterns without significant oblique dysfunction may occur. Inferior oblique overaction and superior oblique paresis result in V-patterns. The oblique muscles are abductors so inferior oblique overaction causes excessive abduction in up gaze causing a V-pattern. Likewise, superior oblique paresis causes a lack of abduction in down gaze and a V-pattern. Superior oblique overaction or rarely inferior oblique paresis can cause A-patterns. Patterns can also be primary or occur in association with cranial facial abnormalities. Patterns in these cases probably represent vertical displacement of the horizontal rectus muscles and/or horizontal displacement of vertical rectus muscles.

Management with Horizontal Rectus Muscle Offsets

The first step in the management of A- and V-patterns is to determine if there is associated oblique muscle overaction or paresis. If there is significant oblique dysfunction then surgically address the oblique muscles. Primary

A- and V- patterns with normal oblique muscle function can be managed by offsetting the horizontal rectus muscles.

The horizontal rectus offset procedure works by moving the horizontal rectus muscles up (supraplaced) or down (infraplaced) to change the vector of the muscle's force. For example, if the medial rectus muscles were infraplaced, they would tighten in up gaze and loosen in down gaze, which would collapse a V-pattern. Conversely, supraplacement would loosen the medial rectus in up gaze and tighten them in down gaze and collapse an A-pattern. Vertically transposing the horizontal rectus muscles, however, does not significantly change the muscle's force in primary position.

Fig. 18-1 shows a method for remembering which direction to move the horizontal rectus muscles for A- and V-patterns. Move the medial recti to the apex of the letter A or V, and move the lateral recti toward the open part of the letter. For a V-pattern, move the medial rectus muscles inferiorly and lateral rectus muscles superiorly. For an A-pattern, move the medial rectus superiorly and the lateral rectus inferiorly. As a rule, a one-half tendon width of vertical displacement results in 10 to 15 PD of pattern correction. A full tendon width vertical displacement produces approximately 20 to 25 PD of correction and is reserved for extremely large patterns. Fig. 18-2 shows a full tendon width inferior transfer of the medial rectus muscle.

INFERIOR OBLIQUE OVERACTION

Etiology

Inferior oblique overaction may be primary and of unknown etiology, or secondary to a congenital superior oblique palsy, as covered in Chapter 19. Primary inferior oblique overaction is commonly associated with congenital esotropia, with the oblique overaction usually presenting after 1 year of age. In addition to congenital esotropia, primary inferior oblique muscle overaction may be associated with exotropia or occur as an isolated inferior oblique overaction without other strabismus.

Clinical Features

Primary inferior oblique overaction is usually bilateral; however, it can be very asymmetric. Clinical signs of primary inferior oblique overaction include an upshoot of the adducting eye on versions, a V-pattern, and extorsion on indirect ophthalmoscopy. If the overaction is symmetric, there will be no significant hypertropia in primary position. Children with primary inferior oblique overaction do not experience subjective extorsion because they have learned to sensorially adapt at a young age. *Bilateral inferior oblique overaction* produces a

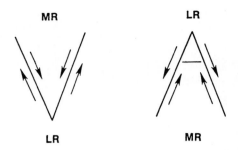

Fig. 18-1   Diagram of how to transpose the horizontal rectus muscles for A- and V-patterns. For V-patterns, move the medial rectus muscles to the apex (down) and the lateral rectus muscles up. For A-patterns, move the medial rectus muscles to the apex (up) and the lateral rectus muscles in the opposite direction (down). (From Wright KW: *Color atlas of ophthalmic surgery,* Philadelphia, 1991, JB Lippincott.)

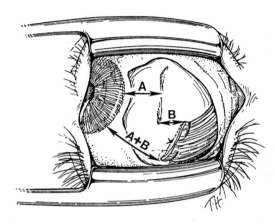

Fig. 18-2   Drawing of a medial rectus muscle recession with infraplacement. "A" represents the distance of the medial rectus insertion from the limbus. "B" represents the amount of recession and "A + B" indicates the measurement from the limbus to the inferior pole of the rectus muscle. When performing supra- or infraplacements it is easy to miscalculate the recession; therefore these measurements are important. (From Wright KW: *Color atlas of ophthalmic surgery,* Philadelphia, 1991, JB Lippincott.)

left hypertropia in right gaze, a right hypertropia in left gaze, and little or no vertical deviation in primary position (Fig. 18-3). Distinguishing primary inferior oblique overaction from overaction associated with secondary superior oblique muscle paresis is largely dependent on the head-tilt test as described in Chapter 19. If the head-tilt test is negative this indicates a primary inferior oblique overaction, whereas a positive head-tilt test (increasing hypertropia with tilt to the side of the inferior oblique overaction) indicates a superior oblique paresis. Differentiating the V-pattern subtype is also helpful. A Y-pattern subtype indicates primary inferior oblique overaction, whereas an arrow pattern indicates a superior oblique paresis. Clinical signs that differentiate pri-

Right   Left

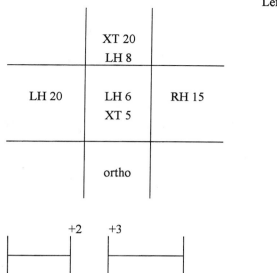

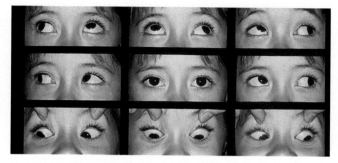

B

Fig. 18-3   **A,** Primary bilateral inferior oblique overaction with left hypertropia in right gaze, and the right hypertropia in left gaze. The left hypertropia in primary position is because of the asymmetry with the left inferior oblique overacting more than the right. **B,** Composite photograph of patient with esotropia and primary inferior oblique overaction. There is a small left hypertropia in primary position that increases in right gaze. In left gaze there is a right hypertropia. There is bilateral inferior oblique overaction, the left eye overacting more than the right eye. Also note that the V-pattern changes more from primary position to up gaze than primary position to down gaze. This is indicative of primary inferior oblique overaction and a Y-pattern subtype.

mary inferior oblique overaction from superior oblique paresis are listed in Table 18-1.

Unilateral inferior overaction is associated with an ipsilateral hypertropia (usually 5 to 15 PD) in primary position that increases in the opposite gaze to the overacting muscle. A left inferior oblique overaction results in a left hypertropia in primary position, which increases in right gaze. A V-pattern may be present but it will be relatively small (usually 5 to 10 PD). Unilateral primary inferior oblique overaction is unusual and many cases may actually represent very asymmetric bilateral inferior oblique overaction.

Differential Diagnosis

Inferior oblique overaction is characterized by an upshoot of the adducting eye on versions, but there are other causes for an upshoot of the adducting eye. *Dissociated vertical deviation (DVD)* can become manifest since the adducting eye is blocked by the nasal bridge, which can mimic inferior oblique overaction. Clinical signs that indicate inferior oblique overaction include the presence of a V-pattern, objective extorsion, and a true hypertropia that increases in lateral gaze (e.g., right hyper increases in left gaze). DVD, on the other hand, is associated with a hypertropia that is the same on lateral gaze, and the hypertropia is not a true tropia since there is no corresponding hypotropia of the fellow eye. It is

Table 18-1   Primary inferior oblique overaction versus superior oblique palsy

Clinical sign	Primary overaction	Secondary overaction
Inferior oblique overaction	Yes	Yes
V-pattern	Yes (Y-pattern)	Yes (arrow pattern)
Head-tilt test	Negative	Positive
Subjective torsion	No	Yes (except in congenital superior oblique palsies)
Objective extorsion (fundus examination)	Yes	Yes
Underaction of ipsilateral superior oblique muscle	No (minimal if any)	Yes

important to remember that DVD and inferior oblique overaction often coexist, making the distinction and relative contribution of each difficult to ascertain.

The presence of a tight lateral rectus muscle can also cause an upshoot of the eye in adduction, which can look like inferior oblique overaction. Such an upshoot is often associated with Duane's co-contraction syndrome, and to a lesser extent, in patients with large-angle intermittent exotropia. A tight or co-contracting lateral rectus muscle acts as a leash to pull the eye up, since it is adducted and slightly elevated. In these patients with a tight or co-contracting lateral rectus muscle, there is often an *X-pattern* with both an upshoot and downshoot when the eye is adducted.

Management

If significant inferior oblique overaction is associated with horizontal strabismus, inferior oblique overaction should be surgically addressed with the horizontal strabismus. Do not alter the amount of horizontal surgery because of oblique surgery. Weakening procedures of oblique muscles do not significantly change the horizontal deviation in primary position. In general, surgery is indicated for inferior oblique overaction of +2 or more. If the inferior oblique overaction is bilateral yet asymmetric, bilateral inferior oblique weakening procedures should be performed even when one eye displays only +1 overaction to avoid unmasking of the minimally overacting inferior oblique. If amblyopia is present (amblyopia greater than 2 lines difference), it is advisable to restrict surgery to the amblyopic eye.

The surgical management of inferior oblique overaction is based on either weakening the inferior oblique muscle by diminishing the muscle tension or changing the vector of mechanical function of the muscle by moving the insertion site. Techniques such as myectomy (Fig. 18-4, *A*) and recession (Fig. 18-4, *B*) act by decreasing the inferior oblique muscle tone. Inferior oblique recession with anteriorization (Fig. 18-4, *C*) diminishes muscle tension and changes the functional insertion. Anteriorizing the inferior oblique muscle insertion anterior to the eyeball's equator changes the inferior oblique muscle from an elevator to more of a depressor. The more the inferior oblique muscle is anteriorized the more it becomes a depressor. Severe inferior oblique overaction is treated with a full anteriorization to the inferior rectus insertion, whereas mild overaction is managed with less of an anteriorization. This author suggests using the "graded anteriorization" protocol listed in Box 18-1.

Graded inferior oblique anteriorization works extremely well for both primary inferior oblique overaction and inferior oblique overaction associated with superior oblique paresis.

It is important to note that full anteriorization of the inferior oblique can be performed with a "J" deformity of the new insertion, which can limit ocular elevation and a produce a postoperative hypotropia worse in up gaze. The J deformity is created when the posterior fibers of

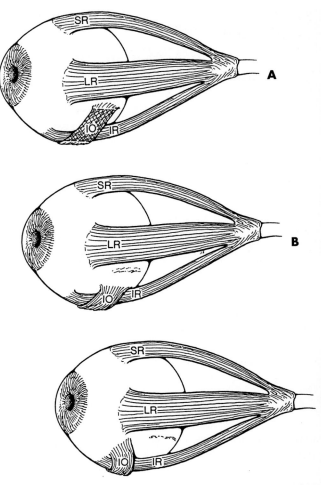

Fig. 18-4   **A,** Drawing of inferior oblique myectomy. The hash marks on the inferior oblique indicate removal of 10 mm of inferior oblique muscle. **B,** Diagram of inferior oblique recession. The inferior oblique muscle is disinserted, then reattached close to the inferior rectus muscle. This produces slack in the inferior oblique muscle, thus weakening the inferior oblique. **C,** Diagram of inferior oblique anteriorization procedure. Inferior oblique muscle is disinserted, then reattached to the globe at the inferior rectus insertion. The posterior fibers of the inferior oblique are, in this case, sutured anteriorly and this is a full anteriorization procedure. In most cases, the author prefers placing the posterior fibers close to the inferior rectus border; thus it becomes a partial anteriorization. The partial anteriorization procedure reduces the complication of induced postoperative hypotropia. (From Wright KW: *Color atlas of ophthalmic surgery,* Philadelphia, 1991, JB Lippincott.)

the inferior oblique are anteriorized parallel or in front of the inferior rectus insertion. Because of this potential complication, the full anteriorization with a J deformity should be avoided for most circumstances. Some have advocated full anteriorization with J deformity for patients with severe (+4) bilateral inferior oblique overaction or bilateral severe inferior oblique overaction with significant DVD.

Box 18-1   Graded Anteriorization Protocol

Full anteriorization for +4 overaction
1 mm posterior to inferior rectus insertion for +3 overaction
3 to 4 mm posterior to inferior rectus insertion for +2 overaction
4 mm posterior and 2 mm lateral to inferior rectus insertion for +1 overaction.

SUPERIOR OBLIQUE OVERACTION

Etiology

The cause of primary superior oblique overaction is unknown. Superior oblique overaction may be associated with a paresis of the contralateral inferior rectus muscle causing the yoke superior oblique to overact, or rarely an ipsilateral inferior oblique paresis.

Clinical Features

Patients with superior oblique overaction show a downshoot of the adducting eye on versions and divergence in down gaze, which produces the characteristic A-pattern (Fig. 18-5). The A-pattern associated with superior oblique overaction is usually a lambda pattern (λ).

In addition to the horizontal and vertical changes, superior oblique overaction also causes intorsion, which increases in down gaze. Since primary superior oblique overaction is congenital, patients adapt to the intorted position and almost never experience subjective torsion in free view or by Maddox rod testing. Indirect ophthalmoscopy, however, will reveal objective intorsion.

Bilateral superior oblique overaction is associated with a small or no hypertropia in primary position, since the bilateral vertical deviations cancel each other. However, reversing hypertropias in side gaze are typical, with a right hypertropia to right gaze and a left hypertropia to left gaze. The lambda type of A-pattern is often quite large measuring greater than 20 PD (see Fig. 18-5). If the bilateral superior oblique overaction is asymmetric, this will cause a hypertropia in primary position. Like inferior oblique overaction, most cases of superior oblique overaction are bilateral with varying degrees of asymmetry. There maybe some limitation to elevation in adduction of both eyes associated with tight superior oblique muscles.

Unilateral superior oblique overaction will result in a hypertropia contralateral to the overacting superior oblique. The hypertropia increases on horizontal versions to the opposite side of the overacting muscle. Note that a small A-pattern less than 10 PD is typical of unilateral superior oblique overaction. There maybe some limitation to elevation in adduction associated with a tight superior oblique muscle.

Differential Diagnosis

Brown's syndrome can usually be differentiated from primary superior oblique overaction, on a clinical basis even without forced ductions (also see Chapter 20). In contrast to superior oblique overaction where the hypertropia is greatest in down gaze, Brown's syndrome is associated with a restriction of elevation thus causing a hypertropia that is greatest in up gaze. Also, instead of an A-pattern as in the case of superior oblique overaction, Brown's syndrome is associated with a Y-pattern with an exotropia in up gaze. Standard forced duction testing, rotating the eye up and in, shows restriction in Brown's syndrome and no restriction in superior oblique overaction. Exaggerated forced ductions as described by Guyton, may show mild tightness of the superior oblique in patients with superior oblique overaction.

Inferior oblique paresis is another entity that may be confused with primary superior oblique overaction. Inferior oblique paresis is rare; it can be congenital or acquired. Patients with inferior oblique paresis show ipsilateral superior oblique overaction, but unlike primary superior oblique overaction, inferior oblique paresis is associated with a positive head-tilt test, and a hypertropia that is greatest when the patient looks up and in. Inferior oblique muscle paresis looks like a Brown's syndrome with ipsilateral superior oblique overaction and a small A-pattern. Table 18-2 compares the clinical features of superior oblique overaction, Brown's syndrome and inferior oblique paresis.

Management

Superior oblique overaction of +2 or more can be dissociating and is reason to consider superior oblique surgery especially if a significant A-pattern is present. If superior oblique overaction is associated with a horizontal strabismus, perform the oblique surgery at the same time as the horizontal surgery. Do not change the amount of horizontal surgery because of simultaneous oblique muscle surgery, since weakening the superior oblique muscles does not significantly change the horizontal alignment in primary position. If the amount of superior oblique overaction is relatively small in comparison to the amount of A-pattern, then consider supraplacement of the medial rectus or infraplacement of the lateral rectus muscles in addition to weakening the superior oblique muscles.

Caution should be exercised when considering supe-

Right   Left

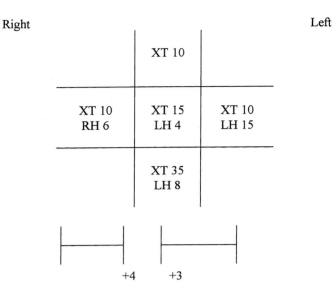

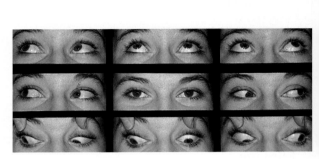

Fig. 18-5   A, Bilateral superior oblique overaction with right overacting slightly more than left. This causes a small left hypertropia in primary position with a right hypertropia in right gaze and a larger left hypertropia in left gaze. **B,** Nine-position composite photograph of patient with bilateral superior oblique overaction and A-pattern. Note that there is bilateral superior oblique overaction resulting in a left hypertropia in left gaze and a right hypertropia in right gaze. An A-pattern is present, which is a lambda subtype. Most of the change in horizontal deviation occurs between primary position and down gaze.

Table 18-2   Differential diagnosis and superior oblique overaction

	Brown's syndrome	Primary superior oblique overaction	Inferior oblique paresis
Bilateral involvement	Rare	Common	Unusual
Pattern	Y (divergence in up gaze)	Lambda (divergence in down gaze)	A (convergence in up gaze)
Superior oblique overaction	No	Yes	Yes
Inferior oblique underaction	Yes	Minimal or moderate	Yes
Standard forced ductions	Positive	Negative	Negative
Head-tilt test	Negative	Negative	Positive
Torsion	None to slight intorsion in up gaze	Intorsion (increasing in down gaze)	Intorsion (increasing in up gaze)
Greatest vertical deviation	Up gaze	Down gaze	Up gaze

rior oblique weakening procedures such as tenotomy and tenectomy in patients with binocular fusion, especially those with high-grade stereopsis. Patients with fusion are at risk for developing postoperative diplopia, if a consecutive superior oblique paresis occurs postoperatively. Patients with intermittent exotropia and A-pattern superior oblique overaction are in this danger category, since these patients usually have high-grade binocular fusion. If superior oblique overaction and A-pattern is present in a fusing patient, consider vertical off sets of the horizontal muscles, or the Wright superior oblique tendon expander rather than a superior oblique

tenotomy or tenectomy to avoid postoperative superior oblique paresis.

Superior oblique weakening will exacerbate *dissociated vertical deviation (DVD)*. If DVD and superior oblique overaction coexists, consider the following options. In patients with significant DVD (greater than 8 PD) and significant superior oblique overaction (+2 to +3) with a large A-pattern, perform simultaneous superior rectus recession and Wright superior oblique tendon expander procedure. If there is a small DVD (<7 to 5 PD), and moderate superior oblique overaction, then use the silicone expander but undercorrect by 1 mm to avoid exacerbating the DVD. If horizontal rectus surgery is planed and the superior oblique overaction and the DVD is mild, vertically shift the horizontal rectus muscles to correct the A-pattern and leave the superior oblique muscles alone.

Patients with *unilateral superior oblique overaction* often have a significant vertical deviation in primary position. If the deviation is less than 8 to 10 PD, a superior oblique tendon weakening procedure (tenotomy, tenectomy, or Wright tendon expander) alone will correct the hypertropia in primary position. Deviations larger than 8 to 10 PD, however, will not be corrected by the single superior oblique weakening procedure, and a surgery on a vertical *rectus* muscle should be added to the surgical plan.

Bilateral superior oblique overaction is usually associated with a large A-pattern and requires bilateral superior oblique weakening procedures. Both the superior oblique tenotomy and the superior oblique tendon expander procedure will eliminate the A-pattern, as well as the superior oblique overaction as seen on versions. If the overaction is asymmetric, perform a larger tendon expander on the side with more overaction. Do not expect asymmetric expander procedures to correct more than 6 to 8 PD of vertical deviation. If a vertical deviation in primary position is more than 8 to 10 PD, consider adding a vertical rectus muscle to the surgical plan.

Patients with *unilateral inferior oblique paresis* will show ipsilateral superior oblique overaction and a large contralateral hypertropia primary position. The hypertropia increases when the patient looks up and in. An ipsilateral superior oblique weakening procedure and a contralateral superior rectus recession best manages these cases.

SUPERIOR OBLIQUE WEAKENING PROCEDURES

Controversy remains regarding the best superior oblique weakening procedure. Berke's *superior oblique tenotomy,* performing a nasal incision and nasal superior oblique tenotomy, is the long-standing classic. The drawback with this incision is that intermuscular septum along the nasal aspect of the superior rectus muscle is disrupted, and it can often lead to scarring and even fat adherence. Parks recommends performing the initial conjunctival incision temporal to superior rectus muscle, then reflecting the incision nasally and performing the superior oblique tenotomy nasally, leaving the intermuscular septum intact. This has resulted in a more controlled tenotomy with less scarring. It also helps prevent secondary superior oblique paresis since the fascial connections around the nasal aspect of the tendon remained more or less intact and prevents large separations of the tendon.

Others have recommended *superior oblique recession.* Superior oblique recession, however, changes the insertion characteristics since it moves the insertion nasal and anterior to the original insertion site. This often creates an anterior leash and limits depression of the operated eye. Other procedures include posterior tenectomy and tenotomy, which involve removing the posterior fibers of the superior oblique but leaving the anterior fibers to keep the intorsion function intact. These procedures have only mild weakening effects and often result in under correction of the superior oblique overaction.

The *Wright superior oblique tendon expander* procedure was developed to allow for a controlled weakening of the superior oblique tendon. Surgery consists of performing a tenotomy, then suturing a segment of 240 silicone retinal band between the cut ends of the tendon to elongate the tendon (Fig. 18-6). The minimal length of the silicone expander should be approximately 4 mm and 1 mm added for each degree of superior oblique overaction to a maximum of 7 mm. It is important to approach the superior oblique tendon per Parks' superior oblique tenotomy with the conjunctival incision being made temporal to the superior rectus muscle; then the conjunctival opening is reflected nasally to expose the nasal aspect of the superior oblique tendon. By performing the initial conjunctival incision temporal to the superior rectus muscle, the nasal intermuscular septum can be left intact, thus preventing the silicone expander from scarring the sclera. The author has reoperated on one superior oblique expander to treat a secondary dissociated vertical deviation and found the expander to be encapsulated, but not adherent to the sclera. The silicone expander has the advantage of promoting a quantitative slackening of the superior oblique tendon while maintaining the functional integrity of the tendon. Additionally, the superior oblique tendon procedure is reversible since the cut ends of the tendon can be found since they are attached to the silicone segment. The surgeon can revise the surgery by increasing or decreasing the length of the silicone tendon expander.

Some have advocated a suture bridge between cut ends of the tendon instead of a firm silicone band. The suture bridge between the cut ends of the tendon does not hold the tendon ends apart and does not prevent postoperative scar contracture from reducing the tendon separation. It is this author's experience that even with superior oblique tenotomy or tenectomy, the cut ends of the tendon can occasionally grow back together and a residual superior oblique overaction will occur several weeks after surgery.

Complications

The most common error when performing superior oblique weakening procedures is missing some of the

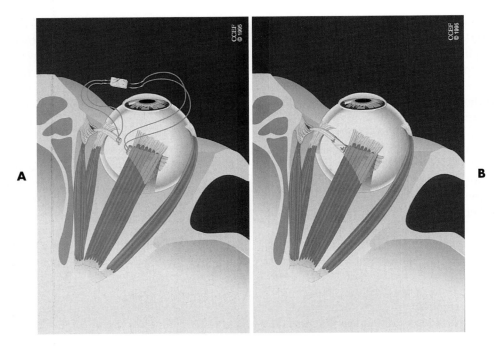

Fig. 18-6   Wright's superior oblique tendon expander for lengthening the superior oblique tendon. **A,** Segment of a 40 or 240 retinal silicone band is sutured between the cut ends of the superior oblique tendon. **B,** The silicone segment has been tied in place to elongate the superior oblique tendon. See color plate.

MAJOR POINTS

For a V-pattern move the medial rectus muscles inferiorly and lateral rectus muscles superiorly, and for an A-pattern move the medial rectus superiorly and the lateral rectus inferiorly.

Distinguishing primary inferior oblique overaction from overaction associated with secondary superior oblique muscle paresis is largely dependent on the head-tilt test.

Bilateral inferior oblique overaction produces a left hypertropia in right gaze, a right hypertropia in left gaze, and little or no vertical deviation in primary position.

Unilateral or asymmetric bilateral inferior overaction is associated with a hypertropia (usually 5 to 15 PD) in primary position, which increases in the opposite field of gaze to the overacting muscle.

Caution should be taken when considering superior oblique weakening procedures such as tenotomy or tenectomy in patients with fusion especially those with high-grade stereopsis.

Superior oblique weakening will exacerbate dissociated vertical deviation (DVD).

The most common error when performing superior oblique weakening procedures is missing some of the posterior tendon fibers, which causes residual superior oblique overaction.

posterior tendon fibers, which causes residual superior oblique overaction. The surgeon can verify a complete superior oblique tenotomy by using the Guyton exaggerated forced duction procedure after severing the superior oblique tendon.

A difficult complication of free tenotomy is a consecutive superior oblique palsy. One approach for correcting this is to reunite the tendon ends. It is technically difficult to find the cut ends of the tendon and exploration can lead to scarring and fat adherence. Mild unilateral superior oblique underaction with inferior oblique overaction can usually be managed by an ipsilateral inferior oblique weakening procedure. Severe superior oblique underaction associated with down gaze esotropia and extorsion, on the other hand, usually requires reuniting of the tendon ends.

Fat adherence and nasal scarring is a complication resulting from surgical technique. Careful dissection and the use of the Parks temporal conjunctival approach to a nasal tenotomy can avoid this. Another uncommon but important technical error is mistaking the superior rectus muscle for the superior oblique tendon. At first thought, this may appear to be difficult to do; however, if part of the superior rectus is hooked and pulled into the surgical field, the muscle will blanch taking on the appearance of a tendon. Inadvertent cutting of part or all of the superior rectus is a well-known complication of superior oblique surgery. It is important to perform careful dissection with avoidance of hemorrhage, so fascial tissue planes can be correctly identified. Superior oblique surgery requires a skilled surgeon who is familiar with the anatomic relationships of the superior oblique and superior rectus.

SUGGESTED READINGS

Apt L, Call NB: Inferior oblique muscle recession, *Am J Ophthalmol* 95:95, 1978.

Berke RN: Tenotomy of the superior oblique for hypertropia, *Trans Am Ophthalmol Soc* 44:304-342, 1946.

Bremer DL, Rogers GL, Quick LD: Primary position hypotropia after anterior transposition of the inferior oblique, *Arch Ophthalmol* 104:229-232, 1986.

Elliot L, Nankin J: Anterior transposition of the inferior oblique, *J Pediatr Ophthalmol Strabismus* 18:35, 1981.

Guyton DL: Clinical assessment of ocular torsion, *Am Orthopt J* 33:7, 1983.

Stager DR, Weakley DR, Stager D: Anterior transposition of the inferior oblique: anatomic assessment of the neurovascular bundle, *Arch Ophthalmol* 110:360, 1992.

Wright KW, Min BM, Park C: Comparison of superior oblique tendon expander to superior oblique tenotomy for the management of superior oblique overaction and Brown syndrome, *J Pediatr Ophthalmol Strabismus* 29:92-99, 1992.

Wright KW: Current approaches to inferior oblique muscle surgery. In Hoyt CS (editor): Focal points 1986: clinical modules for ophthalmologists, *Am Acad Ophthalmol* 1, 1986.

Wright KW: Superior oblique silicone expander for Brown's syndrome and superior oblique overaction, *J Pediatr Ophthalmol Strabismus* 28:101-107, 1991.

CHAPTER 19

Ocular Torticollis and Management of Paralytic Strabismus

Patients with paralytic strabismus and nystagmus often present with a face turn or a head-tilt. This chapter discusses the management of ocular causes of head posturing including nystagmus and extraocular muscle cranial nerve palsies. After an appropriate neurologic evaluation, acquired cranial nerve palsies should be observed for at least 6 months before surgery to allow for muscle function to recover. During this observation period many cases of vascular and traumatic cranial nerve palsies will show significant recovery, so it is important to make surgical decisions after the strabismus has stabilized.

TORTICOLLIS AND FACE TURNS

This section covers the approach to patients who present with an abnormal head posture and ocular torticollis. Torticollis means head-tilt. The first objective is to determine if the torticollis is secondary to a musculoskeletal abnormality of the neck or to an ocular problem compensated for by head posturing (e.g., ocular torticollis). A simple initial test is to have the patient close their eyes and observe them for several seconds to see if the head posturing spontaneously improves. If the face turn improves when eyes are closed, this suggests an ocular cause. Next passively move the patient's head from side to side with both eyes occluded. If the range of motion of the head and neck is normal, this verifies that the head posturing is an ocular torticollis; however, a stiff neck indicates a musculoskeletal problem. The two main ocular causes of compensatory head posturing are listed in Box 19-1.

In addition to torticollis, compensatory head posturing can involve a face turn (horizontal), or a chin elevation or depression (vertical). These forms of head posturing can occur independently or in combination, since a patient with a superior oblique palsy will often have both a head-tilt and a face turn. One of the best ways to evaluate for a chin posture or face turn is to observe the position of the eyes. If head posturing is present, the eyes will be shifted from primary position and away from the direction of the head turn. Thus, if the eyes are shifted up, there is a chin depression; if the eyes are down, there is a chin elevation; and if the eyes are in right gaze, this indicates a face turn to the left (Fig. 19-1).

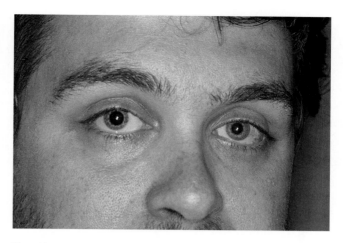

Fig. 19-1   This patient has a large face turn to the left. The left face turn can be identified even without seeing the whole face because the eyes are shifted to the right. This could be a compensatory face turn because of incomitant strabismus or nystagmus.

To identify the cause of the head posturing, straighten the head to place the eyes in primary position and examine for nystagmus or strabismus. If a nystagmus becomes manifest or increases when the head is held erect with eyes in primary position then nystagmus with an eccentric null point is contributing to the head posturing. If the patient has straight eyes and is fusing with a face turn, but strabismus is present when the head is straight with eyes in primary position, then the compensatory head posturing is to allow for binocular fusion.

The amount of face turn can be measured by using an orthopedic goniometer or any protractor placed on the head, and comparing the line of sight to the direction of the turned face (use the nose as a pointer for face position). An alternative method for measuring face turn associated with Duane's syndrome or unilateral limited eye movement is to place a prism over the eye with limited rotation with apex pointing toward the direction of the deviated eye. The prism is progressively increased until the face turn is corrected. The amount of prism required to neutralize the face turn equal is recorded in prism diopters. Prism diopters can be converted to degrees by dividing by 2. Prism correction of head posturing can also be used to measure face turns associated with nystagmus.

Incomitant Strabismus and Compensatory Head Posturing

Head posturing compensates for incomitant strabismus by placing the eyes in a field of gaze where the eyes are best aligned to achieve binocular fusion. For example, a patient with a left sixth nerve palsy will have a large esotropia in left gaze and straight eyes in right gaze. These patients will adopt a face turn to the left to keep their eyes aligned in right gaze as shown in Fig. 19-1. Virtually any incomitant strabismus can cause an abnormal head posture, including cranial nerve palsies, restrictive strabismus, A- or V-patterns, and primary oblique dysfunction. For example, patients with fusion and an A-exotropia or V-esotropia will show a chin depression (eyes straighter in up gaze), whereas an A-esotropia or

V-exotropia will show a chin elevation (eyes straighter in down gaze).

The treatment of an abnormal head posture caused by incomitant strabismus is simply to correct the strabismus in primary position and provide a large field of single binocular vision. If the fixing eye has limited ductions, then move the eye with limited movements to primary position, and the normal eye will follow (Fig. 19-2).

Nystagmus and Compensatory Head Posturing

A compensatory head posture can stabilize nystagmus by placing the eyes at the null point. If the null point is to the right, the patients will shift their eyes to the right and have a face turn to the left. Head posturing associated with nystagmus can take the form of a face turn, chin elevation or depression, and a head-tilt.

A compensatory face turn associated with congenital nystagmus can be treated using strabismus surgery to move the eyes and null point to primary position. Anderson and Kestenbaum and Parks were the first to report that a face turn secondary to nystagmus could be corrected by shifting the eyes (i.e., null point) into primary position with strabismus surgery. This procedure is often referred to as the Kestenbaum procedure but it is correct to acknowledge the other contributors. Box 19-2 gives the general surgical principles for correcting a face turn.

Surgical therapy should be based on the *greatest amount of abnormal head posture* measured at distance and near. For example, if the face turn is obvious at distance, not at near, full correction directed at the face turn at distance should be undertaken. When strabismus coexists with nystagmus, the head posture can be

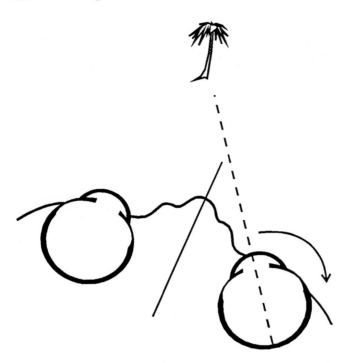

Fig. 19-2 Diagram of a face turn to the right because of a tight right medial rectus muscle of the fixing eye. This face turn can be fixed by moving the restricted fixing eye to primary position (recess the right medial rectus muscle and resect right lateral rectus muscle). The left eye has full ductions and will follow to primary position.

corrected by moving the fixing eye to primary position, then adjusting the fellow eye to compensate for the residual strabismus.

Surgical Treatment of Nystagmus—No Face Turn

Although the Kestenbaum-Anderson-Parks procedure is directed toward eliminating the abnormal horizontal face turn associated with nystagmus, another approach has been described to dampen nystagmus in patients without a face turn. Simultaneous retroequatorial recessions of all the four horizontal rectus muscles have been reported to decrease the amplitude of nystagmus and improve visual acuity. The precise mechanism responsible for dampening the nystagmus is not known and the long-term effect remains an open question. Vision improves in cases of motor nystagmus, not in patients with sensory nystagmus who have an abnormal afferent pathway.

Other Causes of Ocular Torticollis

Other less common mechanisms for head posturing do exist. Rarely, a patient with diplopia adopts a head posture that induces maximal image separation rather than fusion, thus making suppression of the diplopic im-

---

Box 19-2 General Surgical Principles for Correcting a Face Turn

KESTENBAUM-ANDERSON-PARKS PROCEDURE

For example, with a compensatory face turn to the left the eyes will be shifted to the right (Fig. 19-1). To correct the face turn move the eyes to the left into primary position. This is done by moving the right eye "in" (right lateral rectus recession-right medial rectus resection), and the left eye "out" (left medial rectus recession and left lateral rectus resection). The amount of surgery for a specific amount of face turn is listed in **Table 19-1**. Note "Parks Poker straight" 5-6-7-8 (Medial recession 5 mm, medial resection 6 mm, lateral recession 7mm, and medial resection 8 mm) is a way of remembering the amount of surgery for a small face turn, but in most cases larger amounts of surgery are needed. Large recessions and resections are needed to a face turn associated with nystagmus and postoperative limitation of ocular movements are to be expected, an acceptable trade-off.

VERTICAL HEAD POSTURING

Chin depression (eyes up) is treated with large bilateral superior rectus recessions (8 to 9 mm) and inferior rectus resections (6 to 7 mm). This can be done together for large chin depressions or staged, performing superior rectus recessions first, then inferior rectus resections later if necessary. Chin elevations (eyes down) can be treated similarly by recessing the inferior rectus muscles (7 to 8 mm) and resecting the superior rectus muscles (6 to 7 mm).

---

age easier. The authors have seen a few children use the rim of their glasses to cover part of the pupil of their fixing eye to achieve a pinhole effect and improve vision. Other reasons for abnormal head posturing include compensation for visual field defects, ptosis, tilting for monocular torsion, and cosmetic reasons.

SIXTH CRANIAL NERVE PALSY

Etiology

Newborns frequently have transient sixth nerve palsies that resolve spontaneously over a few days to weeks. Persistent isolated congenital sixth nerve palsies on the other hand are extremely rare. In fact, most are probably Duane's syndrome, which is difficult to diagnose in infancy. A common cause of an isolated acquired sixth nerve palsy in early childhood is post viral inflammatory neuropathy. This may occur 1 to 3 weeks after a viral

Table 19-1   Kestenbaum-Anderson-Parks procedure for nystagmus with a face turn to left as seen in Fig. 19-1 (eyes shifted to a right null point)

Face turn (degrees)	Right eye		Left eye	
	Recess lateral rectus (mm)	Resect medial rectus (mm)	Recess medial rectus (mm)	Resect lateral rectus (mm)
<20	7	6	5	8
30	9	8	6.5	10
45	10	8.5	7	11
>50	11	9.5	8	12.5

(Table modified from Archer 1993, Wright 1991.)

Table 19-2   Infranuclear sixth nerve palsy

Localization/accompanying signs*	Etiology
Fascicle Ipsilateral seventh nerve palsy, Horner's, facial analgesia, peripheral deafness, loss of taste from anterior two thirds of tongue; contralateral hemiparesis	Tumor; demyelination; hemorrhage/infarction
Subarachnoid Space Papilledema; other cranial nerve palsies	Meningitis; meningeal carcinomatosis; trauma; increased intracranial pressure causing downward displacement of brainstem; after lumbar puncture, shunt for hydrocephalus, spinal anesthesia, myelography, or halopelvic cervical traction; clivus tumor; cerebellopontine angle tumor; berry aneurysm; abducens neurinoma
Petrous Apex Ipsilateral seventh nerve palsy; pain in eye or face; otitis media; leakage of blood or cerebrospinal fluid from ear; mastoid ecchymosis; papilledema	Mastoiditis; thrombosis of inferior petrosal sinus; trauma with transverse fracture of temporal bone; persistent trigeminal artery, aneurysm, or arteriovenous malformation
Cavernous Sinus/Superior Orbital Fissure Ipsilateral Horner's; ipsilateral third, fourth, fifth nerve involvement; proptosis; disc edema; orbital pain; conjunctival injection	Cavernous sinus thrombosis; carotid-cavernous fistula; tumor; internal carotid aneurysm
Orbit Ipsilateral third, fourth, fifth nerve involvement; proptosis; disc edema; orbital pain; conjunctival injection	Tumor; pseudotumor
Uncertain	Transient abducens palsy of newborn; after febrile illness, immunization, or idiopathic; migraine; toxic

*Any or none of the accompanying signs listed may be present.

illness or immunization, or may occur spontaneously, without obvious cause. These patients should be followed closely to monitor for improvement, and the development of amblyopia. Improvement usually occurs within 6 to 10 weeks. Neuroimaging and a neurologic evaluation is indicated if the sixth nerve palsy does not improve, or if other neurologic signs develop. Other causes of an acquired sixth nerve palsy include closed head trauma, intracranial tumor, Gradenigo's syndrome (mastoiditis and sixth nerve palsy), meningitis, myas-

thenia gravis, and cavernous sinus disease. Table 19-2 lists causes of infranuclear sixth nerve palsies in children.

Clinical Features

Sixth nerve palsy is typically associated with limited abduction, an esotropia in primary position that increases on gaze to the side of the palsy (Fig. 19-3). On attempted abduction there is relative lid fissure widening. This is because both the medial and lateral rectus

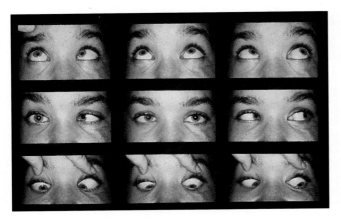

Fig. 19-3   Traumatic sixth nerve palsy right eye.

muscles are relaxed on attempted adduction and orbital pressure proptoses the eye. Remember that on attempted abduction the medial rectus muscle is inhibited (Sherrington's law). Mild sixth nerve paresis may have relatively good lateral rectus function and show only trace limitation of abduction. These patients will, however, have a pattern of *divergence paresis* with an esotropia greater in the distance. Divergence paresis should alert to the possibility of a subtle bilateral sixth nerve paresis.

Treatment

Initial therapy of acquired sixth nerve palsy is observation for 6 months, monitoring the patient for recovery. During the observation period alternate monocular occlusion or press-on prisms can be used to eliminate diplopia if a face turn does not allow fusion. In many cases secondary contracture of the antagonist (i.e., ipsilateral medial rectus) occurs during the observation period. To prevent secondary contracture of the medial rectus muscle some advocate the use of botulinum injection into the ipsilateral medial rectus muscle. Botulinum paralyzes the muscle for 3 to 6 months, thus preventing contracture. The hope is that preventing secondary contracture of the medial rectus muscle will increase the chances of recovery without strabismus surgery. Controversy continues since controlled studies on the efficacy of botulinum injection for sixth nerve palsy are lacking. It should be noted that after a botulinum injection into the medial rectus muscle, both the medial and lateral rectus are paralyzed, resulting in essentially no horizontal movement of the paretic eye. Thus the patient should be warned that the paretic eye will show decreased movement postinjection. In addition, the surgeon should be aware that the effects of botulinum can last over 6 months, and surgery should be delayed until the botulinum has dissipated.

After the 6-month observation period, lateral rectus muscle function should be evaluated since this determines the type of surgery. Lateral rectus muscle function can be measured by saccadic velocity measurement (both clinical estimation and oculography), and the active force generation test. If lateral rectus function is good (approximately 60% to 70% of normal), then a recession of the medial rectus (adjustable suture in adults) and a resection of the lateral rectus should be considered. Adding a recession of the contralateral medial rectus muscle with or without a Faden procedure helps to diminish incomitance. If the saccadic velocities are less than 50% of normal, or the active force generation test is estimated to be half the normal fellow eye, a vertical rectus muscle transposition procedure is indicated.

Transposition procedures act by moving innervated vertical rectus muscles to the lateral rectus insertion to provide lateral force. The lateral force of the transposition does not appropriately activate on attempted abduction, but provides a constant lateral force. Transposition of a rectus muscle can involve the full muscle (full-tendon transfer), or the muscle can be split longitudinally and half the muscle transferred (split-tendon transfer). In addition to a transposition, patients with significant residual paresis almost always require an ipsilateral medial rectus recession to reduce adduction forces. The vertical rectus muscles provide substantial circulation to the anterior segment. Older adult patients, especially those with atherosclerotic disease or hyperviscosity syndromes, are at risk for developing anterior segment ischemia after vertical recti transposition particularly with full-tendon transfers. A partial tendon transfer procedure should be considered in these patients to maintain anterior circulation and prevent anterior segment ischemia (Fig. 19-4). If carefully performed to avoid the trauma to anterior ciliary artery, split-tendon transfer procedures result in long-term good postoperative eye alignment, while reducing the risk of anterior segment ischemia.

Other options include full-tendon transposition with injection of botulinum toxin to the medial rectus muscle. The authors' recommendations for the surgical treatment of sixth nerve palsy are listed in Box 19-3.

DUANE'S RETRACTION SYNDROME

Etiology

The cause of Duane's retraction syndrome (DRS) has been identified to be an agenesis of the sixth nerve and nucleus, with the inferior division of oculomotor nerve splitting to innervate both the medial and lateral rectus muscles. Because both the medial and lateral rectus muscles are innervated by the nerve to the medial rectus muscle, both muscles fire and contract simultaneously on attempted adduction. This co-contraction of the medial and lateral rectus muscles on adduction gives rise to

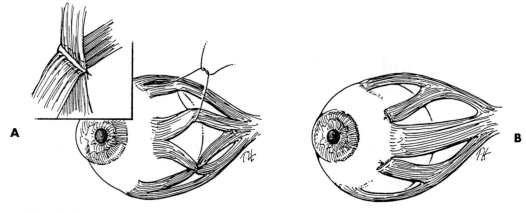

Fig. 19-4 **A,** Diagram of Jensen procedure. Split lateral halves of the superior and inferior rectus muscles are tied to the split upper and lower halves of the lateral rectus muscle. **B,** Diagram of Hummelsheim procedure. Split lateral halves of the vertical recti muscles are transposed and sutured to the sclera adjacent to the lateral rectus muscle. (From Wright KW: *Color atlas of ophthalmic surgery: strabismus,* Philadelphia, 1991, JB Lippincott.)

Box 19-3 Surgical Treatment for Sixth Nerve Palsy

GOOD LATERAL RECTUS FUNCTION

Ipsilateral medial rectus recession (adjustable suture in adults or cooperative children), ipsilateral lateral rectus resection, and a small contralateral medial rectus recession (posterior fixation suture on contralateral medial rectus is optional).

POOR LATERAL RECTUS FUNCTION

Ipsilateral medial rectus recession (adjustable suture in adults or cooperative children), and split-tendon transposition procedure (either Jensen or Hummelsheim).

the term *Duane's co-contraction syndrome.* Fig. 19-5 shows a diagram of various patterns of abnormal innervation possible in DRS. Other oculomotor misdirection syndromes are associated with DRS, such as Marcus Gunn jaw-winking. Duane's syndrome is associated with numerous systemic syndromes, including Goldenhar's syndrome, Klippel-Feil syndrome, maternal Thalidomide ingestion, fetal alcohol syndrome, and oculocutaneous albinism.

Clinical Features

Duane's syndrome is present at birth and is almost always unilateral. Like a sixth nerve palsy limited abduction is almost always present. Only in the rare Duane's syndrome type 2 is abduction intact. Unlike a sixth nerve palsy, the lateral rectus muscle in DRS is innervated,

though by part of the oculomotor nerve. On attempted abduction the lateral rectus muscle does not contract, but on adduction the medial rectus muscle appropriately contracts but the lateral rectus muscle also contracts. Co-contraction of the lateral and medial rectus muscles on adduction causes globe retraction, producing relative enophthalmos and lid fissure narrowing. Co-contraction also explains why some patients with Duane's syndrome (e.g., Duane's syndrome type 3) have limited adduction in addition to limited abduction. The inappropriately contracting lateral rectus muscle prevents full adduction.

Another clinical finding in patients with DRS is the presence of a face turn. The face turn is determined by resting position of the Duane's eye. If the medial and lateral rectus muscles receive comparable innervation from the split oculomotor nerve and the eye is centered in primary position, there will be no significant face turn (type 3). If, however, the medial rectus muscle gets most of the innervation from the oculomotor nerve, then the affected eye will rest in adduction and the patient will have an esotropic DRS with a face turn towards the side of the affected eye (type 1). Less commonly, the lateral rectus will receive most of the innervation from the oculomotor nerve. In these cases, the affected eye will be abducted, causing an exotropic DRS with a face turn toward the opposite side of the affected eye (type 3 with XT).

Classically, Duane's syndrome is classified into three categories, which represent different innervational abnormalities. Table 19-3 lists the characteristics of the three types of Duane's syndromes.

Another rare form of Duane's syndrome is *synergistic divergence.* In this case the nerve to the medial rectus muscle aberrantly innervates the lateral rectus more than

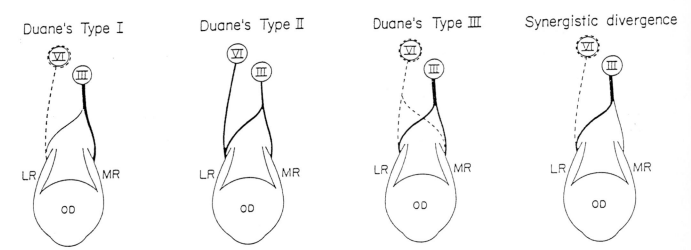

Fig. 19-5   Schematic of anomalies of peripheral innervation that may explain Duane's syndrome and synergistic divergence. The thickness of the line representing the nerve is intended to represent quantitive innervation. Dashed lines indicate hypoplasia or absence of the nerve. *OD*, right eye; *LR*, lateral rectus; *MR*, medial rectus; *III*, oculomotor nerve nucleus; *VI*, abducens nucleus. (From Wilcox LM Jr, Gittinger JW Jr, Breinin GM: *Am J Ophthalmol* 91(1):1-7, 1981.)

Table 19-3   Characteristics of Duane's syndromes

Type 1 Duane's: Most common type	Poor abduction and good adduction	The medial rectus muscle receives most of the medial rectus nerve innervation and the lateral rectus minimal innervation from the medial rectus nerve (Fig. 19-6). Because the medial rectus receives most of the innervation, the Duane's eye is usually fixed in an adducted position, an esotropia in primary position, and there is a compensatory face turn in the direction of the Duane's eye (i.e., left face turn for a left Duane's type 1 syndrome).
Type II Duane's: Least common—extremely rare	Poor adduction and good abduction	EMG recordings show the lateral rectus muscle to contract appropriately on abduction, but it also contracts paradoxically on adduction. This probably represents a partial innervation of the lateral by the sixth nerve nucleus since purposeful abduction is present, in addition to aberrant sixth nerve innervation of the medial rectus muscle. Usually not associated with a face turn.
Type III Duane's: Second most common type	Poor adduction and abduction	Equal innervation of the medial and lateral rectus muscles by the medial rectus nerve (Fig. 19-7). Since the medial and lateral forces are similar the eye will rest in approximately primary position, and there will be no significant face turn. In some cases an exotropia is present in primary position because the lateral rectus receives slightly more innervation than the medial rectus muscle. This causes a face turn away from the Duane's eye.

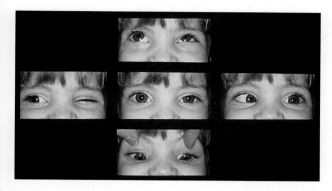

Fig. 19-6   Duane's syndrome. *Type I (left eye):* Good adduction and poor abduction. Note the severe globe retraction.

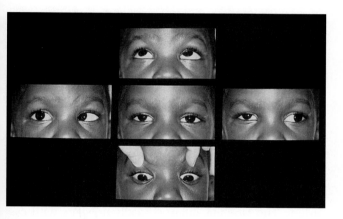

Fig. 19-7   Duane's syndrome. *Type III (right eye):* Poor adduction and poor abduction.

the medial rectus muscle, causing the Duane's eye to paradoxically abducts on attempted adduction. A patient with right synergistic divergence will diverge on attempted left gaze.

Duane's syndrome may be associated with an up-shoot and or a down-shoot on attempted adduction, which may resemble inferior oblique and superior oblique overaction. Studies utilizing EMG has identified a variety of aberrant innervation patterns that explain the vertical movements on adduction. In some cases the up-shoot and down-shoot are caused by strong inappropriate firing of the lateral rectus muscle on adduction. This leash effect pulls the eye up or down as the eye rotates slightly up or down past the horizontal plane. In other cases the vertical recti are aberrantly innervated by part of the medial rectus nerve, so the vertical muscle fires on adduction.

Surgical Treatment

Indications for surgery in DRS are listed in Box 19-4. Usually surgery is electively performed around 3 to 8

Box 19-4 Indications for Surgery in DRS

Significant misalignment of the eyes in primary
  position
Noticeable abnormal head position
Narrowing of palpebral fissure resulting from
  retraction
Significant up-shoot or down-shoot

---

years of age since these patients have excellent fusion and the condition is stable. Rarely a DRS patient will have amblyopia; when present it almost always is associated with anisometropia. Amblyopia should be the first priority in these unusual cases. In general muscle resections should be avoided in DRS, because resections can make the co-contraction and lid fissure narrowing worse.

DRS type 1 with esotropia   The eye is fixed in the adducted position and the face turn is towards the Duane's eye. The medial rectus muscle is usually contracted and tight. The simplest, most effective treatment for DRS type 1 with esotropia is an ipsilateral medial rectus recession (between 5.5 and 7 mm). In adult patients place the medial rectus muscle on an adjustable suture and adjust to a 5 to 10 degree over correction. This results in stable long-term correction of face turn. In contrast a sixth nerve palsy, the lateral rectus muscle is not paretic, but is innervated by a branch of the oculomotor nerve. This tonic innervation provides some abducting force and, thus, a lateral rectus resection or a muscle transposition procedure is not required.

Some advocate a transposition of the vertical rectus muscles laterally for DRS and esotropia. This procedure is more invasive, has a greater risk of anterior segment ischemia, and a vertical deviation is induced in approximately 15% of patients. We prefer the simpler and effective ipsilateral medial rectus recession.

DRS type III with exotropia   The eye is fixed in abduction and the face turn is away from the Duane's eye. There is usually a tight lateral rectus muscle and an ipsilateral lateral rectus recession is indicated.

Globe retraction   Globe retraction can be diminished by recessing both the ipsilateral medial rectus and lateral rectus muscles. In patients with esotropic DRS and severe globe retraction, add a lateral rectus recession but recess the medial rectus muscle more than the lateral rectus to compensate for the esotropia. In exotropic DRS, recess the lateral rectus more than the medial rectus muscle, or for a large exotropia, recess only the lateral rectus muscle (large recession). For orthotropic DRS without a face turn, recess the medial and lateral rectus muscles the same amount.

Box 19-5 Clinical Manifestations of Moebius Syndrome

Facial Weakness
  Partial or complete paralysis, which is typically
    bilateral; occasionally unilateral
Ocular Motor Abnormalities—multiple patterns
    including:
  Straight eyes with no horizontal movements; vertical
    movements preserved
  Esotropia with no horizontal movements; vertical
    movements preserved
  Rarely third or fourth nerve palsies; other vertical
    eye movement disorders; total ophthalmoplegia
  Electromyographic co-contraction of horizontal recti
Other Cranial Nerve Palsies
  Unilateral or bilateral palsy of cranial nerves 5, 8, 9,
    10, or 12
Limb Malformations
  Syndactyly; brachydactyly; absent or supernumerary
    digits; arthrogryposis multiplex congenita; talipes;
    absence of hands or feet
Orofacial Malformations
  Atrophy of tongue; bifid uvula or cleft palate;
    micrognathia; microstomia; external ear defects
Miscellaneous Defects
  Mental retardation; congenital heart defects; absent
    sternal head of the pectoralis major (second major
    component of the Poland anomaly); rib defects;
    Klippel-Feil anomaly; neuroradiologic cerebellar
    hypoplasia; hypogonadotrophic hypogonadism
    with or without anosmia

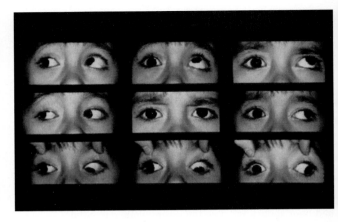

Fig. 19-8 Partial congenital right third nerve palsy with no ptosis.

contraction. The authors have found the Y-splitting procedure more effective than the posterior fixation suture.

MOEBIUS SYNDROME

This is a complex syndrome with the major features being the presence of congenital bilateral sixth and seventh nerve palsies. It is almost always sporadic and there is great variability of findings suggesting the syndrome represent a heterogeneous group of neuromuscular disorders. The Moebius infant typically presents with esotropia, limited abduction, lack of facial expression and difficulty feeding caused by poor sucking reflex. Box 19-5 lists the clinical manifestations of Moebius syndrome.

THIRD NERVE PALSY

Etiology

Congenital third nerve palsy is a common cause of third nerve palsy in childhood (Fig. 19-8). They are often incomplete and may be associated with oculomotor synkinesis. Causes of acquired third nerve palsies include trauma, migraine, associated with viral syndrome, intracranial tumor, or rarely a posterior communicating aneurysm (Table 19-4). An acquired third nerve palsy must be fully worked up with neuroimaging.

Clinical Features

A complete third nerve palsy is associated with a dilated pupil, ptosis, exotropia, and hypotropia (the eye is down and out). There is limited elevation, depression, and adduction. A third nerve paresis is often partial with variable amounts of limited elevation, depression and adduction, and ptosis and pupillary involvement may be absent (see Fig. 19-8).

Up-shoot and down-shoot Approaches to reduce up-shoots and down-shoots associated with DRS include:

1. Y-splitting with recession of the lateral rectus muscle
2. Posterior fixation suture (Faden) of the lateral rectus and appropriate recession of horizontal recti.
3. Inferior oblique recession with anteriorization for up-shoot only, not down-shoot.

The *Y-splitting procedure* of the lateral rectus with recession works by placing some of the lateral rectus muscle above and below the horizontal midline, thus preventing an up-shoot and down-shoot when the eye is in adduction. By combining a recession with the Y-split, the surgeon also reduces the co-contraction. In patients with orthotropic DRS and a severe up-shoot and down-shoot, recess the ipsilateral medial rectus muscle along with a recession and Y-split of the ipsilateral lateral rectus muscle.

The *posterior fixation suture* acts to stop slippage of the lateral rectus muscle when the eye rotates up or down and a concurrent recession reduces co-

Table 19-4 Infranuclear third nerve palsy

Localization/ accompanying signs*	Etiology
Fascicle	
Ipsilateral cerebellar ataxia; contralateral rubral tremor; contralateral hemiparesis; vertical gaze palsy	Demyelination; hemorrhage; infarction (rare in childhood)
Subarachnoid Space	
After papilledema; other cranial nerve palsies	Trauma; meningitis; tumor; Neurosurgery; increased intracranial pressure; uncal herniation
Cavernous Sinus/Superior Orbital Fissure	
Ipsilateral Horner's syndrome; fourth, fifth, sixth nerve involvement; proptosis; disc edema; orbital pain; conjunctival/ episcleral injection mucormycosis	Cavernous sinus thrombosis; tumor; internal carotid aneurysm; carotid-cavernous fistula; Tolosa-Hunt; pituitary apoplexy; sphenoid sinusitis/mucocele
Orbit	
Ipsilateral fourth, fifth, sixth nerve involvement; proptosis; enophthalmos; disc edema; orbital pain; conjunctival/episcleral injection	Trauma; tumor; pseudotumor
Uncertain Localization	After febrile illness, immunization, or idiopathic; migraine

*Any or none of the accompanying signs may be present.

Treatment

The treatment of a third nerve palsy is extremely difficult because there are no vertical muscle forces to move nasally, since all the vertical recti are paretic. Superior oblique tendon transfer to the medial rectus insertion has been suggested as a way of providing medial forces. This procedure, however, limits depression and can result in a large hypertropia in down-gaze.

There is not a good procedure for a complete third nerve palsy; however, an ipsilateral superior oblique tenotomy with ipsilateral recession of the lateral rectus and a large resection of medial rectus can improve alignment. In cases where this procedure has failed the author has split the lateral rectus and transposed the halves to the nasal border of the superior and inferior rectus muscle. This procedure has worked in centering the eye; however, horizontal excursions are minimal. Taylor (1989) reported a good result with a lateral rectus transposition to the medial side of the globe in one case of complete third nerve palsy.

In addition to the difficulty in treating the strabismus, patients with third nerve palsies usually have a ptosis with poor or absent levator function. This should be managed with a frontalis sling procedure with intentional undercorrection of the lid position. Since patients with third nerve palsies have poor Bell's phenomenon, they are at high risk of developing exposure keratitis. The silicone sling procedure has an advantage of being reversible.

INFERIOR OBLIQUE PARESIS

Inferior oblique paresis is rare and can be congenital or acquired. Patients with isolated inferior oblique paresis show ipsilateral superior oblique overaction, but they can be distinguished from those with primary superior oblique overaction (see Table 18-2). Unlike primary superior oblique overaction, inferior oblique paresis is associated with a positive head-tilt test, and a hyperdeviation that is greatest when the patient looks up and nasal away from the affected eye. For example, a left inferior oblique paresis results in a right hypertropia that increases in right gaze and up gaze, and the hyper increases on head-tilt to the right (see head-tilt test in the following discussion). Note that on versions inferior oblique paresis looks similar to Brown's syndrome with limited elevation in adduction, but in Brown's syndrome there is no superior oblique overaction.

FOURTH NERVE PARESIS

A recently acquired superior oblique muscle paresis is usually associated with significant superior oblique underaction, and relatively mild overaction of the antagonist inferior oblique muscle. In long-standing superior oblique muscle paresis, however, there may be significant inferior oblique muscle overaction and little or no superior oblique underaction (Fig. 19-9). Thus the absence of superior oblique underaction does not by itself rule out the diagnosis of superior oblique paresis. The head-tilt test and Parks three-step test described in the following discussion is useful for diagnosing the pareses of a vertical rectus muscle or oblique muscle.

Head-Tilt Test

Patients with a vertical deviation should have the Bielschowsky head-tilt test performed to distinguish primary oblique overaction from a vertical muscle paresis. A positive Bielschowsky head-tilt test is a strong indication that there is a vertical muscle paresis (oblique or vertical rectus muscle), whereas a negative head-tilt usually indicates a primary oblique overaction. If the vertical

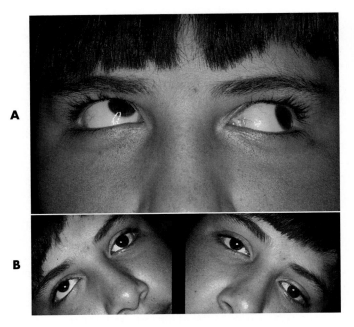

Fig. 19-9   Congenital fourth nerve palsy presenting in a 10-year-old boy. **A,** Right inferior oblique overaction secondary to right fourth nerve palsy. **B,** Forced head-tilt demonstrates clear right hypertropia on right head-tilt.

Box 19-6   Steps of the Parks Three-Step Test and Example

1. Determine the hyperdeviation in primary position
2. Determine where the hypertropia is greatest, right or left gaze
3. Determine whether the hypertropia is greatest in right or left head-tilt

EXAMPLE: WHICH MUSCLE IS PARETIC?
Step 1: Right Hypertropia

Right IR or SO versus Left SR or IO (underacting muscles in right versus left eye).

Step 2: RHT Increases in Left Gaze

Left SR or Right SO (the muscles with field of action in left gaze).

Step 3: RHT Increases on Head-tilt to the Right

Right-tilt induces intorsion of right eye and extorsion of left eye. Both of the two muscles in contention (RSO and LSR) are intorters, but only the RSO produces right intorsion, so the answer is R SO palsy.
ANSWER = R SO palsy

---

deviation changes by more than 5 PD on right-tilt versus left-tilt, then the head-tilt test is considered positive. The Bielschowsky head-tilt test is a critical part of the Parks three-step test used to diagnose oblique and vertical rectus muscle is paretic.

Head-tilting invokes torsional eye movements to correct and maintain the appropriate retinal orientation. A right-tilt, for example, invokes intorsion of the right eye and extorsion of the left eye. The intorters are the superior oblique and the superior rectus muscles, whereas the extorters are the inferior oblique and the inferior rectus muscles. Note that for each pair of torsional muscles there is one elevator and one depressor. For intorsion the superior oblique is the depressor, the superior rectus is the elevator, and for extorsion the inferior oblique is the elevator, the inferior rectus is the depressor. This arrangement keeps vertical forces balanced during the head-tilt. The *Bielschowsky head-tilt test* is based on the premise that if one of the vertical or oblique muscles is paretic, then there will be an imbalance of vertical forces on head-tilting to one side. For example, if the right superior oblique is paretic, then on head-tilt to the right, the right superior oblique and right superior rectus contract to intort the right eye. Since the right superior oblique is paretic, the elevating action of the superior rectus is unopposed and the eye elevates more on head-tilt to the right (creating an increasing right hyperdeviation on head-tilt to the right). Head-tilt to the left

does not cause a vertical change because the right eye extorts on left-tilt and the extorting muscles (inferior rectus and inferior oblique muscles) are in balance and functioning normally.

Parks Three-Step Test

The Parks three-step test incorporates the Bielschowsky head-tilt test with the pattern of incomitance determining which muscle is paretic. When a patient presents with a vertical deviation first perform the head-tilt test to see if a paretic muscle is present. If the head-tilt test is positive (>5 PD difference right-tilt versus left-tilt), then perform the Parks three-step test to determine which oblique or vertical rectus muscle is paretic (Box 19-6). Table 19-5 lists the responses to Parks three-step test for all vertical and oblique muscle palsies.

Problems with the Head-Tilt Test

A positive head-tilt test and the Parks three-step test is not infallible for diagnosing vertical muscle paresis. Some patients with dissociated vertical deviations will show a positive head-tilt, as will some patients with restrictive causes for vertical strabismus. In addition, the head-tilt test is designed to diagnose a single paretic muscle, and it may not reliable when multiple muscles are involved with restriction or paresis.

Table 19-5 Responses to Parks three-step test

Hyper in primary first step	Hyper increases in gaze second step	Increased hyper with head-tilt third step
RSO	RIR	**R** = LIO
RIR	**R or**	**L** = RIR
RHT VS	LIO	
LSR		
LIO		
	RSO	**R** = RSO
	L or	**L** = LSR
	LSR	
RSR	RSR	**R** = RSR
RIO	**R or**	**L** = LSO
LHT VS	LSO	
LSO		
LIR		
	RIO	**R** = LIR
	L or	**L** = RIO
	LIR	

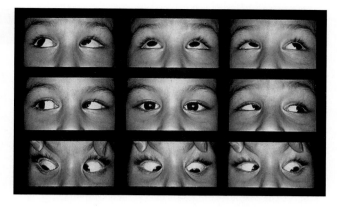

Fig. 19-10 Bilateral superior oblique palsy with a V-pattern arrow pattern subtype. Note the convergence occurs from primary position to down gaze. There is significant bilateral inferior oblique overaction and bilateral superior oblique underaction.

SUPERIOR OBLIQUE PALSY

Clinical Features

Superior oblique palsy is classified as unilateral or bilateral. Typical findings of a *unilateral superior oblique paresis* include an ipsilateral hypertropia increasing on contralateral side gaze and a positive head-tilt test with the hyperdeviation increasing on head-tilt to the ipsilateral shoulder. For example, a right superior oblique paresis shows a right hypertropia, which increases, in left lateral gaze and increases on head-tilt to the right (Fig. 19-9). Usually there is ipsilateral superior oblique underaction, and ipsilateral inferior oblique overaction. In some cases (e.g., congenital superior oblique paresis), there may be relatively little superior oblique under action and mostly inferior oblique overaction. Patients with a unilateral superior oblique paresis adopt a compensatory head-tilt to the side, opposite to paresis, to reduce the hypertropia and fuse. Congenital superior oblique palsy is the most likely diagnosis in patients presenting with a hyperdeviation in primary position and a compensatory head-tilt.

Bilateral superior oblique paresis is associated with bilateral inferior oblique overaction and bilateral superior oblique underaction, which produce a right hypertropia in left gaze and a left hypertropia in right gaze (Fig. 19-10). Other signs include V-pattern, extorsion greater than 10 degrees, and a reversing head-tilt test, with a right hypertropia tilt right, and a left hypertropia tilt left. In down gaze the superior oblique muscle functions of abduction and intorsion counteract the adduction and extorsion of the inferior rectus muscles. If the superior oblique muscles are weak, however, the inferior rectus muscles are unopposed, which causes an esotropia shift and extorsion in down gaze. This type of V-pattern with little change from up-gaze to primary position, but a significant esotropia shift from primary position to down-gaze, the author terms "arrow pattern" (see Fig. 19-10). The presence of an arrow pattern with extorsion increasing in down gaze is diagnostic for a bilateral superior oblique palsy and is often seen with traumatic superior oblique palsies.

A bilateral very asymmetric superior oblique paresis resembles a unilateral superior oblique paresis, and this is termed *masked bilateral superior oblique palsy*. Suspect a masked bilateral paresis if the hypertropia precipitously diminishes in lateral gaze toward the side of the obviously paretic superior oblique muscle. For example, a right superior oblique palsy with a RHT 15 in primary position that diminishes to RHT 2 in right gaze indicates a possible masked bilateral paresis with a mild paresis of the left superior oblique muscle. The left inferior oblique should be examined closely for trace overaction. The presence of a V-pattern, and bilateral extorsion on fundus examination also suggest bilateral involvement in patients with a presumed unilateral palsy. If surgery is performed on only one side of a masked bilateral superior oblique paresis, the contralateral superior oblique paresis will become evident postoperatively. Thus unilateral surgery can unmask a masked bilateral superior oblique paresis. Clinical signs of unilateral versus bilateral superior oblique paresis are shown in Table 19-6.

Fallen eye Significant underaction of the superior oblique muscle and fixation with the paretic eye will produce the classic finding called the *fallen eye*. When a patient with a superior oblique palsy fixes with the paretic eye and tries to look down and nasally into the field of action of the paretic superior oblique muscle, the

Table 19-6 Unilateral versus bilateral superior oblique paresis

Clinical sign	Unilateral	Bilateral
Superior oblique underaction	Ipsilateral underaction	Bilateral underaction
Inferior oblique overaction	Ipsilateral overaction	Bilateral overaction
V-pattern	Less than 10 prism diopters	Greater than 10 prism diopters with arrow pattern (convergence in down-gaze)
Hypertropia	Greater than 5 prism diopters	Less than 5 prism diopters (except asymmetric paresis)
Head-tilt test	Increasing hypertropia on ipsilateral head-tilt (Rt. SOP = RH tilt right)	Positive head-tilt to both sides (RHT on tilt to right and LHT on tilt to left)
Extorsion (combined)	Less than 10°	Greater than 10°

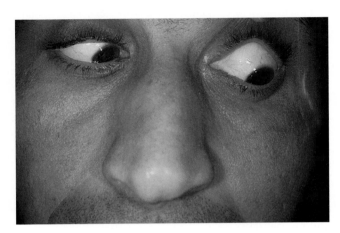

Fig. 19-11 Fallen eye secondary to a severe right superior oblique palsy. The patient is fixing with the paretic right eye. Because of Hering's law the left inferior rectus muscle (yoke to the paretic right superior oblique muscle) overacts as it receives the increased innervation needed to drive the paretic right superior oblique muscle to move the right eye down and in.

weak superior oblique requires a large amount of innervation to make the eye movement down and in. Because of Hering's law, the yoke muscle (contralateral inferior rectus muscle) receives an equally large amount of innervation. Since the inferior rectus has normal function, this increased innervation produces a large secondary hypotropia or fallen eye (Fig. 19-11). A constant hypotropia can lead to secondary contracture of the inferior rectus on the side of the fallen eye, opposite to the superior oblique palsy.

Traumatic Superior Oblique Paresis

Traumatic superior oblique paresis is associated with closed head trauma, often with loss of consciousness, and cerebral concussion. Even very mild head trauma, without loss of consciousness, can cause a superior oblique paresis. Trauma to the trochlear nerve occurs when the brain shifts causing the tentorium to injure the

two trochlear nerves as they exit the posterior midbrain. Since the two trochlear nerves exit the midbrain together only a few millimeters apart, most cases of traumatic superior oblique paresis are bilateral, although the paresis may be asymmetric.

The classic pattern of a traumatic superior oblique paresis is a bilateral paresis with small or no hypertropia in primary position, and esotropia and extorsion in down gaze. Because the strabismus is acquired, patients over 6 years old will complain of torsional, vertical, and horizontal diplopia, which is worse in down gaze. The management of traumatic superior oblique paresis begins with observation for at least 6 months. During this time, serial measurements are taken to establish a pattern of recovery. Alternate patching will eliminate the diplopia and may help to reduce secondary contracture of the ipsilateral superior rectus muscle. If after 6 months significant symptoms persist then strabismus surgery is performed.

Congenital Superior Oblique Palsy

The etiology of congenital superior oblique palsy is unknown. Some cases are associated with superior oblique tendon laxity and rarely, an absent superior oblique tendon. Plager suggests performing the exaggerated forced duction test of the superior oblique tendon at the beginning of surgery to see if the tendon is loose or absent. These authors advocate tightening the superior oblique tendon (S.O. tuck) if forced ductions indicates laxity of the superior oblique tendon.

Classically patients with a congenital superior oblique paresis present with a compensatory head-tilt opposite to the eye with the palsy to minimize the deviation and establish binocular fusion. Congenital superior oblique palsy is most often unilateral or asymmetric bilateral, with a large hypertropia (10 to 20 PD) in primary position. There is usually significant inferior oblique overaction with relatively little superior oblique underaction. Even though the paresis is present at birth, the first clinical sign of congenital superior oblique paresis often pre-

Table 19-7   Treatment of unilateral superior oblique paresis

Clinical manifestation	Procedure
Inferior oblique overaction Hyperdeviation in primary position <15PD Deviation is greater in up-gaze	Inferior oblique graded anteriorization
Superior oblique underaction with minimal inferior oblique overaction Hyperdeviation in primary position <15 PD Deviation greatest in down-gaze	Exaggerated forced duction of SO; If lax SO tendon then: Small superior oblique tuck Or If normal SO tendon laxity then: Inferior oblique graded anteriorization
Inferior oblique overaction with superior oblique underaction Hyperdeviation in primary position >15 prism diopters	Ipsilateral inferior oblique weakening with contralateral inferior rectus recession Or If lax SO tendon then: Ipsilateral superior oblique tuck with contralateral inferior rectus recession

Table 19-8   Treatment of bilateral superior oblique palsy

Clinical manifestation	Procedure
Pure Excyclo-diplopia Minimal hypertropia, <4PD, small V-pattern, and minimal inferior oblique overaction and superior oblique underaction	Bilateral Harada-Ito
Bilateral superior oblique underaction Big arrow pattern (>15PD increase in esotropia from primary to down gaze), >10° extorsion in primary position increasing in down gaze, and reversing hypertropias in side gaze	Bilateral full superior oblique tendon tuck with bilateral medial rectus inferior transposition one-half tendon width
Asymmetric bilateral superior oblique palsy (masked bilateral) Hyperdeviation in primary position >10 prism diopters, asymmetric inferior oblique overaction	Bilateral inferior oblique graded anteriorizations (asymmetric) plus a inferior rectus recession opposite to the hypertropia

sents in late childhood or even adulthood. Normal vertical fusion amplitudes are weak, rarely greater than 3 PD. Patients with congenital superior oblique paresis, however, develop large vertical fusion amplitudes and fuse large hyperphorias up to 35 PD. The presence of large vertical fusion amplitudes is an important clinical sign that the hyperdeviation is long-standing, rather than acutely acquired, and is suggestive of a congenital superior oblique palsy. Over time the fusional control weakens, resulting in a deviation that becomes manifest in later life.

Most patients with congenital superior oblique paresis have excellent stereopsis and show the hyperdeviation intermittently when they are fatigued. Even though patients with congenital superior oblique paresis have high-grade stereopsis, they may also have the ability to suppress, and many do not complain of diplopia when tropic.

Other Causes

The majority of superior oblique pareses are either congenital or traumatic, but other causes include vascular disease, multiple sclerosis, intracranial neoplasm, herpes zoster ophthalmicus, diabetes-associated mononeuropathy, and iatrogenic (after superior oblique tenotomy). If no specific cause of an acquired superior oblique paresis can be found, a neurologic evaluation including neuroimaging is indicated.

Treatment

Cardinal position of gaze measurements are important to determine the pattern of strabismus and where the deviation is greatest. Most treatment strategies identify where the deviation is greatest, then design a surgery to correct the deviation in primary position while reducing

MAJOR POINTS

Two main ocular causes of compensatory head posturing are incomitant strabismus and nystagmus.

Kestenbaum procedure corrects nystagmus-related compensatory face turn by shifting the eyes (i.e., null point) into primary position with recession-resection surgery on each eye.

Post-viral related sixth nerve palsies usually improve over several weeks.

Neuroimaging and an aggressive neurologic evaluation are indicated if the sixth nerve palsy does not improve, or if other neurologic signs develop.

A pattern of divergence paresis with the esotropia being greater in the distance may be indicative of a sixth nerve paresis and/or a neurologic process.

Surgical treatment of sixth nerve paresis is a recession of the medial rectus and a resection of the lateral rectus if lateral rectus function is "good". If lateral rectus function is "poor"/<50% of normal, then a vertical rectus muscle transposition procedure is indicated.

Older adult patients, especially in those with atherosclerotic disease or hyperviscosity syndrome, are at risk for developing anterior segment ischemia after vertical recti transposition particularly with full-tendon transfers.

The cause of Duane's retraction syndrome has been determined to be an agenesis of the sixth nerve and nucleus, with the inferior division of oculomotor nerve splitting to innervate both the medial and lateral rectus muscles.

The treatment for Duane's type l with esotropia is an ipsilateral medial rectus recession.

Moebius syndrome is a complex syndrome with the major features being the presence of congenital bilateral sixth and seventh nerve palsies.

A positive Bielschowsky head-tilt test is a strong indication that there is a vertical muscle paresis (oblique or vertical rectus muscle), whereas a negative head-tilt usually indicates a primary oblique overaction.

Typical findings of a unilateral superior oblique paresis include an ipsilateral hypertropia increasing on contralateral side gaze and a positive head-tilt test with the hyperdeviation increasing on head-tilt to the ipsilateral shoulder.

Bilateral superior oblique paresis is associated with a right hypertropia in left gaze, a left hypertropia in right gaze, arrow type V-pattern, extorsion greater than 10 degrees, and a reversing head-tilt test with a right hypertropia on tilt right, and a left hypertropia on tilt left.

Since the two trochlear nerves exit the midbrain together only a few millimeters apart, traumatic superior oblique nerve palsies are almost always bilateral.

Congenital superior oblique palsy is most often unilateral or asymmetric bilateral, with a large hypertropia (10 to 20 PD) in primary position and a compensatory head-tilt opposite to the eye with the palsy.

the incomitance. For example, a right unilateral superior oblique palsy with a hypertropia less than 10 PD and an inferior oblique overaction, minimal superior oblique underaction can be treated with a simple ipsilateral inferior oblique weakening procedure (e.g., inferior oblique recession or partial anteriorization). If the hypertropia in primary position is greater than 15 PD, then an isolated inferior oblique graded anteriorization may not be enough to correct the hypertropia without limiting up gaze. In this case the surgeon should add a contralateral inferior rectus recession in addition to a partial ipsilateral inferior oblique anteriorization. Late overcorrections after inferior rectus recessions have been known to occur, so be conservative with inferior rectus recessions.

Patients who have a traumatic bilateral superior oblique paresis with extorsion and a large arrow pattern with an esotropia greater than 10 PD in down-gaze should be considered for bilateral superior oblique tucks and bilateral medial rectus recessions with infraplacement. Patients with bilateral traumatic superior oblique paresis after closed head trauma may have partial recovery, and may be left with extorsional diplopia, without significant oblique dysfunction, V-pattern, or hypertropia. In these cases extorsion can be corrected by the *Harada-Ito procedure*, which consists of selectively tightening the anterior one fourth to one third of the superior oblique tendon fibers. These anterior tendon fibers are responsible for the intorsion action of the superior oblique tendon.

Tightening the entire width of the superior oblique tendon (i.e., *superior oblique tuck*), has theoretic utility for improving superior oblique function, but the tight tendon also creates restrictive leash to elevation in adduction (i.e., *iatrogenic Browns Syndrome*). Perhaps the best indication for a superior oblique tuck is bilateral superior oblique paresis associated with esotropia and extorsion in down gaze. The tuck has also been suggested in patients with congenital superior oblique paresis secondary to congenital laxity of the superior oblique tendon. Tables 19-7 and 19-8 list suggested surgical strategies for superior oblique paresis.

SUGGESTED READINGS

Anderson JR: Causes and treatment of congenital eccentric nystagmus, *Br J Ophthalmol* 37:267-280, 1953.

Helveston EM, Ellis FD, Plager DA: Large recession of the horizontal recti for treatment of nystagmus, *Ophthalmology* 98:1302-1305, 1991.

Hotchkiss MG, Miller NR, Clark AW, et al: Bilateral Duane's retraction syndrome, a clinical-pathologic case report, *Arch Ophthalmol* 98:870-874, 1980.

Kestenbaum A: A nystagmus operation, *Proc XVIII Council Ophthalmol* 2:1071-1078, 1954.

Plager DA: Traction testing and superior oblique palsy, *J Ped Ophth Strab* 27:136-140, 1990.

Wright KW: Color atlas of ophthalmic surgery: strabismus, Philadelphia, Lippincott.

Strabismus Syndromes

This chapter covers several types of incomitant strabismus syndromes, most of which are caused by restriction. Restriction can be caused by a tight muscle, such as in congenital Brown's syndrome, congenital fibrosis syndrome, and Graves' disease, or be a result of periocular scarring, such as in fat adherence syndrome. Weak muscle function can also cause incomitant strabismus and slipped/lost muscle, and rectus muscle agenesis are included in the following discussion (see Chapter 19 for cranial nerve palsies). A discussion on the diagnosis of restriction versus paresis can be found in Chapter 14.

CONGENITAL OCULAR FIBROSIS SYNDROME

Congenital ocular fibrosis syndrome is often inherited as an autosomal dominant disorder. It is a restrictive strabismus syndrome caused by fibrous replacement of orbital striated muscle. The etiology is controversial as to whether the characteristic fibrous replacement of muscle is due to myopathy or neuropathy. Patients show positive forced ductions with restriction caused by tight and fibrotic rectus muscles. Five types of congenital fibrosis have been described (Table 20-1). Tight medial rectus muscles and a large angle esotropia are one of the more common presentations (see Fig. 16-5).

Surgical management is directed to relieve the restriction of the extraocular muscles and treat ptosis if present. Recessions, rather than resections, are the preferred procedures. These cases are extremely difficult to manage, and the surgical goal is to straighten the eyes in primary position, realizing that full ocular rotation is often impossible.

GRAVES' OPHTHALMOPATHY (THYROID OPHTHALMOPATHY)

Graves' ophthalmopathy is a symptom complex composed of the responses of the eye and orbit to an inflammatory process, typically associated with autoimmune thyroid disease such as Graves' disease and Hashimoto's disease. There is an initial inflammatory phase with pathologic finding of lymphocytic infiltration of the extraocular muscles and lacrimal gland, which results in enlargement of the extraocular muscle volume and secondary proptosis. Chemosis and injected conjunctiva are also present. These inflammatory changes can spontaneously resolve over the course of one to a few years. In some cases infiltrated swollen muscles undergo cicatricial changes that result in restrictive incomitant strabismus. These processes in children and adolescents seem to be substantially more benign than those in adults.

The most commonly affected muscle is the inferior rectus, followed by the medial rectus, superior rectus, and lateral rectus in decreasing order of severity and frequency. Thus the patients present most commonly with hypotropia, esotropia, or a combination of both. Note that thyroid ophthalmopathy should be considered in the differential diagnosis of acquired vertical strabismus in

Table 20-1   Five types of congenital ocular fibrosis syndrome

	Involved muscles	Heredity	Laterality
General fibrosis syndrome	All extraocular muscles and levator (IR: commonly and most severely affected)	Usually AD; AR; sporadic: less common	Bilateral, but usually asymmetric
Congenital fibrosis of the IR muscle	IR with or without levator	Familial: rare	Unilateral or bilateral
Strabismus fixus	Horizontal recti (MR: more common than LR)	Usually sporadic	Bilateral
Vertical retraction syndrome	Vertical recti (SR: principally confined)	Familial	Bilateral
Congenital unilateral fibrosis with enophthalmos and ptosis	All extraocular muscles and levator on one side	Nonfamilial	Unilateral

AD, autosomal dominant; *AR*, autosomal recessive; *IR*, inferior rectus; *MR*, medial rectus; *LR*, lateral rectus; *SR*, superior rectus.

adults, especially in women. Many patients are euthyroid at the time of diagnosis but they may have a history of thyroid disease in the past.

Indications for treatment are given in Box 20-1. Nonsurgical therapeutic options include high-dose oral corticosteroids and radiotherapy. For relieving acute compressive optic neuropathy, radiotherapy may be more effective than high-dose corticosteroids.

There are three stages of surgical treatment. The first stage is orbital decompression and is indicated for orbital pressure that causes compressive optic neuropathy or severe proptosis. It should be performed before strabismus surgery, because it may cause or aggravate strabismus. The second is extraocular muscle surgery. Prism therapy can be successful in patients with small deviations, but has limited usefulness because of the incomitant nature of thyroid strabismus. Thus surgical treatment of strabismus, principally recession of the restricted muscles, is often necessary after the deviation has stabilized. Usually 6 months to a year follow-up is necessary to document stable measurements before undertaking strabismus surgery. It is important not to operate when the disease is in the active inflammatory phase, or if the strabismus is changing. Adjustable suture surgery has been advocated for this disease. For a hypotropia with limited elevation, recess the inferior rectus muscle; however, late overcorrections are common especially with large inferior rectus recessions. In these cases, initial undercorrection may provide the best long-term results. Another problem associated with large recessions of inferior rectus is marked exotropia in down gaze (A-pattern). This can be minimized by nasal displacement of inferior rectus muscles.

The third stage is eyelid retraction repair. Although eyelid retraction can develop without strabismus surgery, it can develop or be aggravated by strabismus surgery. Thus eyelid surgery should be deferred until strabismus surgery has been completed. Careful dissection of the inferior rectus muscles from the attachment to the lower eyelid retractors lessens postoperative lid retraction.

Box 20-1   Indications for Treatment of Graves' Ophthalmopathy

Threatened vision as a result of impaired optic nerve function
Intractable pain
Exposure keratopathy
Strabismus with diplopia or abnormal head posture

FAT ADHERENCE SYNDROME

Fat adherence syndrome is an acquired, restrictive strabismus. It occurs when posterior Tenon's capsule is surgically or traumatically violated, allowing extraconal fat to prolapse through the rupture. This causes trauma to the highly vascular extraconal fat septae, induces inflammation and fibrosis, and causes adhesions to the extraocular muscles, the sclera, or both (Fig. 20-1). Fat adherence can also occur if the muscle sleeve is traumatized, which can occur during scleral buckle procedures (Fig. 20-2). Remember that the muscle sleeve is a continuation of posterior Tenon's capsule and is where the extraocular muscles penetrate posterior Tenon's capsule.

Parks first described fat adherence syndrome following inferior oblique surgery. Extraconal fat normally is first encountered 10 mm posterior to the limbus. Fat adherence syndrome can occur with virtually any periocular surgery that involves the extraconal fat, including oblique muscle surgery, rectus muscle manipulation with retina surgery (Wright 1986) and trauma.

Successful treatment of fat adherence syndrome is extremely difficult, if not impossible. The best treatment is surgical removal of the fat adherence, and plication of existing Tenon's capsule over the tear in Tenon's capsule. Other methods have been tried, including artificial

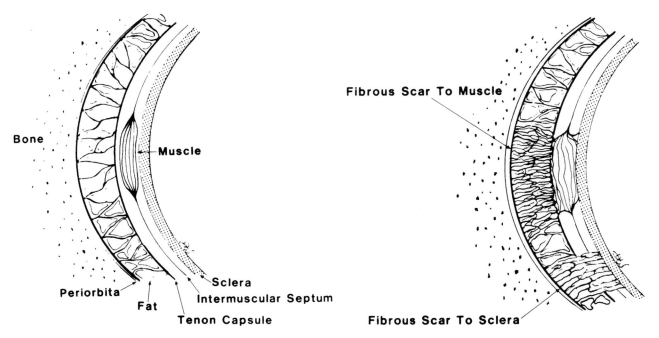

Fig. 20-1   *Left,* Normal anatomic relationship of extraconal fat, Tenon's capsule, muscle, and sclera. *Right,* Diagram of fat adherence syndrome. Fibrous adhesion of periorbita, muscle, and sclera formed after Tenon's capsule had been violated. (From Wright KW: *Ophthalmology* 93:411-415, 1986.)

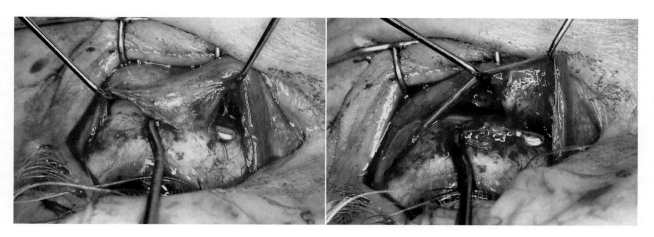

Fig. 20-2   *Left* and *right,* Sequential photographs of the dissection of fat adherence over the rectus muscle following the retina surgery. Prolapsed fat can be seen between the two muscle hooks in the right photograph. See color plate. (From Wright KW: *Ophthalmology* 93:411-415, 1986.)

sleeves and even the use of mitomycin C in the animal model. Artificial sleeves only result in encapsulation of the sleeves with more scarring and fibrosis, and in the animal model, mitomycin C resulted in severe orbital inflammation and increased scarring.

The best treatment is prevention by careful dissection of the extraocular muscles during surgery. Perform a limited posterior dissection on rectus surgery whenever possible. If a large posterior dissection is needed (vertical rectus muscle surgery or oblique muscle surgery), dissect close to the extraocular muscle and avoid penetrat-

ing Tenon's capsule. By conservative and careful surgical dissection, fat adherence syndrome can be avoided.

SLIPPED AND LOST MUSCLES

Slipped and lost muscles are important complications of strabismus surgery. A slipped muscle occurs when a rectus muscle has not been secured properly during strabismus surgery. Instead of securing the muscle fibers, the surgeon inadvertently secures the muscle capsule, and allows the internal muscle fibers to slip posteriorly. This results in an overcorrection with a recession, and an undercorrection with a resection. Initially the alignment may appear acceptable, but over weeks to months the eye will drift. The late overcorrection resulting from a slipped medial rectus muscle is probably not progressive slippage of the muscle, but caused by chronic imbalance of muscle force and secondary contracture of the antagonist muscle. One of the most important signs of a slipped muscle is underaction of the operated muscle (Fig. 20-3). This sign, however, may be subtle, since there are various degrees of muscle slippage. The slipped muscle can be avoided by performing full muscle thickness locking bites at least 2 mm wide at each edge of the muscle.

A lost muscle occurs during strabismus surgery when a rectus muscle is completely detached from the globe and retracts posteriorly. A lost muscle can occur after virtually any rectus muscle surgery, but can also occur during retina surgery, removal of pterygium, or trauma to the extraocular muscles. The medial rectus muscle is the most commonly lost or slipped muscle after strabismus surgery and is the hardest muscle to find. Note that the vertical recti and lateral rectus muscle are connected to an oblique muscle by ligaments, which prevent recoiling of the detached muscle through Tenon's capsule. In fact, Plager and Parks (1990) reported the successful retrieval of only 1 of 10 lost medial rectus muscles, in contrast to retrieving 50% to 75% of other lost rectus muscles. The signs of a lost muscle are more dramatic than a slipped muscle. They include severe underaction of the operated muscle, and lid fissure widening on attempted ductions towards the lost muscle.

If postoperatively a lost or slipped muscle is suspected, an exploration of the suspected muscle is indicated. If in doubt, observe for 7 to 10 days before exploration. This allows time for recovery of muscle function in cases where limited function is secondary to muscle trauma, and not to a lost or slipped muscle. Once a slipped or lost muscle is identified, it should be advanced and replaced anteriorly. A long-standing lost muscle may be very contracted and tight, and contracture of ipsilateral antagonist muscle may coexist. If the antagonist is tight then consider recessing it, in addition to advancing the slipped muscle. A slipped muscle can be converted to a lost muscle during the exploration, thus a careful dissection during the advancement is indicated. A lost muscle, especially the medial rectus, cannot always be found without risking fat adherence syndrome. In these cases where the lost muscle cannot be retrieved, consider a Hummelsheim transposition procedure to provide appropriate muscle forces. Prevention of slipped and lost muscles is the best treatment, and Box 20-2 lists suggested surgical techniques to reduce the likelihood of this complication.

RECTUS MUSCLE AGENESIS

All extraocular muscles have been described as being congenitally absent, but the reports of absent oblique muscles are rare. The most commonly reported absent muscle is the inferior rectus muscle. Rectus muscle agenesis is often associated with craniofacial dysostoses. Other associations include, anencephaly, Axenfeld's anomaly, Moebius syndrome, and congenital ptosis, as well as with absence of other extraocular muscles especially in association with absent superior rectus and superior oblique muscles.

On motility examination, the patients show decreased muscle function, but interestingly, the eye can usually come to midline, probably as a result of tertiary actions of the remaining muscles. Secondary contracture of the unopposed antagonist muscle may develop and result in positive forced duction test in the adult cases. It may be helpful to obtain preoperative coronal CT or MRI scans when absence of a muscle is suspected, since the CT scan may reveal rudimentary rectus muscle in the posterior orbit.

Surgical treatment includes a combination of a Hummelsheim procedure and weakening of the antagonist muscle.

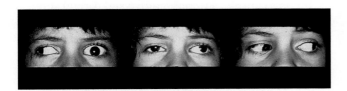

Fig. 20-3   Composite photograph demonstrating the features of consecutive exotropia, limitation of adduction, and widening of the palpebral fissure on adduction in a patient with a slipped left medial rectus muscle following strabismus surgery.

Box 20-2   Surgical Techniques to Prevent a Slipped or Lost Muscle

Careful removal of anterior Tenon's capsule overlying the muscle tendon to clearly visualize full-thickness tendon.

Full-thickness locking bites at each edge of the muscle tendon, making sure to incorporate tendon fibers in the locking bite.

Conservative posterior dissection of check ligaments and intermuscular septum, especially in case of the medial rectus muscle.

STRABISMUS ASSOCIATED WITH ORBITAL FLOOR FRACTURE

Blunt trauma to the inferior orbital rim can cause a floor fracture with or without associated rim fracture. A pure "blow-out fracture" is caused by trauma to the eyeball, which increases orbital pressure, which fractures the orbital floor. Typical signs of blow-out fracture are listed in Box 20-3. Some surgeons have advocated immediate exploration of the fracture; however, many ophthalmologists suggest waiting for approximately 2 weeks before surgery, monitoring for clinical improvement. Late repair of fracture, however, may produce less desirable results since this allows time for permanent scarring. Indications for surgery at approximately 2 weeks post trauma include significant enophthalmos, large fractures greater than one half the floor, and restrictive strabismus.

After repair of the orbital fracture with removal of herniated fat from the maxillary sinus and placement of a synthetic floor replacement such as silicone or Teflon, you should wait at least 6 weeks to 2 months before correcting the strabismus. Correction of strabismus depends on the residual restriction after the floor has been repaired.

The vertical motility deficit most commonly associated with a floor fracture is limited elevation. This is caused by entrapment of extraconal fat and/or muscle within the "trap door" of the fractured bone. Entrapment of extraconal fat and/or muscle can result in scarring of the muscle to the floor. This creates a leash so the eye cannot elevate. It can also create a deficit in depression since the inferior rectus pulls against the floor of the orbit rather than the eyeball. Thus large floor fractures can cause limited elevation, as well as limited depression. Fig. 20-4, *A* shows a young child with a left orbital fracture. Note the left eye does not elevate well and also shows some limitation of depression. Fig. 20-4, *B* shows a computed tomography (CT) scan with extraconal fat herniating into the maxillary sinus through a fracture of the floor of the orbit.

Patients with limited elevation can be managed by a recession of the ipsilateral tight inferior rectus muscle, with or without a recession of the contralateral superior rectus. If the major problem is in down gaze with limited depression, the ipsilateral inferior rectus can be tucked or resected slightly and the contralateral inferior rectus recessed. The most important fields of gaze are primary position and down gaze, so it may be necessary to trade off some diplopia in up gaze to achieve single binocular vision in primary position and down gaze. In many cases, adequate repair of the floor fracture will release most of the restriction. The first effort should be directed towards repairing the floor fracture and releasing the herniation of extraconal fat and inferior rectus muscle. It is important to realize that the depression deficit seen with floor fractures is usually not secondary to a paralysis of the inferior rectus muscle. It is secondary to adhesions of the inferior rectus muscle to the floor, which isolate the inferior rectus from pulling on the globe.

Box 20-3   Typical Signs of Blow-Out Fracture

Enophthalmos
Diplopia with limited vertical eye movements
Positive forced ductions with the eye limited to elevation
Numbness in the infraorbital nerve region (cheek and upper teeth)

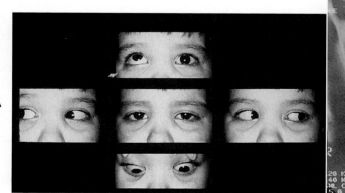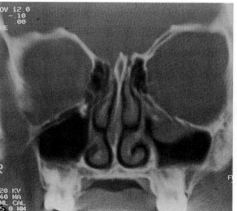

Fig. 20-4   A, Left blow-out fracture with limited elevation of left eye. **B,** CT scan showing fat herniation into the maxillary sinus associated with floor fracture.

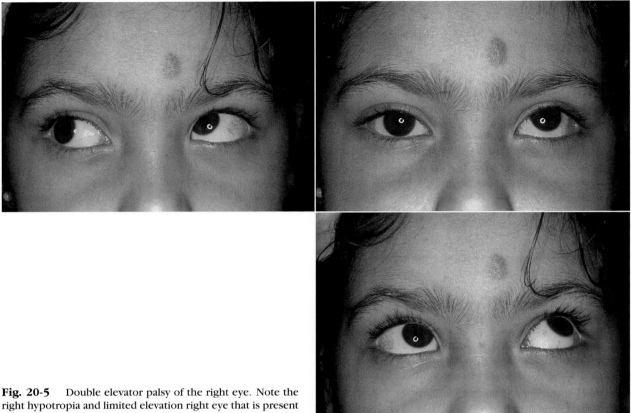

Fig. 20-5   Double elevator palsy of the right eye. Note the right hypotropia and limited elevation right eye that is present in adduction but worse in abduction.

DOUBLE ELEVATOR PALSY

The term *double elevator* (DEP) implies paresis of superior rectus and inferior oblique muscle. This is, however, a misnomer since in 70% of cases the deficient elevation is due to restriction, secondary to a tight inferior rectus, and only 30% as a result of true paresis of the superior rectus and inferior oblique muscles. Because of this many ophthalmologists prefer the term *monocular elevation deficiency* over double elevator palsy. Both types, (inferior rectus restriction, and vertical muscle palsy) show limited elevation of one eye "across the board" (in adduction, as well as abduction) on version testing. In many cases, elevation in adduction is worse than abduction (Fig. 20-5). This is important since double elevator palsy may be mistaken for Brown's syndrome. In Brown's syndrome there is limited elevation but it is worse in adduction (see the next section on Brown's syndrome).

Patients with double elevator palsy present with a unilateral hypotropia, often with a chin elevation and ptosis. True ptosis because of levator weakness is present in 50% to 60% of cases, whereas pseudo-ptosis occurs in almost all patients with a large hypotropia. Associated innervational abnormalities include Marcus Gunn jaw winking,

Duane's syndrome, and other misdirection syndromes.

Surgery is indicated if vertical strabismus is present in primary gaze and there is a significant chin elevation. If supraduction forced ductions are positive indicating a tight inferior rectus and there is a good up-gaze saccade, then the diagnosis is restriction of the inferior rectus muscle, and the procedure of choice is a recession of the inferior rectus muscle. If forced ductions do not show a significant restriction and the up-gaze saccade is absent then the diagnosis is superior rectus–inferior oblique paresis, and a rectus muscle transposition is indicated. The Knapp procedure is a full-tendon tansfer of the medial and lateral rectus muscles up to the superior rectus insertion. This works well but this author prefers a split-tendon transfer such as a vertical Hummelshiem or Jensen procedure to spare the anterior ciliary arteries and reduce the chances of anterior segment ishchemia.

BROWN'S SYNDROME

Etiology

Brown's syndrome is a restrictive strabismus characterized by limitation of elevation, which is worse when the eye is in adduction (Fig. 20-6). There are many etiologies of Brown's syndrome. The term *true* or *congen-*

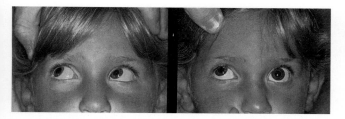

Fig. 20-6   Acquired Brown's syndrome left eye. *Left,* elevation in adduction is pretty good: no limitation. *Right,* taken a few minutes later and now shows a marked limitation to elevation in adduction a −3. This case demonstrates the intermittence and variability of acquired Brown's syndrome.

ital Brown's syndrome indicates a congenitally tight superior oblique muscle tendon-complex in contrast to acquired Brown's syndrome, which has many etiologies.

Causes of acquired Brown's syndrome are given in Box 20-4. Some patients will develop an acquired Brown's syndrome of unknown etiology. If the cause of an acquired Brown's syndrome is not known, then orbital imaging studies are indicated. Acquired Brown's syndrome is often intermittent and sometimes associated with a click, which is felt by the patient in the superior nasal quadrant when the patient looks "up and in" (Fig. 20-6). In some cases, the click can be heard with a stethoscope localized in the superior nasal quadrant. The cause of the click and limited elevation is not known, but may represent inflammation or an abnormality of fascial tissue around the superior oblique tendon. In many cases, acquired Brown's syndrome will spontaneously resolve over several months. Surgery should only be considered after the patient has been observed for at least 6 months to 1 year.

Another form of acquired Brown's syndrome is *inflammatory Brown's syndrome.* It is associated with superior nasal orbital pain and tenderness. It is hypothesized that trochlear or peritrochlear inflammation is the cause. Rheumatoid arthritis has been reported as a rare cause of inflammatory Brown's syndrome but in the majority of cases the cause of the inflammation is unknown. The treatment of inflammatory Brown's syndrome includes a trial of systemic nonsteroidal anti-inflammatory agents (e.g., indomethocin 25 to 50 mg TID), or a local steroid injection in the area of the trochlea. Acquired Brown's syndrome of unknown etiology should be worked up with orbital imaging as a variety of local or systemic diseases around the trochlea may cause Brown's syndrome. Medical therapy, not surgery, is the treatment of choice for most cases of inflammatory Brown's syndrome.

Clinical Features

The hallmark of Brown's syndrome, regardless of the cause, is limited elevation in adduction. In congenital Brown's syndrome this occurs because the tight posterior tendon fibers prevents the back of the eye from rotating down, so the front of the eye cannot elevate. This is a constant limitation and does not improve. On clinical examination there is typically an ipsilateral hypodeviation, limited elevation worse in adduction, minimal to no superior oblique overaction, and divergence (Y-pattern) in up gaze (Fig. 20-7). There is often some limitation of elevation in abduction but the key is that the limitation is much worse in adduction. Patients with Brown's syndrome usually have excellent binocular fusion, and adopt a compensatory chin elevation and a face turn away from the Brown's eye. A patient with a right Brown's syndrome will have a chin elevation and a face turn to the left.

Standard forced duction testing shows a restriction to elevation in adduction. If the Brown's syndrome is caused by a tight superior oblique tendon, then Guyton's exaggerated forced ductions of the superior oblique muscle will reveal restriction to moving the eye up and in.

Differential Diagnosis of Congenital Elevation Deficit

Congenital causes for limited elevation include double elevator palsy, inferior oblique paresis, and superior oblique overaction. Double elevator palsy can be distinguished by the presence of similar limitation in abduction and adduction, whereas primary superior oblique overaction and inferior oblique paresis may be more difficult to differentiate since they have a greater elevation deficit in adduction. Table 18-2 compares the clinical finding of Brown's syndrome primary superior oblique overaction and inferior oblique paresis.

Surgical Indications for Congenital Brown's Syndrome

In general, surgery should be considered for Brown's syndrome if there is a hypodeviation in primary position

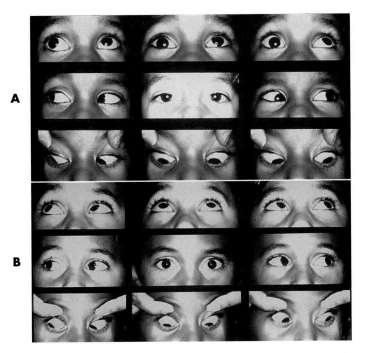

Fig. 20-7 **A,** Congenital Brown's syndrome of the right eye. The right eye shows −4 limitation to elevation to adduction and −2 limitation of elevation in abduction. In up gaze there is divergence (Y-pattern), straight left gaze a large right hypotropia; however, there is no significant superior oblique overaction. Note that in primary position (center frame) the eyes are in down gaze indicating the presence of a chin elevation. **B,** Patient from **A** after a Wright superior oblique silicone expander 6 mm right eye. Note the much improved elevation in both abduction and adduction of the right eye. These photographs demonstrate essentially normal postoperative versions and the patient no longer has chin elevation head posturing.

that causes a significant face turn. Patients with a minimal restriction and no significant face turn can be managed conservatively. Except for a few exceptions, surgery should be reserved for children older than 4 years of age. Older children are less likely to develop postoperative suppression and amblyopia. Rarely, a surgeon may be forced to operate on a child under 4 years of age if the hypodeviation is large enough to disrupt fusion.

Surgery for Congenital Brown's Syndrome

Management of congenital Brown's syndrome is based on lengthening the superior oblique tendon. Procedures such as tenotomy and tenectomy release the restriction but are not controlled since the cut ends of the tendon can separate widely, resulting in a superior oblique paresis. In contrast to superior oblique overaction, in Brown's syndrome, the superior oblique is not overacting and therefore procedures such as tenotomy or tenectomy often result in a secondary superior oblique paresis. In a study by Eustis, et al., 85% of patients with

Brown's syndrome demonstrated some degree of post-tenotomy superior oblique paresis with one third requiring a second operation. Recently, Sprunger, et al., reported that 50% of patients required further surgery because of an ipsilateral superior oblique paresis after superior oblique tenotomy. To address this problem, Parks has previously suggested performing an ipsilateral inferior oblique recession at the same time as the superior oblique tenotomy. This approach, however, results in prolonged underaction of the inferior oblique and a persistence of Brown's syndrome.

To achieve a controlled elongation of the superior oblique tendon the author has developed a new procedure—the Wright superior oblique silicone expander (see Chapter 18, Fig. 18-6). A segment of retinal silicone band (usually 6 mm long) is carefully sutured between the cut ends of the superior oblique tendon 3 mm nasal to the superior rectus muscle. The initial conjunctival incision, however, is made temporal to the superior rectus. The temporal incision is stretched nasally to expose the nasal aspect of the superior rectus muscle. The maneuver preserves nasal intermuscular septum so the silicone segment does not scar to sclera. The silicone is actually placed within the superior oblique tendon capsule with capsule floor intact. Parks, the authors, and others have found excellent results using the superior oblique silicone expander (see Fig. 20-7, *B*). The superior oblique silicone expander allows for controlled, and reversible elongation of the tendon while maintaining the functional integrity of the superior oblique muscle tendon complex. In trained hands complications of the procedure are rare but include extrusion of silicone and scarring of the silicone to the sclera with postoperative limitation of depression. These complications can be limited by meticulous technique and limiting the maximum length of the silicone segment to 7 mm. Many ophthalmologists now consider the superior oblique silicone expander the procedure of choice for Brown's syndrome.

SUGGESTED READINGS

Brooks SE, Ribeiro GB, Archer SM, et al: An animal model of fat adherence syndrome and treatment with mitomycin C, (abstract) *ARVO* 28, 1993.

Cuttone JM: Absence of the superior rectus muscle in Apert's syndrome, *J Pediatr Ophthalmol Strabisamus* 16:349-354, 1979.

Eustis HS, O'Reilly C, Crawford JS: Management of superior oblique palsy after surgery for true Brown's syndrome, *J Pediatric Ophthalmol Strabismus* 24:10, 1987

Guyton DL: Exaggerated traction test for the oblique muscles, *Ophthalmology* 88:1035, 1981.

Helveston EM, Merriam WW, Ellis FD, et al: The trochlea: a study of the anatomy and physiology, *Ophthalmology* 89:124-144, 1982.

Mets MB, Parks MM, Freeley DA, et al: Congenital absence of the inferior rectus muscle: a report of three cases and their management, *Binocular Vision* 2 (2):77-86, 1987.

Parks MM: Causes of the adhesive syndrome. In Symposium on Strabismus: Transactions of the New Orleans Academy of Ophthalmology, St Louis, 1978, Mosby.

Plager DA, Parks MM: Recognition and repair of the "lost" rectus muscle, *Ophthalmology* 97:131-137, 1990.

Sprunger DT, von Noorden GK, Helveston EM: Surgical results in Brown syndrome, *J Pediatric Ophthalm and Strabismus* 28(3) 164-167, 1991.

Wilson ME, Eustis HS, Parks MM: Brown's syndrome, *Surv Ophthalmol* 34(3):153-172, 1989.

Wright KW: Color atlas of ophthalmic surgery: strabismus, Philadelphia, 1991, Lippincott.

Wright KW: The fat adherence syndrome and strabismus after retina surgery, *Ophthalmology* 93:411-415, 1986.

Wright KW: Superior oblique silicone expander for Brown's syndrome and superior oblique overaction, *J Pediatr Ophthalmol Strabismus* 28:101-107, 1991.

Index